Electrodiagnosis, Toxic Agents and Vision

Documenta Ophthalmologica
Proceedings Series volume 15

Editor H. E. Henkes

Dr W. Junk bv Publishers The Hague/Boston/London 1978

Electrodiagnosis, Toxic Agents and Vision
15th I.S.C.E.V. Symposium
Ghent, Belgium, June 20-23, 1977

Edited by J. François & A. De Rouck

Co-editors: J. T. Pearlman & J. Kelsey

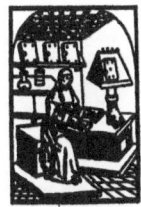

Dr W. Junk bv Publishers The Hague/Boston/London 1978

Cover design: Max Velthuijs

© Dr W. Junk b.v. Publishers 1978

Softcover reprint of the hardcover 1st edition 1978

ISBN-13: 978-94-009-9959-6   e-ISBN-13: 978-94-009-9957-2
DOI: 10.1007/978-94-009-9957-2

CONTENTS

OPENING ADDRESS

Mr. President, Ladies and Gentlemen, my dear Friends,

Since the International Society for Clinical Electroretinography was founded in Brussels in 1958 under the sponsorship of Prof. Karpe, Prof. Franceschetti, Prof. Henkes, Prof. Burian and myself, it is the second time that it has its congress in Ghent, the preceding one having been held in 1966.

Our first president, Prof. Karpe, with the collaboration of his secretary general, Prof. Henkes, who is our president at the present time, gave a great impulse to our society, which became more and more important, the number of members increasing greatly. Under the presidency of Prof. Henkes, assisted by our very active secretary general, Dr. Van Lith, our society still more enlarged its objectives in order to promote interest in every field of visual electrophysiology.

Today I am very thankful to many people. Firstly, I should like to impart my greatest gratefulness to the members of the organizing committee, Prof. Henkes, Prof. Van der Tweel, Prof. De Smedt and Dr. Van Lith for their constant efforts in supervising the scientific part of our meeting. Nevertheless, I should like to thank more particularly and very warmly my collaborator and active secretary, Dr. Alfred De Rouck, for his efficient, hard and continuous work in organizing so beautifully our symposium. I thank also very sincerely Mrs. Caluwaerts-De Coninck, Miss Agnes Van Gerven, Mrs. Dhaenens, Mr. André Uvijls and Mrs. Christine Ghesquière, who helped us as much as possible and with great efficacy.

I should also like to thank the chairmen of the various sessions as well as the invited speakers, who have kindly accepted to present a report with the conclusions of their research work. Thanks to them and also to the participants, who will present interesting papers, this congress will be able to realize its purpose, which should be the aim of every scientific meeting, namely the better understanding and the elucidation of one or other specific or complex problem by the addition of new information to the data already known and by the discussion of recent viewpoints and interpretations, so that we know where we are exactly, and from where we can start for further research and wider learning.

My dear friends, it is my great pleasure to bid a very hearty welcome to each of you, who came from more than twenty different countries and in fact from all parts of the world. I hope that the important and rather heavy scientific programme will not diminish the pleasure, which the social programme intends to give you. Belgium, traditional country of freedom, labour and culture, and Ghent, the oldest city of our country with its artistic and historical heritage, want to present to you the best of their warm hospitality, so that this symposium will leave an excellent souvenir in your heart and in your mind. The scientific discussions as well as the human contacts during this meeting will consolidate and enlarge the ties of friendship between ophthalmologists of different countries throughout the world for the greatest benefit of science, humanity and peace.

Ladies and gentlemen, I wish the whole of you a pleasant and fruitful meeting. It is my privilege to open this 15th International Symposium on Electroretinography.

Professor Jules François
President of the Congress

THE MODE OF ACTION OF NEUROTOXINS AND SOME COMMON CHEMICALS UPON THE ELECTROPHYSIOLOGICAL PROPERTIES OF PERFUSED MAMMALIAN RETINAS

YOSHIHITO HONDA

(Kyoto, Japan)

INTRODUCTION

Prior to the appearance of the in vitro retina as an experimental preparation, intravenous administration of chemicals was a common way of studying retinal toxicology of mammals. However, intravenous administration may bring about unexpected changes in general physiological conditions and is, therefore, limited as a toxicological method. When an in vitro preparation was desired, eyes of cold-blooded animals have been employed. In vitro studies on mammalian retinas originated from a combination of these two approaches; in vivo study of mammalian eyes and in vitro experimentation on tissues from cold-blooded animals.

METHODS
(BIOCHEMICAL AND PHYSIOLOGICAL CONDITIONS)

The following are important factors in maintaining high activity of mammalian retinas in vitro:
1. Composition of perfusates (Table 1).
2. Temperature regulation during the stage of preparation and during the stage of incubation.
3. pH of perfusates,
4. Osmotic pressure.
5. Oxygen supply.
6. Photic conditioning.
7. Surgical procedures.

ADVANTAGES OF PERFUSED MAMMALIAN RETINAS AS EXPERIMENTAL MATERIALS FOR TOXICOLOGY

Wide selection of materials

A wide selection of materials is possible, including tissue from cone-dominated, rod-dominated and mixed retinas. Experiments can be performed during all seasons of the year. The eyes of some mammals are larger in size than those of most cold-blooded animals and, therefore, are more easily

INVESTIGATOR MATERIAL	Ames et al. rabbit	Sickel et al. rabbit, cat, human, rat	Honda rabbit, human, cat guinea pig	Nagayama I rabbit	Weinstein, Hobson & Dowling rat	Winkler rat	INVESTIGATOR MATERIAL
Na+	145.7		143	142.5	146.4	145	Na+
K+	3.6		3.6	3.6	3.1	5	K+
Ca++	2.3	modified	1.15	1.15	0.8	2	Ca++
Mg++	2.4	Tyrode	1.20	1.06	1.2	1	Mg++
Cl-	125.4	Solution	125.4	125.4	125.4	129	Cl-
HCO3-	22.6	+	25.0	22.6	24.4	25	HCO3-
HPO4--	0.8	horse	0	0.1	0	0	HPO4--
H2PO4-	0.1	serum	0.5	0.4	0.5	0	H2PO4-
SO4--	2.4		1.2	1.06	1.2	1.0	SO4--
glucose	1.0		1.0	26	28 (dextrose:22)		glucose
serum	2-10%		none (mEq)	none	2%	2-5% (mEq)	serum

Table 1. Perfusates for mammalian retinas.

handled. Materials in vitro may be selected from among (a) the retina with pigment epithelium and choroid (eye-cup), (b) the retina without pigment epithelium and choroid (isolated retina) or (c) the retina with pigment epithelium (difficult).

Chemicals may be delivered to their site of action by perfusion from either the ganglion cell or the receptor cell side or from both.

Direct reaction of chemicals

Studies in vitro make it possible for toxins to act directly on the retina, independent of in vivo regulation systems. Environmental concentration of chemicals can be precisely controlled. To an in vitro retina, toxins of high concentrations, which would be lethal to intact animals, can be applied locally, and direct effects on the retina can be observed. Photic stimuli are delivered directly to the retinal preparation and can be exactly controlled, since there are no optic media.

Essential nutritional demands

Mammals have more complicated nutritional demands than cold-blooded animals. Some chemicals might be expected to be effective or toxic only for mammalian retinas, but not for retinas of cold-blooded animals. Even when the modes of action are the same, effective doses may be different.

Mechanical stability

In the excised retina, fine manipulations, such as microelectrode techniques, can be employed thanks to the mechanical stability possible with such preparations. An experimental retina in vitro is free from the movements of limbs, respiration and circulation.

Component isolation

Fragility of mammalian retinas in vitro provides many important clues for the analysis of toxic mechanisms. Sodium aspartate and glutamate isolate a stable P III in mammalian retinas in vitro as well as in those of cold-blooded animals. P III, or a P III-resembling potential may be isolated without chemicals, simply by cooling the retina. Characteristics of ERG components appear magnified relative to those in vivo. This feature is convenient for toxicological studies.

Electrophysiology combined with histological observations

In in vitro studies, it is possible to directly relate electrophysiological responses to histological observations. Experimental materials have already been excised in vitro when responses are recorded. Time loss occurring during fixation is quite short and essentially negligible.

COMMON MODES OF ACTION OF TOXIC CHEMICALS ON THE ERG

Effects should always be discussed in relation to chemical dosage in toxicological studies. Several metabolic inhibitors increase some of the electrophysiological activities of tissue when applied in low concentrations. On the retina, several toxins, for example, iodoacetate (Noell, 1959; Honda, 1970), dimethylaminopentane (Nakajima, 1958b), dinitrofluorobenzene (Nakajima, 1958a), malononitrile (Nakajima, 1958a) and ouabain (Honda, 1972), have been shown to temporarily increase the ERG amplitude at an initial stage when applied in very low concentrations. Such temporary enhancement of the ERG amplitude has also been reported by an experimentally or clinically induced mildly hypoxic condition of the retina (Henkes, 1957; Karpe & Uchermann, 1955).

Based on in vitro studies, we reached the following conclusions: the dose-response curve provided important clues for the analysis of the mode of action (Honda, 1972). The mode of action of toxic chemicals on the retina is fundamentally biphasic. A transient increase of the ERG amplitude might exist prior to inhibition. The implicit time of the b-wave is prolonged. P III, or a P III-resembling potential remains unaffected, even when the b-wave is markedly decreased in amplitude. Isolation of this slow potential is frequently observed during the course of a toxic action. Modes of action of toxic chemicals on the b-wave and the oscillatory potentials are sometimes different. It is important to determine whether the affected ERG will recover or not. In in vitro studies, it is easy to rinse the once-poisoned retina in fresh medium without toxin and examine recovery of responses.

CHEMICALS INDUCING A PARADOXICAL INCREASE
OF THE ERG AMPLITUDE

Fig. 1 shows the effect of pentobarbital sodium (6×10^{-5}M) on the ERG of rabbit retina in vitro. Time courses of the b-wave and P III amplitude changes (per cent of pre-administration level) are shown in Fig. 2. The b-wave ampli-

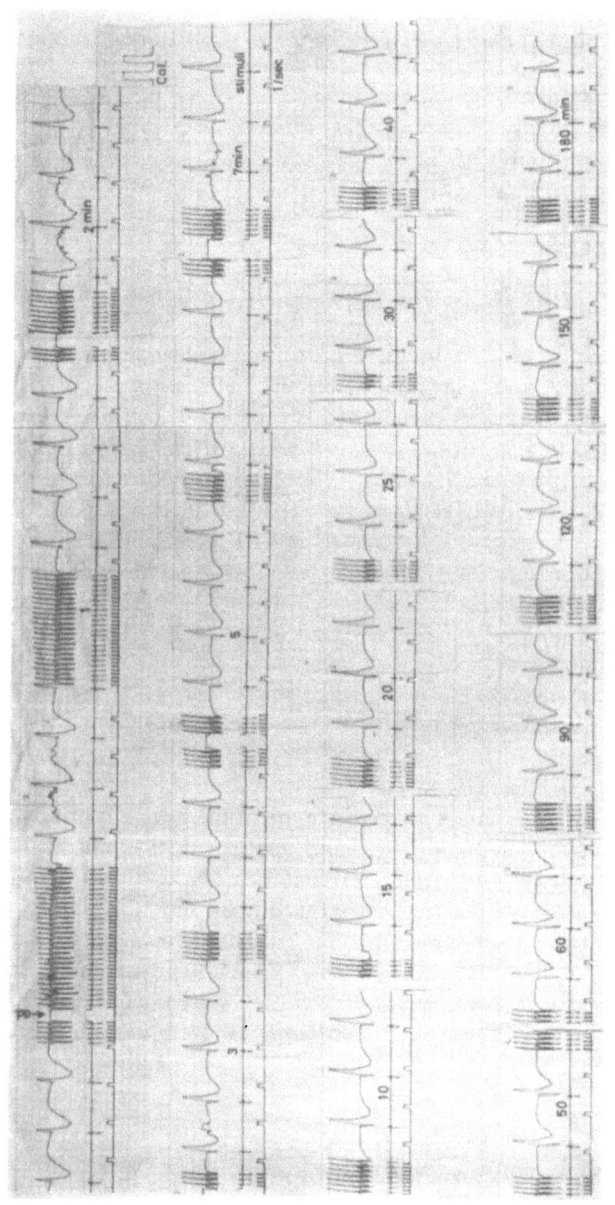

Fig. 1. Examples of responses evoked by photo-stimuli indicating the effect of 6 x 10^{-5} M pentobarbital sodium on an in vitro rabbit retina. Calibration mark represents 0.1 mV.

tude increased immediately after administration and reached a maximum in 10–20 minutes. The implicit time was prolonged. The time course of the P III amplitude change was affected by prolongation of the implicit time of the b-wave. The effects were reversible. When the retina was immersed in a medium without barbiturates, the ERG amplitude recovered to near the pre-administration level. It has been observed by several investigators that barbiturates increase the b-wave amplitude. In 1956, Wohlzogen reported that kemithal (thialbarbital sodium) increased the b-wave of cat ERGs in vivo. This phenomenon has been observed both in cold-blooded animals and in mammals (Table 2). Recent studies of Bornschein et al (1966), Rockstroh & Hanitzsch (1966), Honda & Nagata (1972), and Honda (1977) revealed that enhancement occurs in retinas in vitro. There can be no centrifugal influence through the optic nerve in this preparation. It is, therefore, established that barbiturates directly affect retinal cells, or synapses among them, resulting in ERG enhancement.

Cephaloridine is also an interesting chemical which increases the ERG amplitude. Both a- and b-wave increased in amplitude immediately after administration of cephaloridine (Honda & Nagata, 1975). The effect appeared more prominently in high drug concentrations, and was maintained until the end of incubation with cephaloridine. The phenomenon was shown to be reversible.

Diphenylhydantoin (DPH) also increases the ERG amplitude. The mean time courses of the b-wave and P III amplitude changes for each concentration of DPH have been described in our previous reports (Honda et al., 1973). The implicit time of the b-wave was delayed by the administration of effective doses of DPH. As the potassium concentration of the medium was increased, the prominent DPH-induced enhancement of the b-wave amplitude observed in the standard medium was inhibited (Honda et al., 1973b). When the potassium concentration was reduced to the standard level, the amplitude of the b-wave immediately increased.

A relationship between the DPH-effect on the retina and potassium concentration is suggested. This phenomenon can be interpreted in two ways: that the Müller cells are the origin of the b-wave of ERG (Miller & Dowling, 1970); and that they act as potassium channels, inducing spreading depression of the retina (Mori et al., 1976).

Alcohols are also known to enhance the ERG amplitude (Honda & Okada, 1974). Figs. 3 and 4 show the time courses of the effect of ethanol and methanol on ERGs from in vitro rabbit retinas. The effects of alcohol on the ERG in vivo have been studied in detail by Potts and his associates in the 1950's (Potts, 1955), and do not require comment, except to note that even methanol increased the b-wave amplitude in vitro and that the effect was reversible. The prominent inhibition of ERGs in vivo might be produced by metabolic products of methanol.

Besides these, we know several other chemicals which increase the ERG amplitude during application but also show reversibility (Zimmerman et al., 1973). Among chemicals increasing the ERG amplitude, a structural similarity can be pointed out. In Fig. 5, barbiturates have a ring structure combined in -1-2-3-4-5-6-. DPH has a structure similar to the lactam ring. The

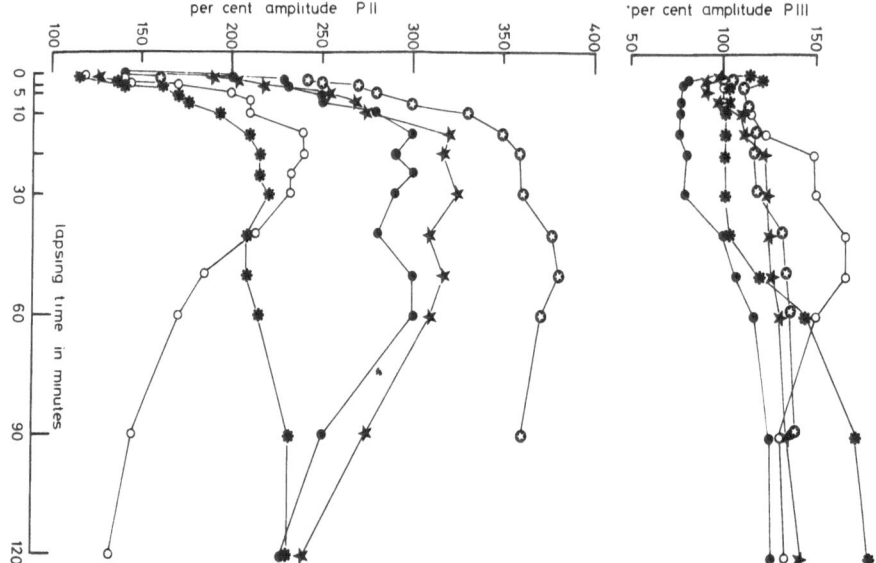

Fig. 2. Time courses of change in amplitude (per cent of pre-administration level) of the b-wave and P III after administration of 6 x 10⁻⁵ M pentobarbital sodium.

(investigator)	(material)	(status)	(barbiturates used)	(year)
Wohlzogen	cat	in vivo	Kemithal (=thialbarbital sodium)	1956
Jacobson	cat,monkey	in vivo	pentobarbital	1958
Noell	rabbit	in vivo	nembutal (=pentobarbital sodium)	1958
Arden,Granit & Ponte	cat	in vivo	nembutal	1960
Ogawa	rabbit	in vivo	nembutal	1961
Mita, Suzuki, Nikara & Ogawa	rabbit	in vivo	nembutal thiopental sodium	1961
Masuda	rabbit	in vivo	nembutal	1963
Bornschein, Hanitzsch & Lützow	rabbit	in vitro	pentobarbital sodium	1966
Rockstroh & Hanitzsch	frog	in vitro	pentobarbital sodium	1966
Yonemura, Kawasaki & Tuchida	rabbit	in vivo	nembutal	1966
Honda & Nagata	rabbit	in vitro	thiopental sodium phenobarbital sodium	1972
Wündsch	cat, rabbit	in vivo	nembutal	1975
Honda	rabbit	in vitro	diabutal (=pentobarbital sodium)	1976

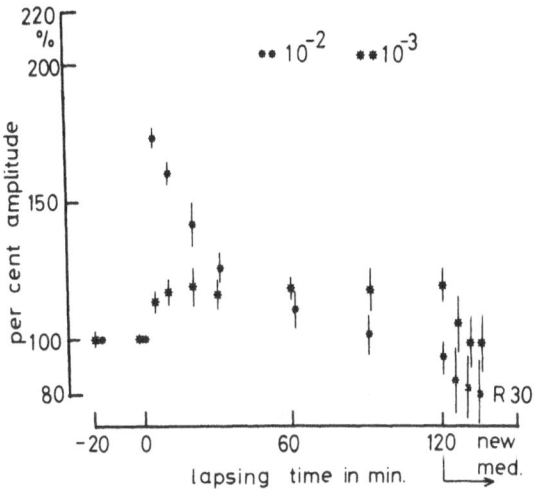

Fig. 3. Time course of the per cent amplitude of the b-wave, using an average of four cases for each concentration. The retina was incubated with ethanol for 120 minutes. Then, the incubating chamber was drained and filled with fresh medium.

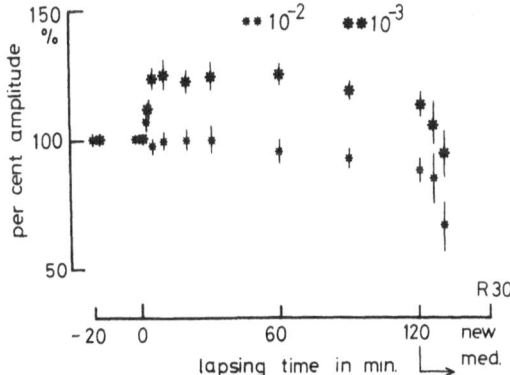

Fig. 4. Time courses of the per cent amplitude of the b-wave. The retina was incubated with methanol for 120 minutes. Then, the incubating chamber was drained and filled with a fresh medium.

nucleus of cephaloridine is closely related to that of penicillinic acid, which is made by connection of -2-3-4-5-oxygen-. Including penicillin derivatives, all of these chemicals are anti-convulsants. The mode of action of each chemical on the retina has not yet been clarified. However, we are inclined to consider chemicals having a lactam ring or allied structures to be capable of increasing the ERG amplitude, especially the b-wave amplitude, by depressing function of inhibitory pathways within the retina. Further studies are now in progress.

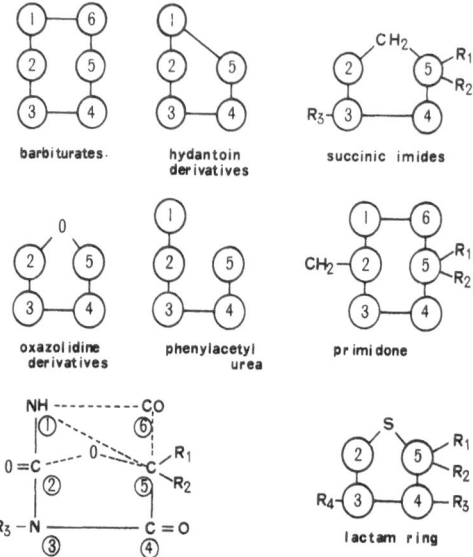

Fig. 5. Structure of anti-convulsants.

REFERENCES

Bornschein, H., R. Hanitzch & A. von Lützow. Der Nachweis der Barbiturateffektes an der isolierten Warmbluternetzhaut. *Experientia* 22: *98–99* (1966).

Henkes, H.E. Electroretinography. An evaluation of the influence of the retinal and general metabolic condition on the electrical response of the retina. *Am. J. Ophthal.* 43: *67–86* (1957).

Honda, Y. The mode and site of action of iodoacetic acid upon the in vitro preparation of rabbit's retina. *Acta Soc. Ophthal. Jap.* 74: *302–316* (1970).

Honda, Y. Quantitative analysis of some effects of ouabain upon the electrical activity of mammalian retinas. *Invest. Ophthal.* 11: *699–705* (1972).

Honda, Y. Chemicals increasing the b-wave amplitude of the in vitro ERG. *Acta Soc. Ophthal. Jap.* 81: *372–378* (1977).

Honda, Y. & M. Nagata. Some observations of the effects of barbiturates upon the electroretinogram of rabbits. *Ophthal. Res.* 4: *129–136* (1972).

Honda, Y. & M. Nagata. A neurological side effect of cephaloridine: enhancement of the electroretinogram. *Ophthal. Res.* 7: *395–400* (1975).

Honda, Y. & K. Okada. Some observations of the effects of alcohol on the ERG of rabbits. *Acta Soc. Ophthal. Jap.* 78: *1164–1169* (1974).

Honda, Y., S.M. Podos & B. Becker. The effect of diphenylhydantoin on the electro-retinogram of rabbits. I. Effects of concentration. *Invest. Ophthal.* 12: *567–572* (1973a).

Honda, Y., S.M. Podos & B. Becker. The effect of **diphenylhydantoin** on the electro-retinogram of rabbits. II. Effects of hypoxia and potassium. *Invest. Ophthal.* 12: *573–578* (1973b).

Karpe, G. & A. Uchermann. The clinical electroretinogram. VII. The electroretinogram in circulatory disturbances of the retina. *Acta Ophthal.* 33: *493* (1955).

Miller, R.F. & J.E. Dowling. Intracellular responses of the Müller cells of mud-puppy retina: their relation to the b-wave of the electroretionogram. *J. Neurophysiol.* 33: *323–341* (1970).

Mori, S., W.H. Miller & T. Tomita. Microelectrode study of spreading depression in frog retina. Part I. *Jap. J. Physiol.* 26: *203–217* (1976).

Nakajima, A. The effect of inhibitors of carbohydrate metabolism on the rabbit electroretinogram. *Ophthalmologica* 136: *99–107* (1958a).

Nakajima, A. The effect of amino-phenoxyalkanes on rabbit ERG. *Ophthalmologica* 136: *332–344* (1958b).

Noell, W.K. The visual cell: electric and metabolic manifestations of its life processes. *Am. J. Ophthal.* 48: *344–370* (1959).

Potts, A.M. The visual toxicity of methanol. VI. The clinical aspects of experimental methanol poisoning treated with base. *Am. J. Ophthal.* 39 (II): *86–92* (1955).

Rockstroh, W. & R. Hanitzsch. Der Einfluss von Barbituraten auf das ERG der isolierten Froschnetzhaut. *Experientia* 22: *100–101* (1966).

Wohlzogen, F.X. von. Beeinflussung des Säuger-ERG during zentralnervös wirksame Substanzen. *Z. Biol.* 108: *217–233* (1956).

Zimmerman, T.J., W.W. Dawson & C.R. Fitzgerald. ERG in human eyes following oral adrenocorticoids. *Invest. Ophthal.* 12: *777–779* (1973).

Author's address:
Department of Ophthalmology
Faculty of Medicine
Kyoto University
Sakyo-ku
Kyoto 606
Japan

Docum. Ophthal. Proc. Series, Vol. 15

ON THE EFFECT OF URETHANE AND HALOTHANE®
ON THE ERG OF RATS*

A. STUTE, J.G.H. SCHMIDT & E. WEBER

(Cologne, Fed. Rep. Germany)

Earlier experiments with rats have shown the considerable effects of urethane on the ERG (Tamaki, 1967; Schmidt & Weber, 1970) and mitochondria of the pigment epithelium (Amemiya, 1968). The long effect of urethane on the potentials and on the condition of the animals are disadvantages, especially for frequent examinations within a time interval of a few days. Therefore, we have used Halothane® (bromochlorotrifluoroethane) to obtain better procedure.

The results of Perdriel et al. (1964), Nye (1968) and Whitten & Brown (1973), stating that Fluothane® does not change the amplitudes and profile of the ERG are in contrast to those of François & De Rouck (1963) who found that the a-amplitude remains unchanged, but that the b-amplitude is reduced. Under scotopic conditions, De Molfetta et al. (1965) have shown in clinical investigations an extension of the b-wave peak time and an increase of the a- and b-wave amplitudes. Using vectorelectroretinography, Norren & Padmos (1973) found a dramatic effect on dark adaptation with apes. The considerable deviations can partly be explained by differing experimental conditions.

METHOD

Electroretinographic recordings and anaesthesia correspond to those in earlier experiments with urethane (Weber, 1975) and Halothane® (Schmidt & Stute, 1972; Stute 1978). 10% urethane solution (1 ml/100 g body weight) was injected intraperitoneally 2 hours before the beginning of the experiments.

In our investigations with increasing Halothane® concentrations the animals were exposed to nitrous oxide and oxygen in a proportion of 3:1; the flow remained constant at 1,2 l/min. Following each increase of Halothane® concentration, the respiration frequency was measured for half a minute. After 1.5 more minutes, the ERG readings were taken. By observing respiration anaesthesia was prevented from slipping into stage IV, which, according to Guedel, preceeds a depression of the respiratory and circulatory centers.

* This research was supported by the Deutsche Forschungsgemeinschaft, Bonn/Bad Godesberg.

Deep breath or gasps quickly signalled the immediate need for reducing the depth of the narcosis.

The time lapse from the end of the anaesthesia to the reawakening of the excitation stadium was about 10 min. in the average.

RESULTS

These experiments with urethane and Halothane® were performed to find out the effects of intravitreal foreign bodies on the ERG. The results for this publication are taken from the control eyes. As the changes of the potentials occur rapidly in the first stage, we have taken our recordings in short periods of time, later in larger intervals.

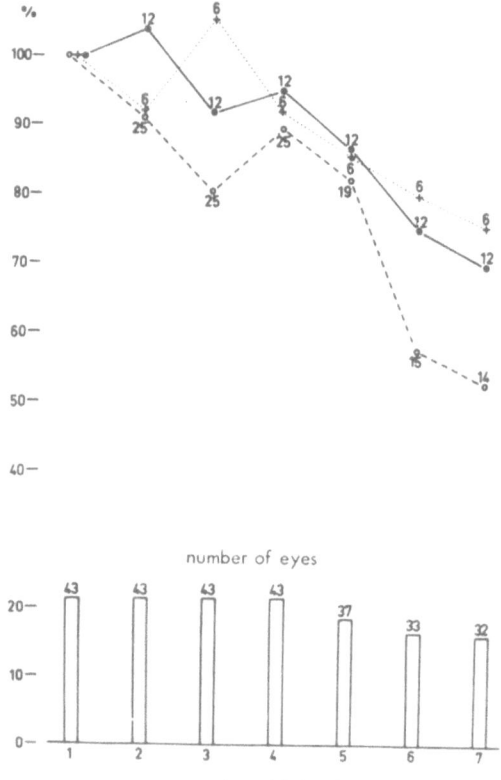

Fig. 1. Effect of urethane. Mean values of uninjured fellow eyes. Solid line (12 eyes): first eye uninjured; dashed line (25 eyes): first eye with an implanted metal particle; dotted line (6 eyes): first eye with an implanted glass splinter; 1st to 5th injection: 18 days; 1st to 7th injection: 80 days.

Urethane

Fig. 1 shows the effect of urethane on the b-wave amplitudes of rat eyes. Summarizing these results the values after the 2nd and 4th injection did not differ significantly from those after the first one. However, significant differences were found for the 3rd anaesthesia as well for the 5th to the 7th. The period of time between the first four injections was 3 or 4 days.

The strong toxic effect of urethane could be seen already in the general behaviour of the rats. The stage of complete anaesthesia lasted for several hours; as a rule, the rats regained normal standing and running abilities and eating habits after 24 hours.

Halothane®

1. With increasing Halothane® concentration during anaesthesia, the a-wave amplitude of the rat remained almost constant (Fig. 3a), while the b-wave amplitude fell sharply (Fig. 3b). These values are statistically significant (95.5% level). We suggest that this b-wave change is the result of hypoxia due to respiratory impairment (Fig. 2). It is possible that, in addition, a lowering of the blood pressure may play a role as has been noted in dogs, rabbits and cats. Therefore, hypoxia and ischaemia may be responsible for the b-wave fall.

2. In the experiments on the influence of repeated, flat anaesthesias the Halothane® concentration was kept at 2% during the ERG recordings.

For a long period of our observation time — i.e., up to 98 days — we did not get any significant differences in comparison to those of the first anaesthesia. Only after 125 days we got a deviation, which was significant for most amplitudes and peak times of the a- and b-wave (Fig. 4a+b). At the

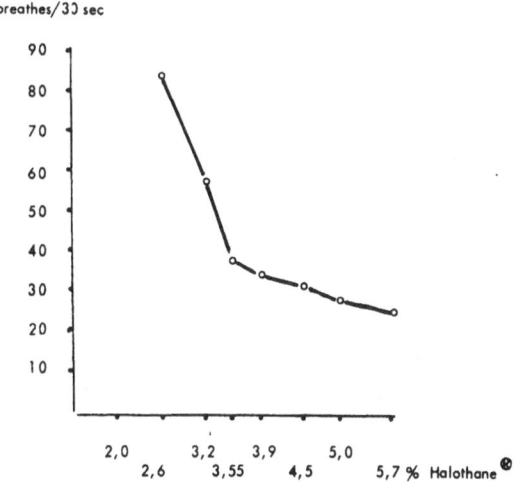

Fig. 2. Effect of increasing Halothane® concentrations. Mean values of 5 rats.

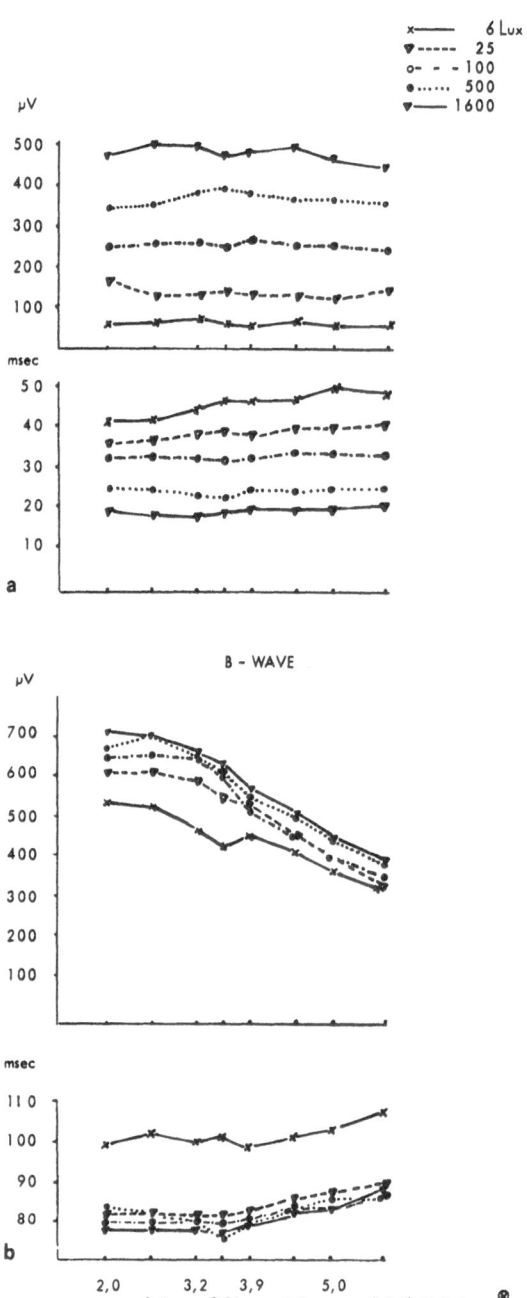

Fig. 3a+b. Effects of increasing Halothane® concentrations. Mean values of 5 rats.

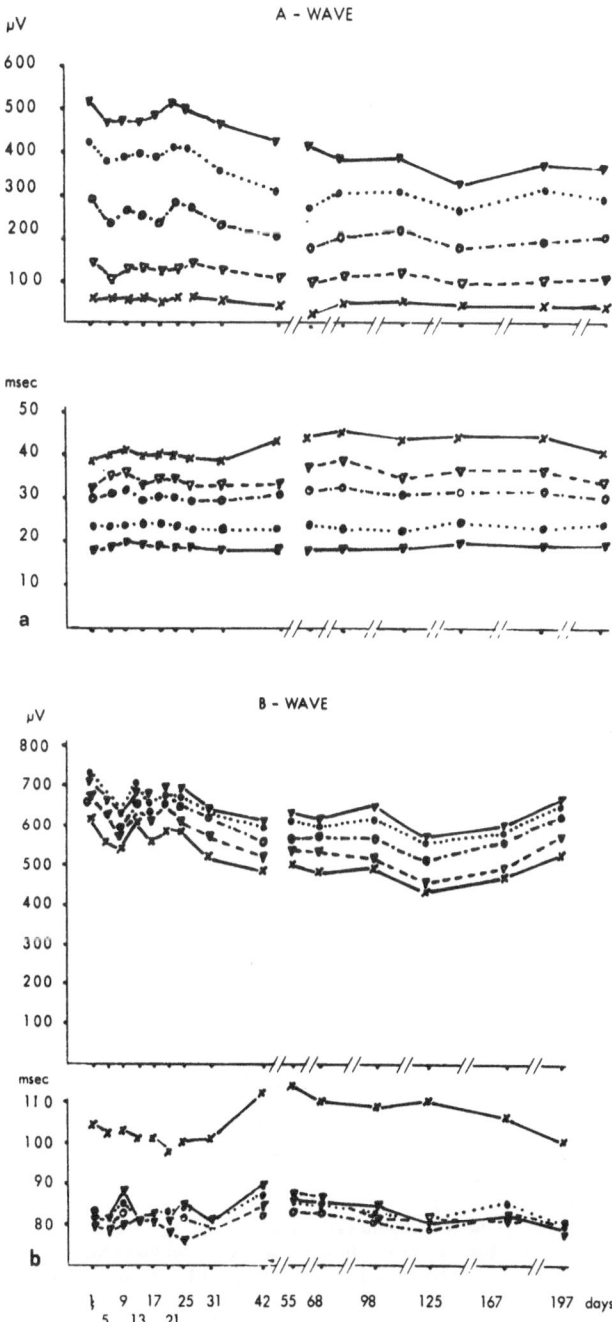

Fig. 4a+ b. Effects of repeated flat anaesthesias. Mean values of 8 uninjured eyes (8 rats). First eye with an implanted iron particle.

17

end of the observation time of 197 days the data did not again show any significant deviation. Probably we have to explain this phenomenon from the different intervals of the anaesthesias. Until the recordings on the 68th day the periods of time were relatively short, so there might be a cumulation effect, whereas after this time the long intervals permit a recovery of the retina.

CONCLUSION

The negative effect of Halothane® on the ERG potentials applying the conventional concentration of this drug is much less as compared with urethane. We find significant changes of the a- and b-wave only if we repeat the Halothane® narcosis very often and after short intervals. If we consider these data, we are able to study chronic or slowly developing ERG changes without influence of repeated anaesthesis.

In case of urethane the investigated side effects appear much more intensive and earlier. The distinct difference between the toxic effect of the two drugs is not only demonstrated by these ERG changes and the behaviour of the animals. Using urethane we lost nearly 25% of the animals up to the 7th narcosis. By using Halothane®-nitrous oxide, we only had one casualty during the 627 periods of narcosis carried out on 72 rats at intervals ranging from 4 hours to 30 days; and this casualty was due to incorrect proportions of the gas mixture.

We are grateful to Mrs. Hertha Keßler and Miss Annegret Weege for technical assistance.

REFERENCES

Amemiya, T. Electron microscopic study of the retina of rats repeatedly treated with urethane. *Acta Soc. Ophthal. Jap.* 72: *293–298* (1968).

Amemiya, T. Fine structure of Bruch's membrane in vitamin A deficiency and urethane intoxication. *Acta Soc. Ophthal. Jap.* 73: *1008–1015* (1969).

De Molfetta, V., P.G. Sironi & D. Spinelli. Rapporti tra narcosi e risposta elettroretinografica. *Ann. Oftalm.* 91: *1385–1393* (1965).

François, J. & A. De Rouck. L'électroretinogramme normal des jeunes enfants. *Ann. Ocul.* 196: *570–583* (1963).

Norren, D.V. & P. Padmos. Halothane retards dark adaptation. In: XIth ISCERG Symposium, Bad Nauheim, 1973. Junk, The Hague (1974).

Neye, P.W. An examination of the electro-retinogram of the pigeon in response to stimuli of different intensity and wavelength and following intense chromatic adaptation. *Vision Res.* 8: *679–696* (1968).

Schmidt, J.G.H., V. Micovic & A. Stute. Surface area sizes of intravitreal copper particles: their effects on the ERG of rabbits and rats. Paper presented at the 15th ISCERG Symposium, Ghent, Belgium (1977).

Schmidt, J.G.H. & A. Stute. Electroretinogram and ophthalmoscopic findings in intravitreous iron, copper and lead particles. In: XIth ISCERG Symposium, Los Angeles, 1972. Junk, The Hague (1973).

Schmidt, J.G.H., A. Stute & E. Weber. Elektroretinographische und ophthalmoskopische Befunde bei intraocularen Metallfremdkörpern der Ratte. *Ber. dtsch. Ophthal. Ges.* 71: *391–396* (1972).

Schmidt, J.G.H. & E. Weber. The effect of intra-ocular copper alloys on the ERGs of human and rat retinas. In: VIIIth ISCERG Symposium, Pisa (1970).

Stute, A. Elektroretinographische und ophthalmoskopische Veränderungen bei intra-vitrealen Eisen-, Kupfer- und Blei-Fremdkörpern der Ratte unter Berucksichtigung des Narkose-Einflusses. Thesis, Cologne (1978).

Tamaki, S. Electroretinographic studies on the experimental hypervitaminosis A and vitamin A deficiency. *Acta Soc. Ophthal. Jap.* 71: *2102* (1967).

Walsh, F.B. Clinical Neuroophthalmology. Williams & Wilkins, Baltimore (1957).

Weber, E. Der Einfluss intra-okularer Kupfer-Fremdkörper auf das Elektroretinogramm der Ratte. Thesis, Cologne (1975).

Whitten, D.N. & K.T. Brown. The time courses of late receptor potentials from monkey cones and rods. *Vision Res.* 13: *107–135* (1973).

Wirth, A., G. Tota & A. Vagelli. The effect of fluothane anaesthesia on the electro-retinogram of the rabbit. In: VIIth ISCERG Symposium, Istanbul (1969).

Authors' address:
Universitäts-Augenklinik
5000 Cologne 41
Fed. Republic of Germany

THE EFFECTS OF ANESTHETICS ON THE ERG AND EOG

IKUO WATANABE & KIICHI TOYAMA

(Hamamatsu, Japan)

ERG recording in experimental animals without general anesthesia is ideal, because it is well known that the anesthetics seriously influence the ERG. However, the quantitative studies regarding this point are scarce.

The effect of commonly used anesthetics, i.e. Urethane and Nembutal, on the ERG components was studied for the purpose of determining the safety-dose, with which the ERG components remained unchanged.

RESULTS

Rabbits

The effect of Nembutal (Fig. 1)

1. Repeated injections of 5 mg/kg Nembutal i.v. (30 min interval). With an additive administration of Nembutal (each dose: 5 mg/kg), no change was observed in the b-wave after the first and second injections. With the third and fourth injections, a transient increase and decrease in the b-wave amplitude was observed. Until the fourth injection, the oscillatory potentials were unchanged in amplitude, but the peak latency was shortened. No changes in the V/I curves were found after the first, second or fourth injections.

2. 10 mg /kg Nembutal i.v. The amplitude of the b-wave increased and the peak latency of the oscillatory potentials was shortened after a single injection of 10 mg/kg Nembutal i.v. The V/I curve shifted towards the left, 0.7 log units 30 min after the injection.

3. 15 mg/kg Nembutal i.v. A transient increase in the b-wave amplitude was observed after an injection of 15 mg/kg Nembutal i.v. However, it returned rapidly to baseline and the V/I curves measured at 30 min and 75 min after the injection were similar to the control. The oscillatory potentials showed no change in the peak latency but a decrease in the amplitude.

4. 20 mg/kg Nembutal i.v. A transient increase in the b-wave was also observed; but the duration of the increase was longer than that of 15 mg/kg. The V/I curve, measured 30 min after the injection, was 0.5 log units shifted towards the right. The oscillatory potentials showed a delay of the peak latency and remarkable decrease in amplitude especially for the second wavelet (O_2).

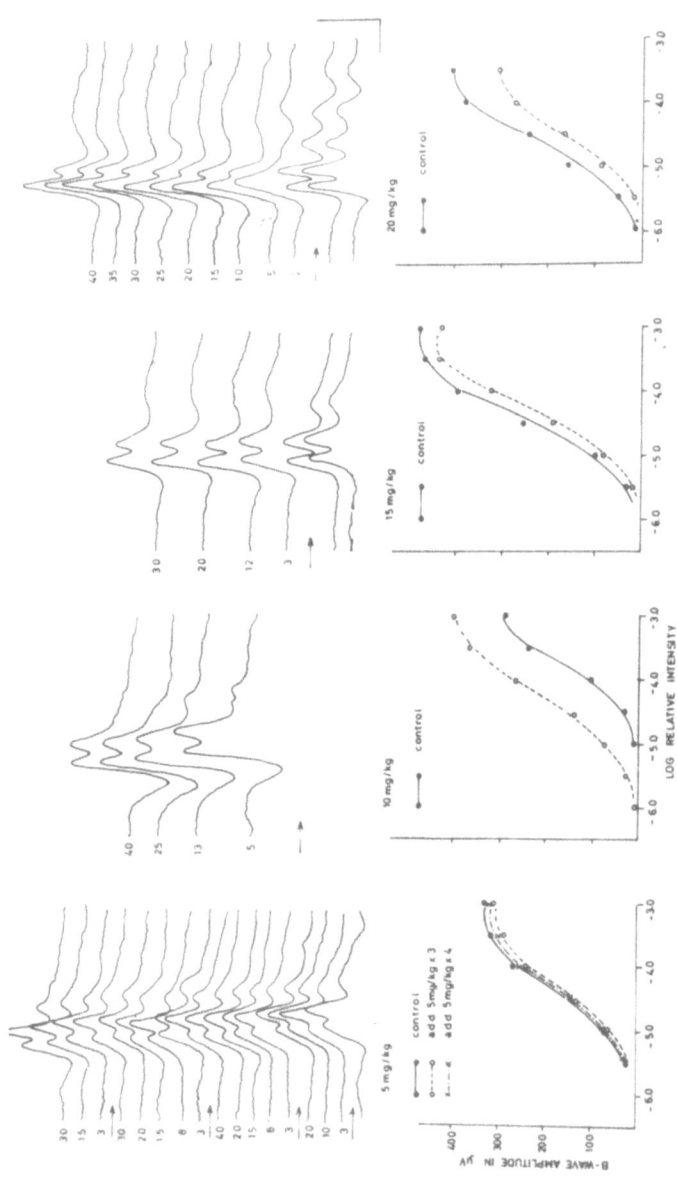

Fig. 1. Top: oscillatory potentials after Nembutal injection i.v. The y-axis numbers refer to minutes after the injection. Bottom: changes of the V/I curves after injection of Nembutal. Black dots: control; white circles; after the injection of nembutal. (Rabbits.)

The effect of Urethane (Fig. 2)

1. Repeated injections of 100 mg/kg Urethane i.p. No changes in amplitude and in peak latency of the oscillatory potentials were observed until the fifth injection (total dose: 500 mg/kg). The V/I curve at the fourth injection shifted towards the left by less than 0.5 log units.

2. 400 mg/kg Urethane i.p. An increase of the b-wave amplitude without change in the peak latency of the oscillatory potentials was observed with the second injection (total dose: 800 mg/kg). With the third injection, a decrease in amplitude and with the fourth injection (total dose 1600 mg/kg) disappearance of the oscillatory potentials was observed. The V/I curve shifted towards the left, 0.5 log units, after the third injection.

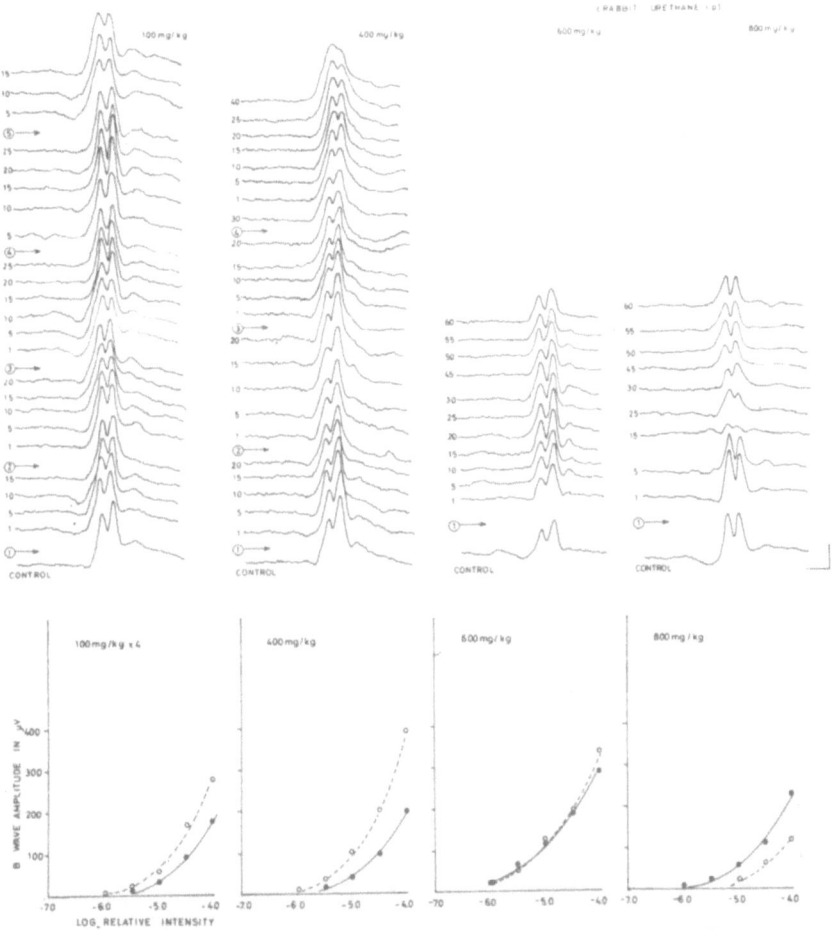

Fig. 2. Top: changes in the oscillatory potentials after injection of Urethane (i.p.). Bottom: V/I curves of the b-wave. Black spots: control; white circles: after injection of Urethane. (Rabbits.)

23

3. 600 mg/kg Urethane i.p. With a single injection of 600 mg/kg Urethane no change of the b-wave amplitude was observed, and the oscillatory potentials were still unchanged. With a repeated injection, the V/I curves were the same until the fourth injection (total dose: 2400 mg/kg). With the third injection, the oscillatory potentials disappeared.

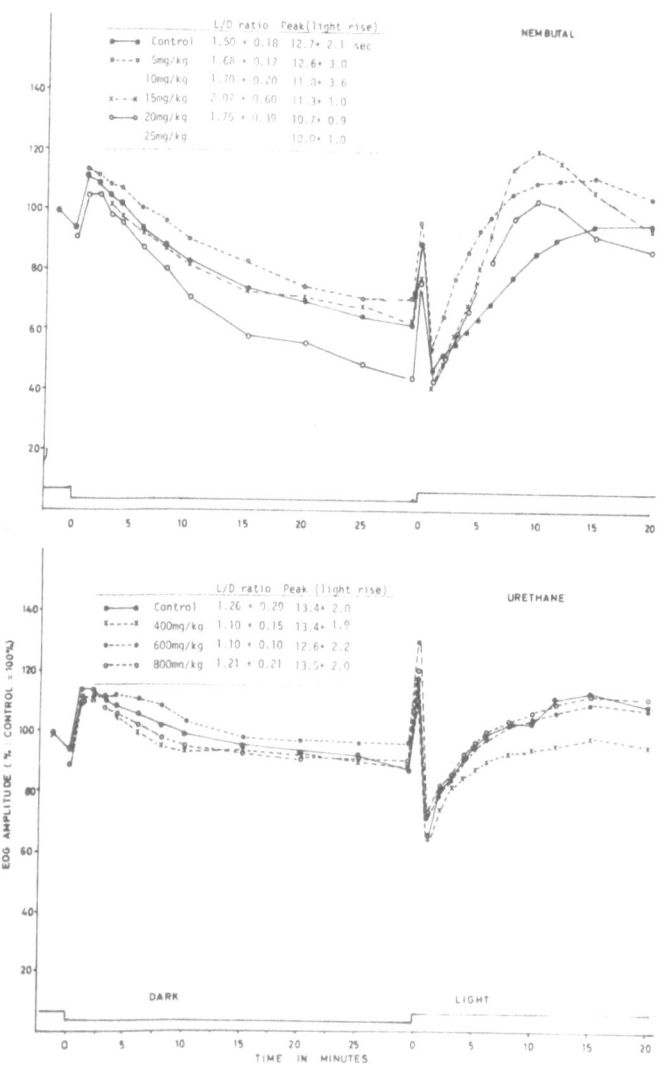

Fig. 3. Effects of Nembutal i.p.(top) and of Urethane (bottom) on the EOG of rabbits. Insertions give the L/D ratio and the time from 'light on' to the peak of light rise.

4. 800 mg/kg Urethane i.p. A decrease of the b-wave after the injection of 800 mg/kg Urethane i.p. was observed, and the V/I curve shifted towards the right 0.5 log units. The oscillatory potentials disappeared 10 min after the injection, and then recovered. The peak latency of the O_1 and O_2 was unchanged throughout.

EOG change (Fig. 3)

No change in L/D ratio was observed between the group injected with 400, 600 and 800 mg/kg Urethane i.p. and the control group. The L/D ratio was 150 ± 18 in the control group; 168 ± 17 in the group with 5 mg/kg Nembutal i.p.; 170 ± 20 with 10 mg/kg; 207 ± 60 with 15 mg/kg, and 175 ± 39 with 20 mg/kg Nembutal i.p., respectively.

The time from 'light on' to the peak of light rise was shortened with an in-

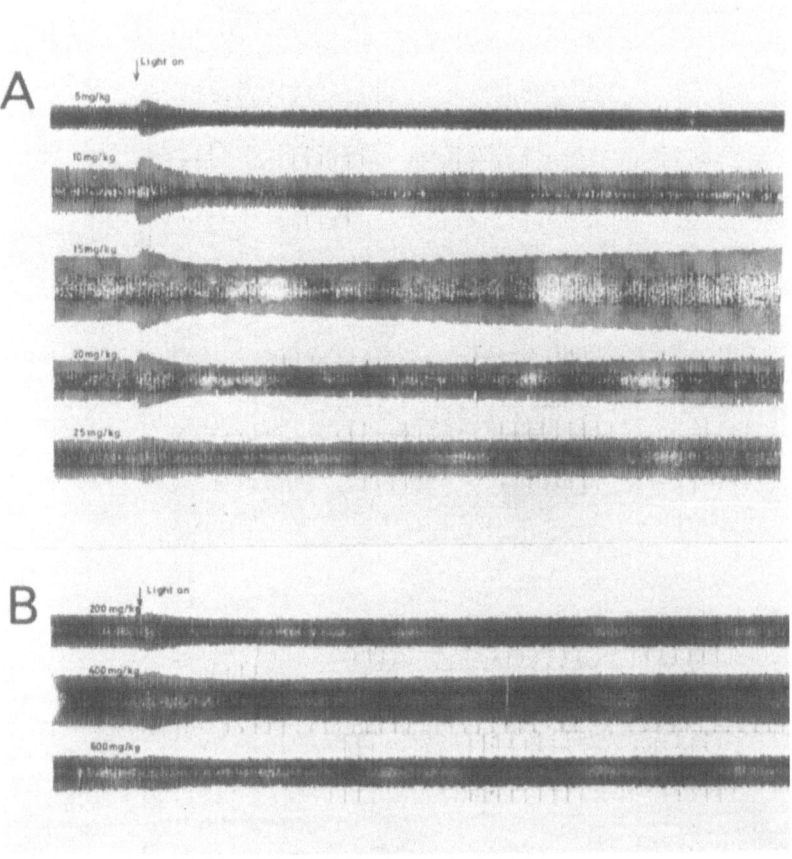

Fig. 4. Top: transient phenomena at 'light on' after several doses of Nembutal i.p. injections. Bottom: after Urethane i.p. (Rabbits.)

creased dose of Nembutal. There was, however, no significant difference ($\alpha = 0.05$) between the control and the treated group by F-test.

No remarkable changes in the transient phenomenon at 'light on' were found in the group with Nembutal i.v., but when Urethane was injected intraperiotonealy, the increase of the EOG amplitude at this point was slower as compared with the control group (Fig. 4).

Rats

The effect of Urethane i.p.

The V/I curves of the b-wave were measured repeatedly at 15 min intervals after injection of 100 mg/kg Urethane i.p. The difference between the first and fourth V/I curves was about 0.5 log units.

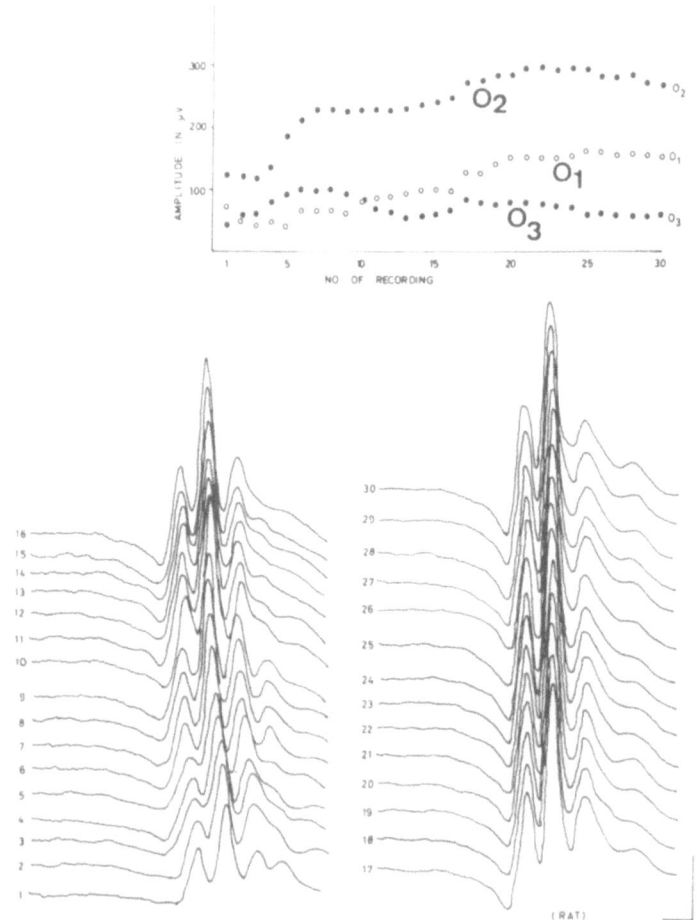

Fig. 5. Changes of the oscillatory potentials at repeated stimuli of 0.1 Hz. (Experimental animal: rat; basic anesthesia: 1000 mg/kg Urethane i.p.).

The oscillatory potentials showed small amplitudes just after dark adaptation. After repeated stimuli of 0.1 Hz, the amplitude increased during the first five to six recordings and after that the increase of the amplitude was slower (Fig. 5).

Under the basic anesthesia of 1000 mg/kg Urethane, additional injections of Urethane (each dose: 500 mg/kg) showed an increase of the b-wave amplitude. The degree of the increase was 60 to 70% of the initial value, even after a total dose of 2000 mg/kg. The shift of the V/I curve towards the left was at maximum 0.7 log units after two additional doses of Urethane (see Fig. 7).

Under the same conditions as above, the oscillatory potentials increased in amplitude. The increase of the O_1 amplitude was four times the initial value; that of O_2, however, was less than half (Fig. 6). The off-effect reacted in a fashion similar to the b-wave. The injection of over 2000 mg/kg Urethane i.p., even in divided doses, resulted in the death of the animals.

The effect of Nembutal i.p.

Following repeated injections of Nembutal i.p., the amplitude of the b-wave showed an increase. The V/I curve of the b-wave shifted towards the left by more than 1.2 log units. The oscillatory potentials also showed an increase of the amplitude; the peak latency was, however, unchanged until the third injection (total dose 120 mg/kg). Another injection caused death in the animals.

Under basic anesthesia with Urethane (1000 mg/kg) an additional injection of Nembutal also caused an increase in the amplitude of the b-wave, and the shift of the V/I curve was 1.5 log units (Fig. 7).

Under the same conditions, the additional injection of Nembutal subcutaneously (each dose: 25 mg/kg) caused some increase in the b-wave amplitude, but the shift of the V/I curve towards the left was 0.5 log units and it was the same value with the experiment using Urethane only, at 1000 mg/kg i.p.

DISCUSSION

There is well documented evidence that a small dose of Nembutal enhances the ERG amplitude. Earlier papers (Jacobson & Gestring, 1958) explained this phenomenon by the suppression of the centrifugal inhibitory process with the anesthetics. However, later papers (Bornschein et al., 1966; Yonemura et al., 1966; Honda & Nagata, 1972, 1973) denied such a hypothesis because with an intravitreal injection of Nembutal or in the experiment with isolated retina an enhancement of the ERG amplitude was also recorded. They concluded that this phenomenon was due to the direct effect of Nembutal upon the retina. Honda & Nagata stated that the enhancement of the ERG amplitude might be induced by the abolition of any inhibitory synaptic pathways at the retinal level.

Concerning Urethane, we could not find any studies which showed enhancement of ERG amplitude. Danis (1959) could not find any change in

ERG when Urethane was injected intra-arterially. Van Norren & Padmos (1977) demonstrated retardation of dark adaptation of the cone ERG.

In this work, distinct enhancement of the ERG under Urethane anesthesia was confirmed, but the degree of the enhancement was less than that of Nembutal.

A subcutaneous injection of Nembutal caused less enhancement than an intraperitoneal injection, even when the total dose was the same. These results confirmed the findings in Levett's paper (1974) on the rabbit's ERG.

These results suggest that the speed of absorption of the drug might be an important factor. The divided administration of the drug caused less enhancement than that of a single administration, even when the total dose was the same.

Changes in the EOG were very small, and the difference between the test

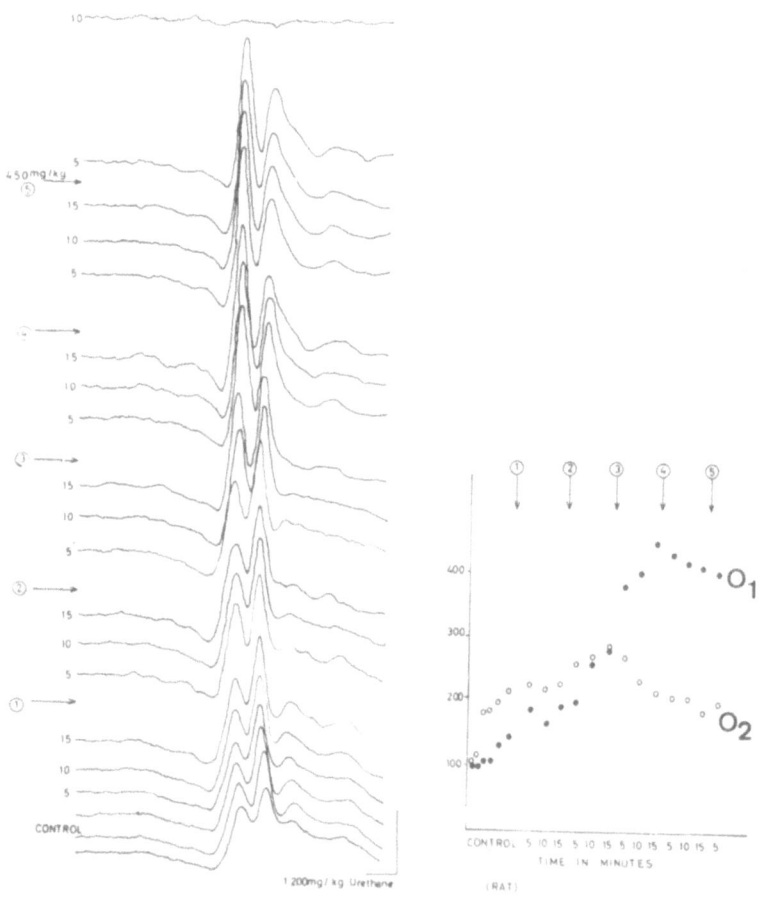

Fig. 6. Effect of additive administration of Urethane on the oscillatory potentials. (Experimental animal: rat; basic anesthesia: 1200 mg/kg Urethane i.p.).

group and the control was negligible in the group with Urethane. On the other hand, Nembutal, even with such a small dose as 5 mg/kg, caused an increase in the L/D ratio, but there was no significant difference between the control and the treated group by F-test.

From our experimental results, it was impossible to determine the safety-dose of anesthetics which caused no ERG change as even small doses of the anesthetics caused, more or less, alterations in some or all components of the ERG recording.

When we employed commonly used doses of anesthetic, ERG and EOG changes were generally smaller with Urethane than with Nembutal. Therefore, the authors recommend the use of Urethane anesthesia in ERG and EOG experiments and, furthermore, the divided administration of the drug.

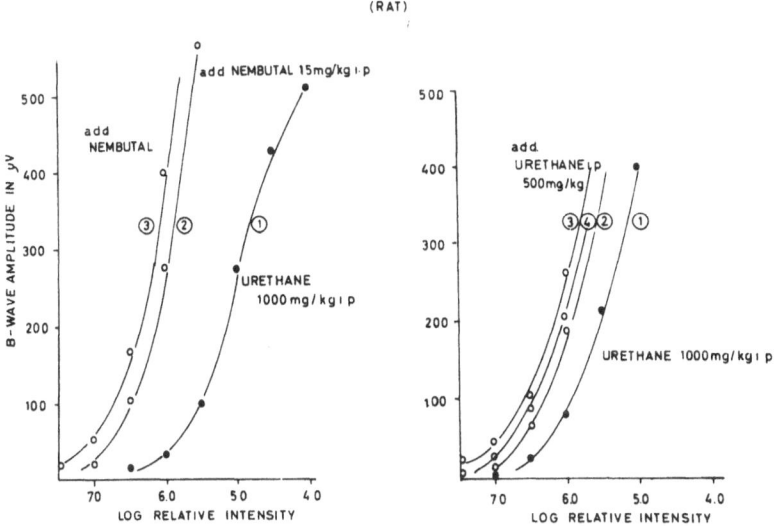

Fig. 7. Changes of V/I curves after additive injection of Nembutal i.p. (left) and of Urethane i.p. (right). (Experimental animal: rat; basic anesthesia: 1000 mg/kg Urethane i.p.).

SUMMARY

The effect of Nembutal and Urethane on the ERG and EOG of the rabbit and rat was tested with intravenous, intraperitoneal and subcutaneous injections. The changes of the ERG and EOG were smaller with Urethane i.p. than with Nembutal i.v. or i.p. Subcutaneous injection of Nembutal induced the same degree of change in the ERG as that of Urethane i.p.

The authors recommend Urethane i.p. anesthesia in animal ERG and EOG experiments, where there is a choice.

REFERENCES

Bornschein, H., R. Hanitzch & V. Lützow. Der Nachweis des Barbiturateffektes an der isolierten Warmblüternetzhaut. *Experientia* 22: 98–99 (1966).

Danis, P. Contribution à l'étude électrophysiologique de la rétine. Impr. Méd. et Sci., Brussels (1959).

Honda, Y. & M. Nagata. Some observations of the effect of barbiturates upon the electroretinogram of rabbits. *Ophthal. Res.* 4: *129–136* (1972, 1973).

Jacobson, J.H. & G.F. Gestring. Centrifugal influence upon the electroretinogram. *Arch. Ophthal.* 60: *295–302* (1958).

Levett, J. An examination of Nembutal as a reasonable anesthetic in electro-retinography. *Ophthal. Res.* 6: *320–327* (1974).

Norren, D. van & P. Padmos. Influence of anesthetic, ethyl alcohol, and freon on dark adaptation of monkey cone ERG. *Invest. Ophthal.* 16: *80–83* (1977).

Watanabe, I. & K.A. Hellner. Threshold of the oscillatory potentials in mice. Docum. Ophthal. Proc. Series 4: 471–476 (1974).

Yonemura, D,. K. Kawasaki & Y. Tuchida. Differential vulnerability of the ERG components to pentobarbital. pp. 155–166, in: Proc. 4th ISCERG Symp. Jap. J. Ophthal. 10, Supplement, Tokyo (1966).

Authors' address:
Department of Ophthalmology
School of Medicine, Hamamatsu University
Handa-cho 3600 Hamamatsu -shi
Shizuoka-ken,
Japan 431 31

Docum. Ophthal. Proc. Series, Vol. 15

EFFECT OF ANESTHETICS ON RATS' ERG IN VIVO

YOSHIMI SUGIMACHI, MAKOTO INATOMI & AKIRA NAKAJIMA

(Tokyo, Japan)

INTRODUCTION

Small rodents such as mice, rats and guinea pigs are often used for experiments to learn about the influence of some drugs on the visual system, especially for screening purposes. General anesthetics are used, but there are many reports on the influence of anesthetics themselves, such as barbiturates, urethane and others on the ERG (Noell, 1958; Ogawa, 1961; Yonemura et al., 1965; Honda et al., 1972; Van Norren et al., 1977). On the other hand, it is not easy to record stable ERGs in small rodents in vivo without general anesthesia.

This study has a two-fold purpose: one, to find the best method of recording the ERG in small rodents under topical anesthesia alone, and, secondly, to find out the condition having the minimum influence on the ERG under general anesthesia.

MATERIAL AND METHODS

Preliminary experiments were carried out to record the ERG of rats, mice and guinea pigs under topical anesthesia. Rats seemed to be the easiest of the three for obtaining the ERG. Guinea pigs were difficult to fix without general anesthesia, and the ERG was of low amplitude and contaminated with EMG artefact. In the case of mice it was difficult to set the electrode in a dark room because the eye was so small. Therefore, this experiment was performed on rats.

ERGs were recorded from the same eye at 1 or 2 minute intervals in each animal, and recorded ERGs were reproduced as shown in Figure 1.

Albino rats, approximately 200 g in body weight, were used. The pupils were dilated by mydriatics (mixed solution of 0.5% Tropicamide and 0.5% Phenylepherine hydrochloride). Prelight adaptation of 1000 lux for 10 min and complete dark adaptation for 2 hours were routinely used. After dark adaptation, subsequent experiments were done under dim red light. The animal was fixed to a wooden plate, and the fixation became nearly perfect by fixing the upper canine teeth to a fixing pole with a string. The canine teeth had been topically anesthetized slightly with 0.4% oxybuprocaine. After fixing the animal to the wooden plate, the animal's eye was anesthe-

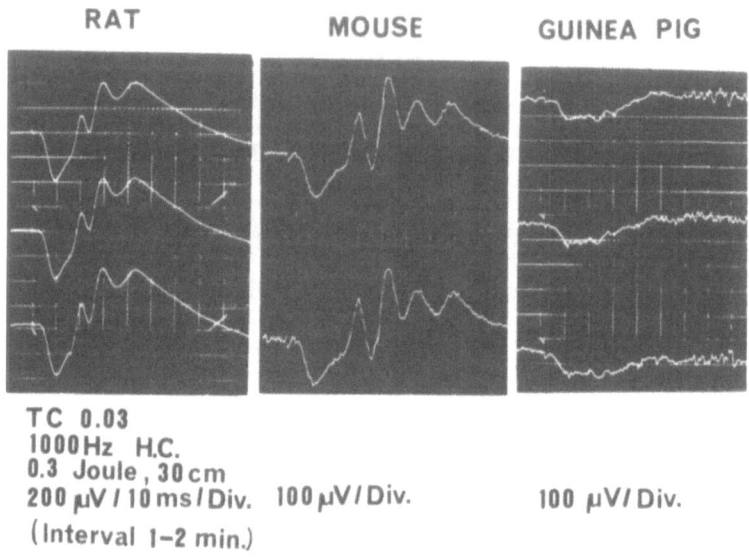

RAT **MOUSE** **GUINEA PIG**

TC 0.03
1000Hz H.C.
0.3 Joule , 30 cm
200 µV / 10 ms / Div. 100 µV / Div. 100 µV / Div.
(Interval 1–2 min.)

Fig. 1

tized topically with 0.4% oxybuprocaine, and the eyeball was semi-luxated
without canthotomy. ERG, EKG and EEG electrodes were then set on the
animal. Needle electrodes for EEG and EKG were introduced into the sub-
cutis of the front legs and in two places on the mid-line of the scalp.

Heart rate and EEG were monitored during the experiment. The electrodes
of the ERG were made of platinum wire, 0.5 mm in diameter. The tip of the
direct electrode was dull, and it was attached perpendicularly to the center

THE LIST OF ANESTHETICS

AMOBARBITAL SODIUM ----	50 mg/kg
PENTOBARBITAL SODIUM -----	30 mg/kg
URETHAN ----------	1000 mg/kg
KETAMINE ---------	20 mg/kg
CHLORAL HYDRATE ----------	100 mg/kg
ALFAXALONE ----------	3.6 mg/kg
DROPERIDOL ----------	1 mg/kg
PROPANIDID ----------	40 mg/kg
CHLORPROMAZINE ----------	12 mg/kg
DIAZEPAM ----------	1 mg/kg

Fig. 2.

of the cornea by a mechanical manipulator. The indirect electrode was ring-shaped and used both as an electrode and as an eyelid retractor.

The ERGs were recorded on polaroid film by a Cathode Ray Oscilloscope VC7a (Nihon Kooden KK, Tokyo). The time constant was 0.03 second and 1000 Hz high cut-off. Light stimuli were delivered by a Xenon flash, 0.3 joule, 30 cm from the cornea with 1 or 2 minute intervals.

The list of general anesthetics and their doses, tested in this study, are shown in Fig. 2. When suitable doses of intraperitoneal injection of the drugs were not known, the doses tested in this study were calculated to be about 4 to 5 times the amount of clinical doses by intra-venous administration or one-tenth of LD_{50}.

The amplitude of a+b wave was measured as the perpendicular height from the bottom of the a-wave to the slow hump of long duration after the wavelets. Therefore, there are many cases where the peak of the b-wave was lower than that of the wavelets (Fig. 3).

RESULTS

Mean values

The mean values of ERGs obtained before the administration of general anesthetics in 39 rats are shown in Figure 4.

Amplitude

The amplitude of a- and a+b waves against time in minutes after injection of

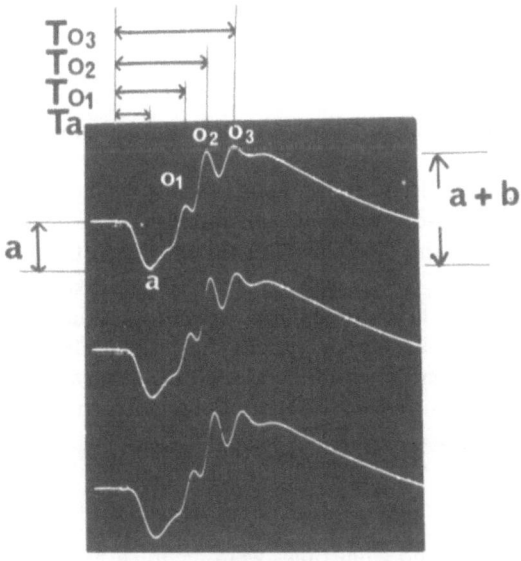

Fig. 3.

$$\left\{
\begin{array}{l}
\text{LIGHT ADAPTATION : } 1000 \text{ LUX, } 10 \text{ MIN.} \\
\text{COMPLETE DARK ADAPTATION : } 1 - 2 \text{ HOUR} \\
\text{T.C. : } 0.03 \text{ SEC , HIGH CUT : } 1000 \text{ HZ} \\
\text{LIGHT STIMULUS : } 0.3 \text{ JOULE, } 30 \text{ CM}
\end{array}
\right\}$$

AMPLITUDE

A – WAVE	$486 \pm 73.8\ \mu V$
A + B WAVE	$1076 \pm 212.4\ \mu V$
$\dfrac{A}{A+B}$	0.46 ± 0.06

IMPLICIT TIME

T_A	11.4 ± 0.9 MSEC
T_{O1}	22.8 ± 2.0 MSEC
T_{O2}	30.3 ± 2.3 MSEC
T_{O3}	42.6 ± 3.2 MSEC

Fig. 4.

anesthetics are expressed as a percentage of that of before the injection (Figs. 5, 6). At the level of doses tried, almost all anesthetics tested had a tendency to increase the amplitdue of a- and a+b wave with the exception of the a+b wave in barbiturate administration, although the results of the experiments showed large variations.

Chlorpromazine showed the most remarkable changes. The amplitudes increased to more than 150% at 30 minutes after injection. Chloral hydrate, Diazepam, Alfaxalone and Droperidol also increased them.

Implicit time

The implicit time of components of ERG showed less variation than amplitude.

In the case of barbiturates, the implicit times of the a-wave and wavelets were prolonged, especially on the O_3 component after the administration of drugs (Fig. 7). On the other hand, in the case of Ketamine, almost all implicit times of wavelets were shortened in all cases (Fig. 8). Urethane, Diazepam and Alfaxalone have shown slight elongations of implicit times. Propanidid and Chlorpromazine failed to show a constant effect on implicit times. In the case of Droperidol and Chloral hydrate, changes in implicit times of a-, O_1 and O_2 were minimum among the anesthetics tried in this study (Fig. 9).

SUMMARY

ERGs in rats, mice and guinea pigs were recorded under topical anesthesia successfully, but with effort. Barbiturates decreased the height of a+b waves.

RELATIVE AMPLITUDE

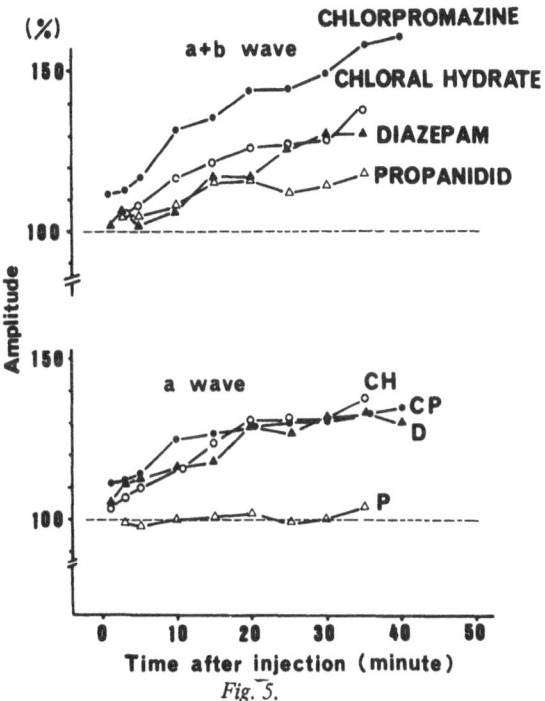

Fig. 5.

RELATIVE AMPLITUDE

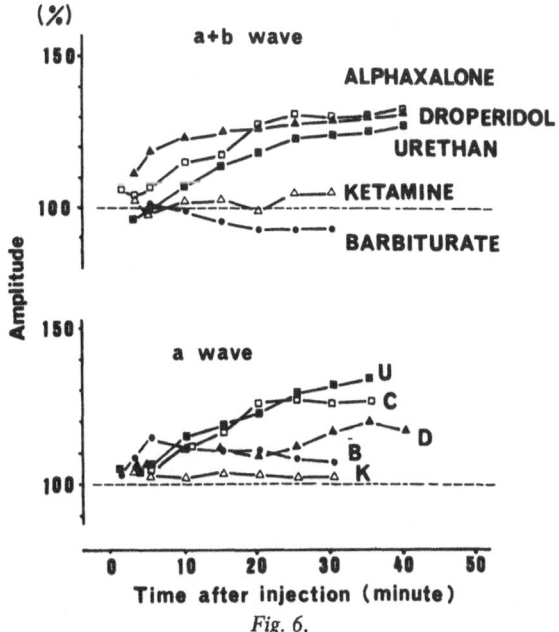

Fig. 6.

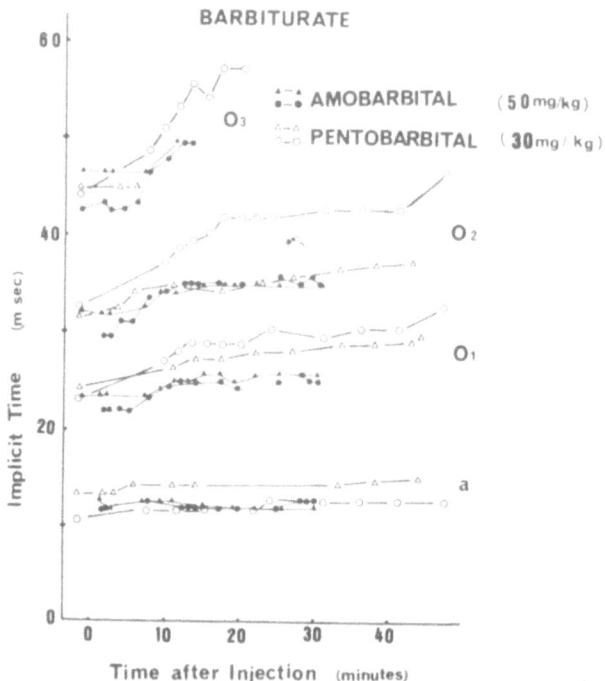

Fig. 7.

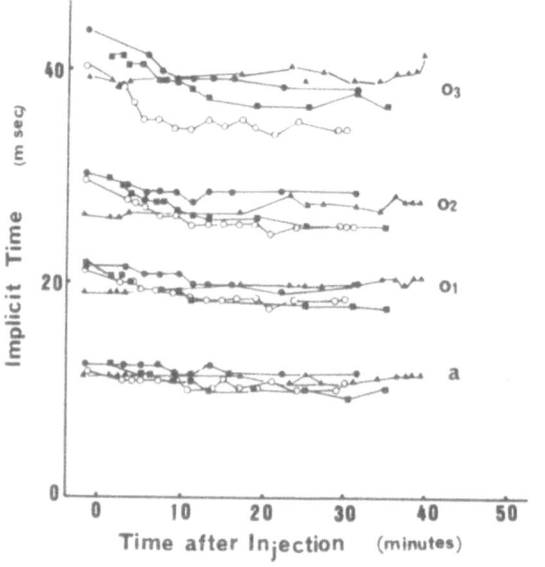

Fig. 8.

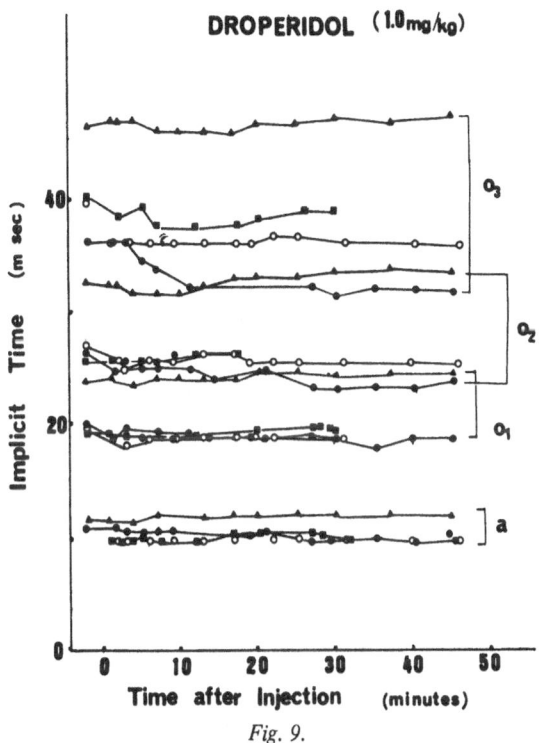

Fig. 9.

All other drugs tried increased it. Ketamine shortened, the other drugs prolonged the implicit times of ERG. Chloral hydrate and Droperidol had the least effect on the implicit time among the drugs tried in this stydy.

ACKNOWLEDGEMENTS

This work was supported by a Grant of the Ministry of Health and Welfare. The author wishes to thank Dr. K. Matsuki for his kind suggestions for this study and Mrs. E. Kawara for her assistance.

REFERENCES

Honda, Y. et al. Some observations of the effects of barbiturate upon the Electro retinogram of rabbits. *Ophthal. Res.* 4: *129* (1972).

Noell, W.K. Differentiation, metabolic organization and viability of the visual cell. *Arch. Ophthal.* 60: *702* (1958).

Norren, D. van, et al. Influence of anesthetics, alcohol and Freon on dark adaptation of monkey cone ERG. *Invest. Ophthal. Vis. Sci. 16: 80* (1977).

Ogawa, T. Effects of nembutal on ERG. *J. Iwate Med. Assn* 13: *822* (1961).

Yonemura, D., et al. Differential vulnerability of the ERG components to pentobarbital. Proc. 4th ISCERG Symposium, p. 155 (1965).

Authors' address:
Department of Ophthalmology
Juntendo University
School of Medicine
Hongo, Tokyo
Japan

DRUG EFFECTS ON B—WAVE AMPLITUDE
AND ON READAPTATION AFTER GLARE

J. SCHULZE & E. APPEL

(Dortmund, Fed. Rep. of Germany)

Recent official surveys have shown that 30% of all patients are given barbiturates and 40% tranquilizers by the medical administrations. So we have to expect that more than half of the adult population take these drugs in a more or less uncontrolled manner. General cautions of the producers concern only the possibly affected psychological reactions, for instance in driving a car or occupational situations. Our aim was to find out if there might be any influence on the sensory organ itself, especially on the retinal function, and to prove it by the ERG. Starting such investigations, we prefer to use animal experiments (cats) for several reasons- drug administrations to healthy volunteers for experimental reasons only can be avoided and not so much attention has to be paid to some restrictions with regard to the dosage, even in case of repeated administration. In pharmacological experiments on the ERG a greatmany physiological parameters have to be observed, e.g. blood pressure, heart rate, respiration, body temperature etc., because we know that the b-wave is very sensitive to the general physiological condition. To get statistically evaluable results very long lasting experiments of several hours and an optimal signal-to-noise ratio are necessary.

Fig. 1 shows the modifications in the ERG after 15 and 20 minutes of infusion of a small dose of barbiturate. The b-amplitude is progressively reduced, the peak-latency increases and an a-wave appears. On the other hand, similar reducing of the b-amplitude by slight light-adaptation shows the well-known decrease in peak-latency and does not produce an a-wave.

A detailed investigation shows that the peak-latency is rapidly increasing in the early phase of amplitude reduction after administration of barbiturates and is more distinct than the decreasing effect of light adaptation. In order to study the time-course of these effects we have realized an automatic measurement of b-amplitude and peak-latency of sequentially evoked ERG's.

For these measurements, the ERG is processed in the following way:
1. Triggered by the test-flash a gated amplifier is opened with a delay of some ms for about 200 ms, in order to eliminate stimulus artefacts as well as spontaneous base-line shifts and the potential of the ERG induced by the glare stimulus.
2. The dc-level at the start of the test-ERG is measured and used for baseline corrections.
3. While the gate is open, amplitude and latency of the absolute maximum

Comparison between Background Illumination
and Barbiturate Infusion

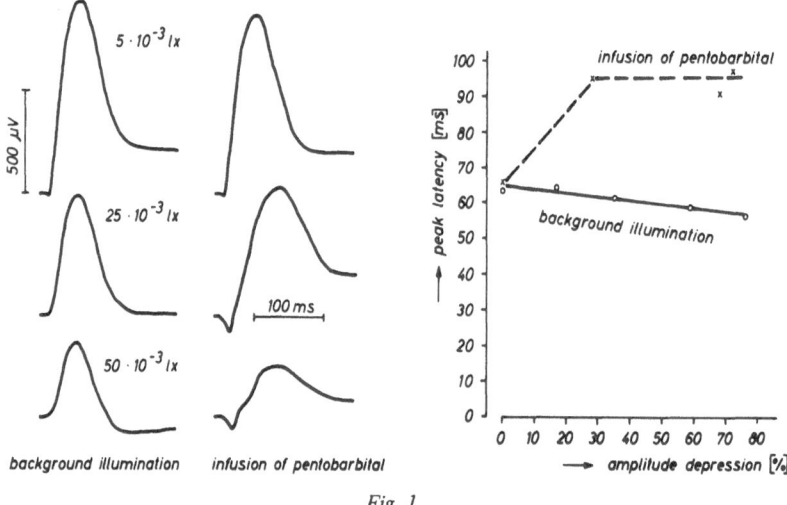

Fig. 1.

are measured and stored, until they are transferred to the computer at the end of the gate.

This procedure allows the continuous analysis of a series of test-ERG's and so the time-course of pharmacologically induced modifications in b-amplitude and peak-latency can be studied simultaneously.

Fig. 2 shows the time-course of these phenomena after injection of barbiturate. After about 30 testflashes, one per second, producing an ERG of about half the maximum amplitude, pentobarbital is injected. The b-amplitude decreases within 25 sec to about 20% of the initial value, while peak-latency increases by more than 50%. The decay of the effect on the peak-latency is delayed compared to recovery of b-amplitude.

In Fig. 3 the effects of a tranquilizer of diazepam-type are compared with the barbiturate effect. The main differences are a prolonged depression of the b-amplitude by the tranquilizer and quite a different reaction of the peak-latency. It is more or less unaffected or even shortened during the initial phase of amplitude reduction.

Modification in peak-latency caused by barbiturate in comparison to the light adaptation as well as the different influence of barbiturate and valium show that b-amplitude and peak-latency are affected independently in different ways. Simultaneous measurement of b-amplitude and peak-latency, therefore, might lead to additional information on retinal function and its affection by drugs. In order to investigate the drug influence on dynamic processes in the retina we have studied the recovery time course after glare.

Influence of Barbiturate on
b-amplitude and Peak-latency

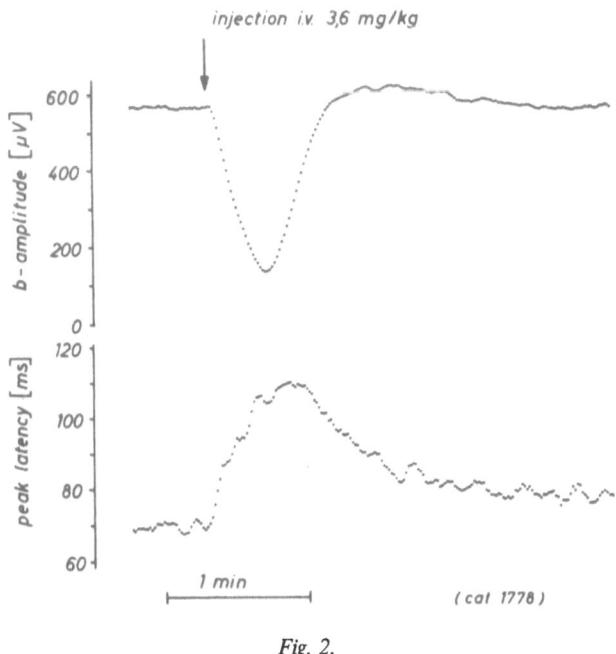

Fig. 2.

Recovery of the sensitivity of the retina after glare can be described by the re-increasing of the b-amplitude after its extinction by a glare stimulus.

Fig. 4 demonstrates a remarkable prolongation of readaptation time after administration of a tranquilizer in two different experiments. In single experiments retardation of recovery of more than 50% might occur. But a statistical evaluation of this effect does not prove such a strong modification.

Fig. 5 demonstrates the continuously recorded readaptation time, each bar representing mean and variation of 50 measurements of that time, necessary to reach 50% of the initial sensitivity. Means and variations of all measurements in a period of one and a half hour before and after injection of drug or placebo are marked by horizontal lines. It is shown, that after injection of placebo no sudden reaction can be observed but the readaptation time increases slightly with time. The injection of valium, however, is followed by a sudden retardation of the readaptation by about 10%. Compared with the results of single experiments, the statistical analysis shows a relatively small effect. This might be caused by differences in individual sensitivity to the drug, also known from patients who sometimes even react with an excitation after administration of a tranquilizer.

41

Different Influence of Barbiturate and Diazepam
on b-amplitude and Peak-latency

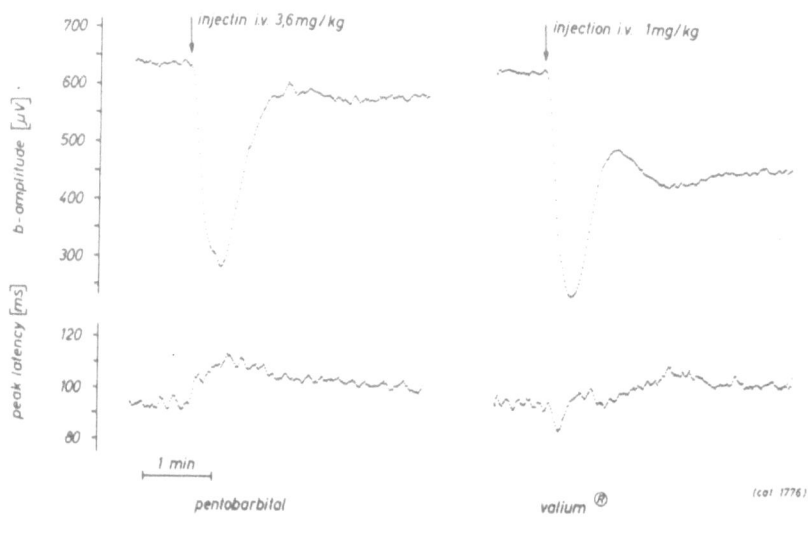

Fig. 3.

Readaptation Time Course after Glare
before and after Injection of Valium ®

(injection i.v. 1 mg/kg ; cat 1689)

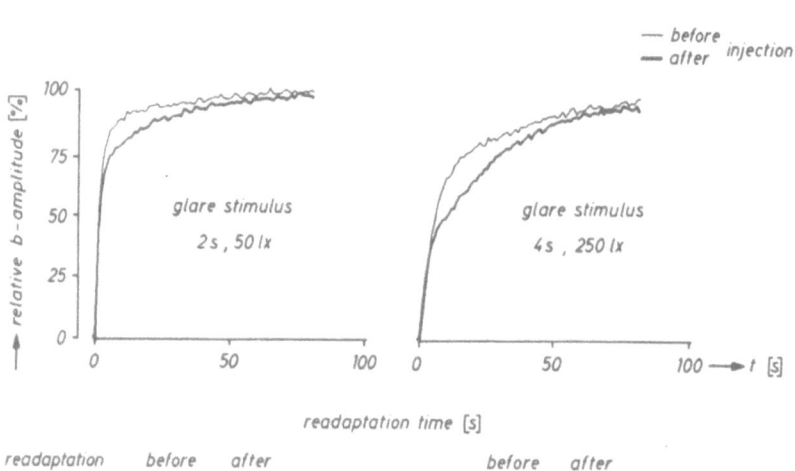

readaptation level [%]	before	after injection	before	after injection
50	1,9	2,4 (+26 %)	6,2	9,9 (+62 %)
75	3,8	6,7 (+77 %)	16,6	28,3 (+79 %)

Fig. 4.

Readaptation Time after Injection of
Valium® and Placebo

(glare stimulus : 1,6s , 125 lx ; readaptation level 50%)

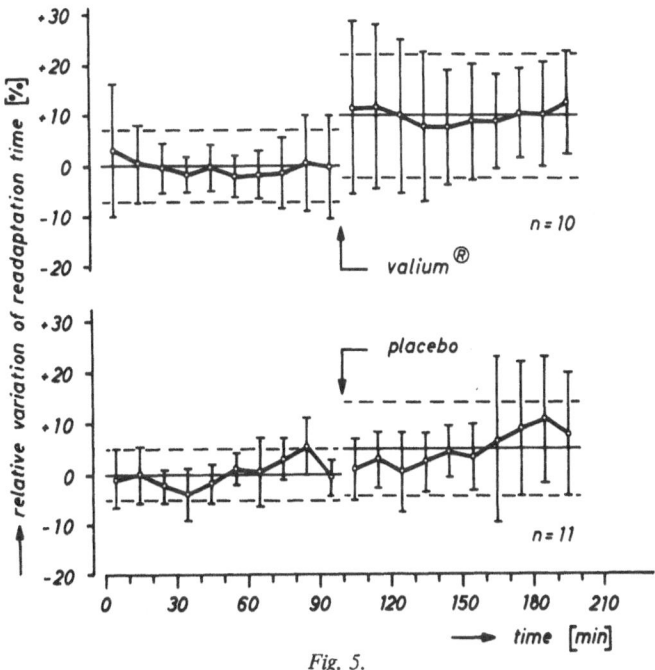

Fig. 5.

Retarding effects, caused by pharmacological influence are superimposed by spontaneous modifications of readaptation time. Its mean and variation grow with the duration of the whole experiment. This is shown in Fig. 6 which demonstrates an average of eleven experiments lasting 5 hours of continuous measurement of readaptation unaffected by drugs or any other experimental interference.

This short communication could be no more than a rough survey of the possible influence of tranquilizing or analgesic drugs on the ERG and on sensory function. With our ERG-investigations we could show that very common drugs may disturb the retinal function and delay the readaptation after glare to different extent. This means that ingestion of such drugs might bear some impairment in visual information, for instance in car driving or occupational situations by night.

On the other hand, when performing ERG-examinations under tranquilizing or sedative treatment we should beware of misleading results.

Spontaneous Variation of Readaptation Time
(glare stimulus . 1,6 s , 125 lx ; readaptation level 50 %)

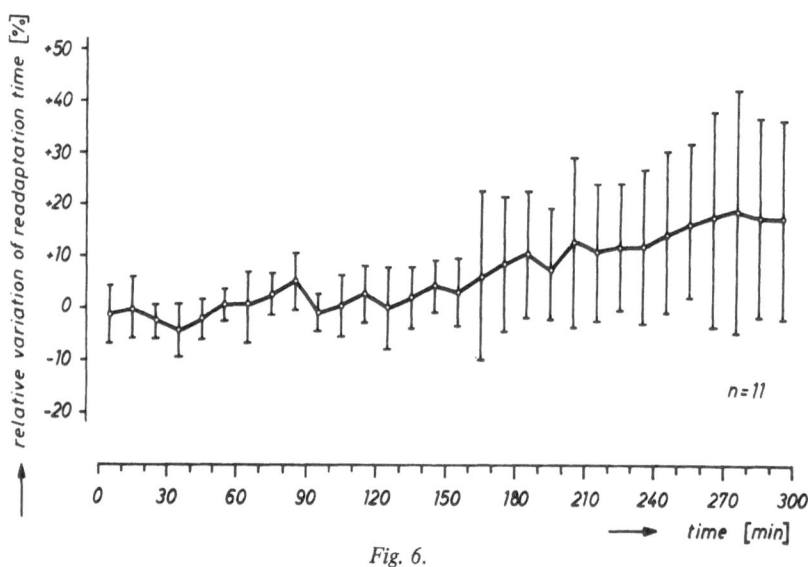

Fig. 6.

Authors' address:
Institut für Arbeitsphysiologie an der
Universität Dortmund
Ardeystr. 67
4600 Dortmund
W. Germany

Docum. Ophthal. Proc. Series, Vol.15

INTRAVITREAL INJECTION OF GENTAMICIN–EXPERIMENTAL FINDINGS

G. PALIMERIS, M. MOSCHOS, E. CHIMONIDOU, E. PANAGAKIS, D. ANDREANOS & T. SMIRNOF

(Athens, Greece)

ABSTRACT

In this experimental investigation, the authors study the electroretinographic alterations and the histological lesions of the retina of rabbits following the intravitreal injection of different doses of Gentamicin.

Gentamicin is a broad-spectrum antibiotic which belongs to the aminogluco-
cides and acts satisfactorily against a great variety of bacteria, especially a-
gainst Pseudomonas and certain strains of Staphylococcus.

Since the penetrance of Gentamicin into the vitreous body is small following local instillation, subconjunctival injection or systemic administration,
the intravitreal injection of the drug ensures better therapeutic results in cases of severe endophthalmitis.

The purpose of the present study, is to investigate in rabbits both by
means of ERG and histologically the toxic effect of Gentamicin on the retina and to determine the non-toxic dosage of the drug after intravitreal injection.

MATERIAL AND METHOD

Our study involved 40 eyes of 20 rabbits weighing from 1.5 to 3 kg. A further 12 eyes (6 rabbits) were used as controls.

The test animal was immobilized on a special table and locally anaestheti-
zed for intervention in the eye by means of instillation of Propacaine and
Tetracaine-Adrenaline eyedrops. The anterior chamber was then subjected
to paracentesis in order to achieve adequate hypotony, whereupon a Gentamicin solution (commercial brand name 'Garamycin') of various concentrations was introduced into the vitreous cavity. This injection was performed by means of a 30 gauge needle on a tuberculin-syringe, the location of
the insertion of the needle being 3 mm from the sclerocorneal limbus towards the cornea.

The Gentamycin solutions used varied between 4.00 mg and 0.01 mg/0.1
ml (Table 1). Into the vitreous of the control-eyes o.1 ml sterile saline was
injected.

All eyes were clinically examined by means of indirect ophthalmoscopy,
the slit-lamp and ERG. For the electroretinographic investigation a MEDE-

Table 1.

Eyes	Dose of Gentamicin
4	4.0 mg
6	2.0 mg
8	0.5 mg
8	0.1 mg
10	0.05 mg
4	0.01 mg

LEC NR6 apparatus was employed which was equipped with an electronic averager.

The ERG was taken after dark adaptation for 5. The source of light was placed at a distance of 2 cm from the pupils, which were dilated.

Prior to the injection of Gentamicin an ERG was taken of all the rabbits, and the ERG was subsequently studied on the 1st, 2nd, 3rd, 6th, 15th, 30th, 60th and 90th day after the start of the experiment.

RESULTS

In the 4 eyes of Group 1, which had received a Gentamicin injection of 4 mg/0.1 ml, ERG disturbances were observable already after the lapse of 24 hours. After one week the ERG was extinguished. The vitreous body was clouded and the retina showed diffuse pigment deposits (Fig. 1).

Of the 16 eyes of Group 2, in which the injected dose amounted to 2 mg/0.1 ml, 2 eyes presented no ERG changes after the first 24 hours, whereas the remaining 4 eyes showed a diminution of the b-wave. After a lapse of 3 days the ERG alterations were clearly discernible in all eyes and one week after the injection, the ERG was extinguished (Fig. 2). Clinically, the retinal alterations resembled those observed in Group 1.

As regards the 8 eyes of Group 3, the ERG taken 24 hours after the injection of the drug proved normal. Subsequently, however, the amplitude of the b-wave showed a reduction with the result that two weeks later its value amounted to only 50% of the normal value. After a period of 3 weeks its value was down to 10% of normal and 4 weeks from the beginning of the experiment the ERG was extinguished (Fig. 3).

Of the 8 eyes of Group 4, into which 0.1 mg/o.l. ml of the drug had been injected, the ERG was normal in 6 eyes at the end of the first week and remained so for up to 3 months. In the remaining 2 eyes a progressive diminution of the ERG value was noted, which after 3 months amounted to 50% of the normal value in the one eye while the other was flat. After 3 months, the ERG became flat in the other eye also, whereas in the remaining 6 eyes the bioelectrical activity remained good (Fig. 4).

In Group 5, comprising 10 eyes which had received an injection of 0.05 mg/0.1 ml, the ERG remained normal three months later for 8 eyes, while in 2 eyes a diminution of the ERG value by about 50% was established.

46

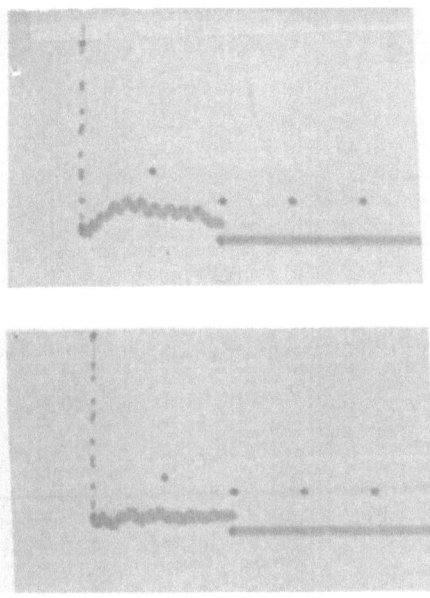

Fig. 1. ERG of Group 1 (4 mg). ERG flat after 1 week.

Finally, in the eyes into which a dose of 0.01 mg/0.1. ml had been injected, the ERG remained normal until 3 months had elapsed since the Gentamicin administration (Fig. 5).

It should be pointed out that no ophthalmoscopic findings were established in the eyes of the last two groups. The ERG results of the eyes into which Gentamicin solution had been injected are summarized in Table 2.

Histological findings

All Gentamicin concentrations which caused manifest disturbances of the ERG also produced anomaly in the structure of the layers of the retinal cells accompanied by a pigment disruption. (Fig. 6). This pigment disruption was noted particularly in cases of high concentrations of the drug (4 mg/ml — 0.1 mg/ml), whereas with smaller concentrations such a disturbance did not occur.

DISCUSSION

The primary question with which the present experimental investigation has been concerned was to establish a non-toxic Gentamicin dose for the human retina. According to previous publications of Peyman et al. (1974) Gentamicin was considered to be toxic for the retina when injected into the vitreous

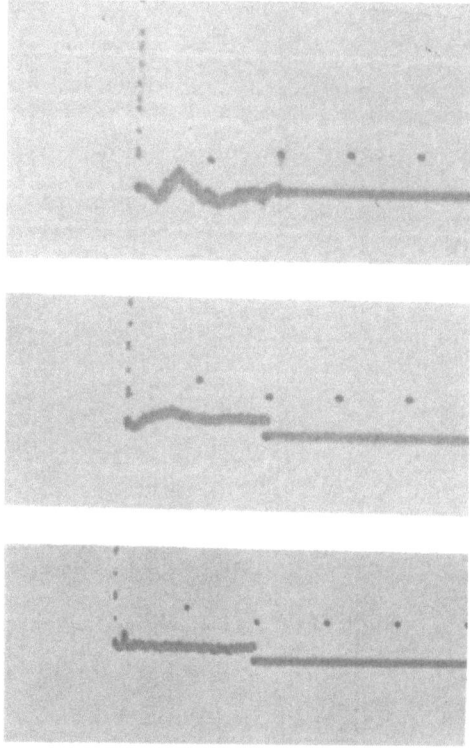

Fig. 2. ERG of Group 2 (2 mg). Flat after 1 week.

at a dose of 1.0 mg. It was also known that a dose of 2.0 mg − 10.0 mg is likely to cause cararact.

Furthermore, we are aware of the nephrotoxic effect of the drug in the human if the daily administered dosage exceeds 5 mg/kg.

In cats the nephrotoxic action manifests itself upon the administration of doses of 20 mg/kg, while disturbances of the labyrinth appear when the drug is given at a dosage of 40 mg/kg daily over a period of 11 days (Leopols, 1976).

Previous experimental studies by Zachary-Forster (1976) have demonstrated that the injection of Gentamicin into the vitreous body in a dose of 0.4 mg/ml or more causes lesions to the retina of rabbits, finally resulting in functional necrosis, the time of the onset of which is dependent on the quantity of the drug injected.

Our own experiments demonstrate that with the injection of a dose of 0.5 mg/ml the ERG, which for about 2 weeks remains normal, after a lapse of 3 months shows a diminution of the value by up to 70% of normal in 20% of the eyes. Moreover, even with a dose of 0.1 mg the ERG is dimished

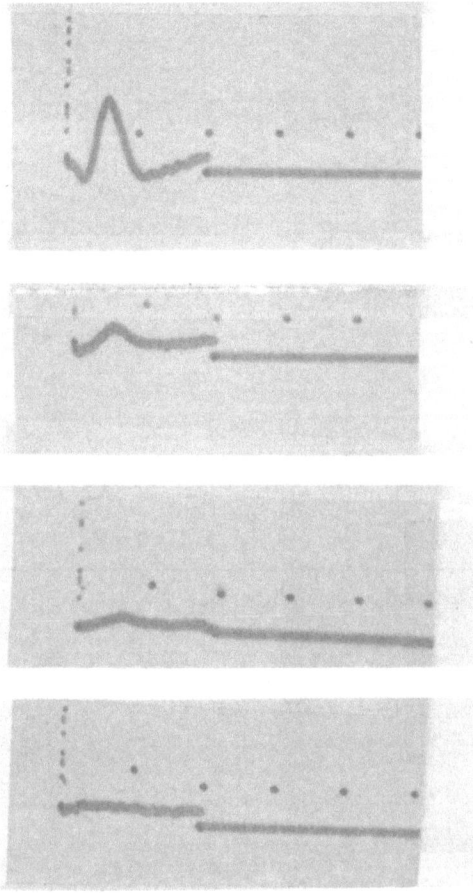

Fig. 3. ERG of Group 3 (0.5 mg). Normal 1st day, reduced the 2nd and 3rd weeks and flat in the 4th week.

to such an extent that after 3 months 40% of the eyes show reduced values by up to 70% of the normal value. On the other hand, we can say that doses under 0.05 mg/ml may be considered as safe, seeing that no disturbance of the ERG or of a histopathological nature was observed 3 months after the injection of this dosage.

As regards the precise mechanism of the toxic action of Gentamycin upon the retina as well as the question whether the drug has any special affinity to the pigment epithelium, we are no more able to say anything definite than concerning numerous other retinotoxic substances, such as e.g. Sodium iodate, Chloroquin or Indomethacin. Besides, it is not easy to detemine exactly the alterations of the photopic or scotopic elements of the retina of rabbits (Palimeris 1972).

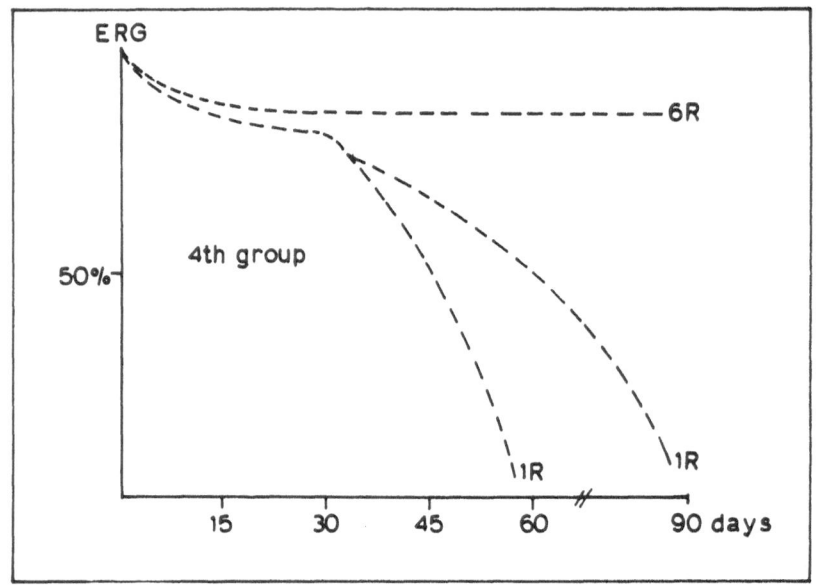

Fig. 4. Mean values of the ERG of Group 4.

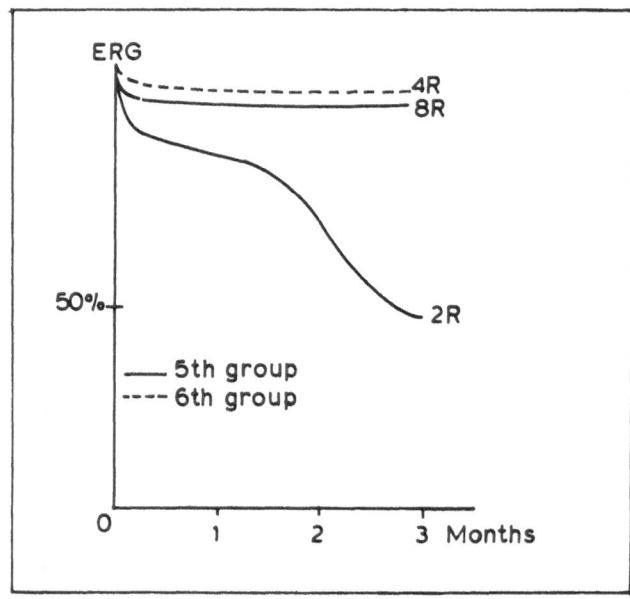

Fig. 5. Mean values of ERG of Groups 5 and 6.

Table 2.

Eyes	Dose	Normal	ERG after 3 months Subnormal	Flat
4	4.0 mg	–	–	4
6	2.0 mg	–	–	6
8	0.5 mg	–	–	8
8	0.1 mg	6	2	–
10	0.05 mg	8	2	–
4	0.01 mg	4	–	–

From a clinical point of view the injection of 0.05 mg Gentamicin into the vitreous of rabbits, which has a volume of 1.4 ml, or into the human vitreous, the volume of which is 4 ml, will result in a temporary concentration of the drug of approximately 35 mg/ml and 12.5 mg/ml respectively, i.e. a concentration which is bound to exert an inhibitory effect upon numerous bacteria (Jao & Jackson, 1964).

Taking into account the gravity of an endophthalmitis, we may conclude that a dose of 0.1 mg, which would result in a concentration of 25 mg/ml in the vitreous of the human eye, may be regarded as the optimal indication, even if we make due allowance for a certain toxic effect upon the retina.

REFERENCES

Jao, R.L. & G.G. Jackson. Gentamicin sulfate. A new antibiotic against gram negative bacilli. *J. Am. Med. Assn* 189: *817* (1964).

Leopold, I. Ocular Pharmacology. Mosby, St Louis (1976).

Palimeris, G., J. Koliopoulos & P. Velissaropoulos. Ocular side effects of Indomethacin. *Ophthalmologica* 164: *339* (1972).

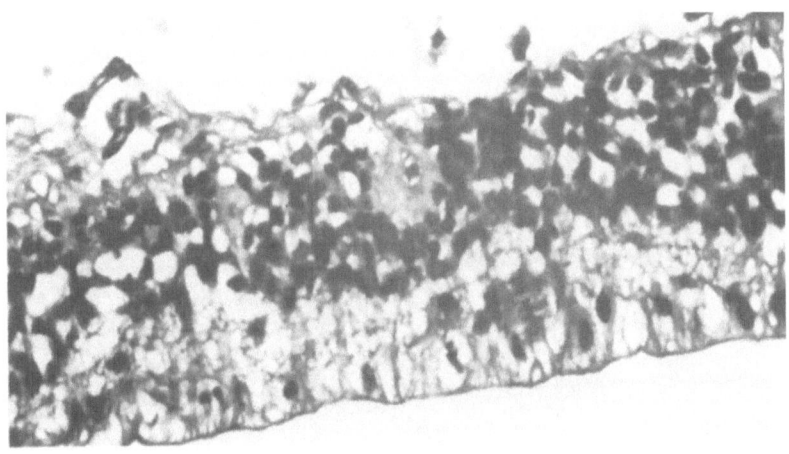

Fig. 6. Histological lesions. Pigment deposits and structural alterations of the cell layers.

Peyman, C.A., D.R. May, E.S. Ericson & D. Apple. Intraocular injection of Gentami-
cine. Toxic effects and clearance. *Arch. Ophthal.* 92: *42* (1974).
Zachary, G. & K.R. Forster. Experimental intravitreal gentamicin. *Am. J. Ophthal.* 82:
604 (1976).

Authors' address:
Athens University Eye Clinic
National Ophthalmological Center
170 Messoghion Street
Cholargos (Athens)
Greece

Docum. Ophthal. Proc. Series, Vol. 15

ZINC – ITS EFFECT ON THE OSCILLATORY POTENTIAL

G. STEPHENS, A. CINOTTI, H. J. WHITE &
E. VELTRI
(Newark, N. J., USA)

Intraocular copper foreign bodies oxidize and lead to generalized chalcosis, affecting the retinal cells with their high metabolic activity. This is followed by pigmentary degeneration of the retina and ends with obliteration of its blood vessels (Hogan, 1962). The severity of this damage has been found to depend on the surface size of the Cu particule (Schmidt et al., 1972).

Attempts at removal of such foreign bodies (f.b.) are rarely successful, therefore, an alternative method of treatment would be useful in preserving sight.

Many substances have been tried in order to halt the destructive effect of the copper, e.g. sodium thiosulfate (Dambite, 2959, 1960), sodium hyposulfate (Delbequet et al., 1966), bal &2–3 dimercaptopropanol (Habiget et al., 1951), penicillamin (Rouher, 1958), etc. But none of these have been retained as a universal treatment of intraocular copper foreign body in everyday practice. In our experiments we decided to try zinc as a new protective substance. The following incited us to use zinc:

1. Last summer we observed a family with sex linked tapeto-retinal degeneration, in which the affected members of the family have a low zinc:copper ratio – below 1, in their blood plasma. In contrast, the healthy members had a zinc:copper ratio – above 1 (Bastek et al., 1973). This evoked the thought that zinc might inhibit the toxic effect of the copper which could affect, besides the retinal structure, the different biochemical components present in the retina.

2. In cases of metallosis there are descriptions of deterioration of the light sense. In metallosis of copper and iron there is an extinguished ERG response as in tapeto-retinal degeneration. (In some cases of metallosis concentric constricted field was found, see Knave, 1969.) In advanced R. P. constricted field could be found.

3. Zinc is known to be an indispensable component of enzymes (Valle, 1976), e.g. carbonic anhydrase, carboxypepitdase, alcohol dehydrogenase, etc. One of these enzymes, namely, alcohol dehydrogenase, is important in the rhodopsin cycle (Wald, 1960). In cuprosis, a disturbance of the enzymatic systems cannot be ruled out.

4. Itoi (1937) (quoted by Knave, 1969), found that placing an iron particle in a rabbit's eye and connecting it to a zinc block placed subcutaneously

produced galvanic coupling and no rust could develop. A similar effect could result in the case of copper and zinc in the eye.

METHOD AND MATERIALS

This is a preliminary report. Eight albino rabbits have been used. All animals, at the start, have had ERG examination of both eyes. After this, in the left eye of each animal, a particle or particles (Cu or Zn, or Cu and Zn) were inserted. In order to avoid the surface differences factor (Schmidt et al., 1972), all particles were of about 1 cgr in weight, slender metallic rods of 3.5 mm long and 0.35 mm diameter. They were pushed inside the eye in the vitreous through the pars plana by a plunger through a 20 gauge needle.

Ophthalmoscopically, and a check-up with X-ray later, showed that most of the foreign bodies migrated toward the retina.

The foreign bodies were inserted as follows: Rabbits (R 1–2) copper alone (Cu). Rabbits (R 3–4) zinc alone (Zn). Rabbits (R 5–6) copper and zinc (Cu and Zn). Rabbits (R 7–8) copper alone (Cu), –then iontophoresis with zinc was done for this last group*.

After the insertion of such a foreign body or bodies, the ERG was done on the third day and then once a week. (On 2 rabbits with a Cu particle in the eye iontophoresis with zinc was done on the second day, and then once a week). During the ERG recording each animal was restrained in a wooden box. No anesthesia was used except topical proparcaine 1%. The Grass PS electronic flash, intensity 16, at an 18 inch. distance, provided the stimulation light. The retinal potentials from the rabbit's eye were led to high gain amplifiers of the Grass EEG machine, model 8–10, and from it to the multi-channel tape recorder; then, after passing a semi-automatic electronic analyser were led to CAT (Mnemotron) for summation and averaging.

A pre-set automatic counter coupled with the CAT stopped the summation at the desired number. Permanent visual recordings were made on a Hewlett-Packard X-Y recorder. The right eye (which was without a f.b.) of each animal served as control. This was done because of variation of rabbit's ERG, day-to-day, as reported by Spivey et al. (1983) and Lawwill (1972).

In rabbits (R 7-8) with a copper particle in the left eye, iontophoresis with zinc was applied. The iontophoresis treatment was done as follows: a piece of cotton was soaked with prepared zinc glucontate solution (in 100 ml distilled water 10 mg of zinc glucontate was dissolved). The soaked cotton was placed on an electrode which was affixed to the cornea of left eye. The other end of the electrode was connected to the positive pole of the apparatus. The negative pole was applied by means of a silver needle on the back of the animal's head. A 2 volt 1.6 ma was applied for 22 minutes, which activated the passage of the zinc ion in the eye.

All ERG tracings given from now on are of oscillatory potential of rabbit's eyes obtained by white light stimulations 1.5 x 10 f.c. in D.A. state. The ERG's were registered on Mnemotron, sweep duration 0.0625 sec. summation 30, magnification 10 (Dambite, 1959, 1960).

* A more detailed description of the method of ionophoresis will be sent on request.

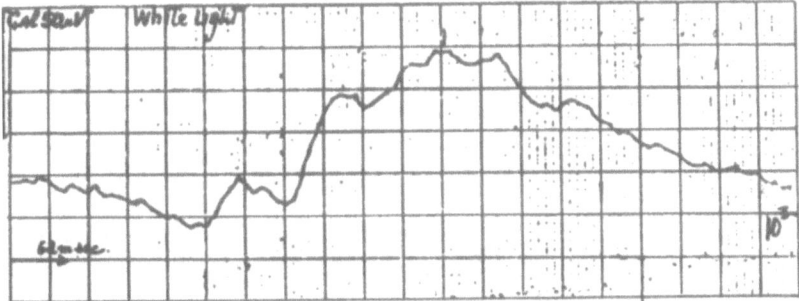

Fig. 1. ERG oscillatory potential (average response) of a rabbit's eye for control (no f.b. in it).

The changes of the ERG b-waves amplitude and oscillatory potential due to different foreign bodies gave the following data:

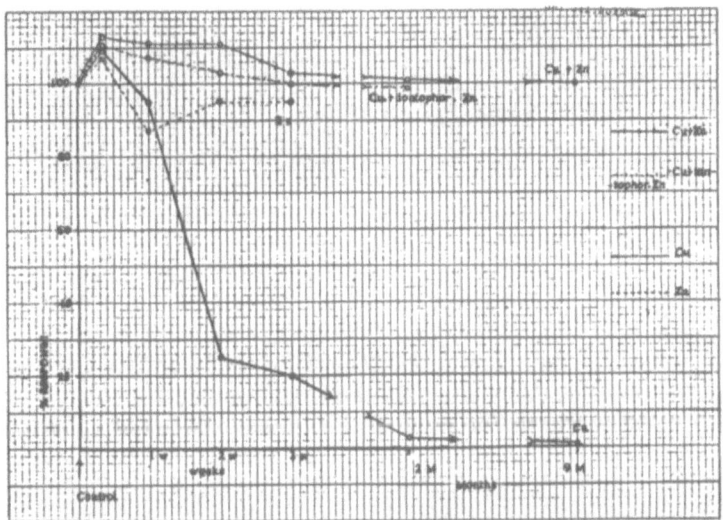

Fig. 2. The curves of the ERG response b-wave in Uv of rabbit's eyes with Cu, Zn, Cu and Zn and Cu plus iontophoresis with Zn at different length of time. At the 3rd day all responses were above the base line.

At the end of the first week the ERG response (b-wave and oscillations) of the eyes with Cu and Zn (R 4-5) and iontophoresis with Zn (R 6-7) were still above the basis line. The ERG response of the eyes (R 1-2) with Cu particle alone and the eyes with Zn particle (R 3-4) alone were slightly below the base line. The latencies of the oscillatory potential of the eyes having Zn particle or having iontophoresis with Zn were slightly shorter (about 5 m sec) than the latencies of the eyes with Cu. (Knave (1970) noted after the first 5 days increase in the latency of the oscillatory potential of rabbits eyes with intraocular Cu f.b. and the amplitude of the oscillations reduced.)

At the end of the second week the response of the eyes with Cu and Zn (R 5-6) and the response of the eyes with Cu and iontophoresis with Zn (R 7-8) were still above the base line. The response of the eyes with Zn alone (R 3-4) in the second week was slightly increased. At the same time the ERG response (b-wave) of the rabbit's eyes with Cu alone (R 1-2) plunged 77% and the oscillatory potential disappeared almost completely. The ERG response was very small.

At the end of the third week, the b-wave and the oscillatory potential of the eyes with Cu alone (R 1-2) plunged down further to 20% of its base response.

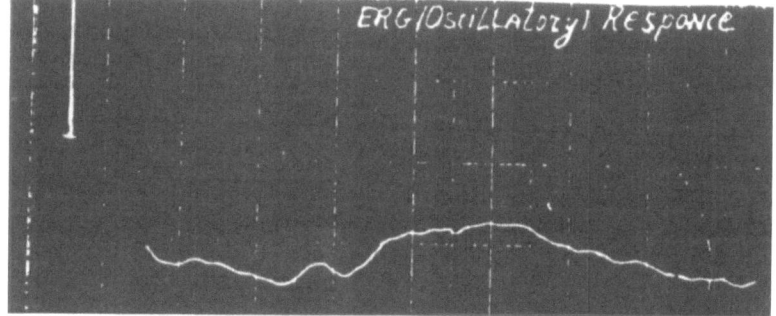

Fig. 3. ERG oscillatory potential of an eye 3 weeks after implantation Cu F.B. in it. Cal. 50 μV.

The response of the eyes with Cu and Zn (R 5-6) and the eyes with Cu and iontophoresis with Zn (R 7-8) were still slightly above the base line.

The response of the eyes with Zn alone (R 3-4) had stabilized at a level 5% below the base line. Soon after the third week one of the rabbits with Zn particle in his eye, died. The other rabbit with Zn in his eye died long after.)

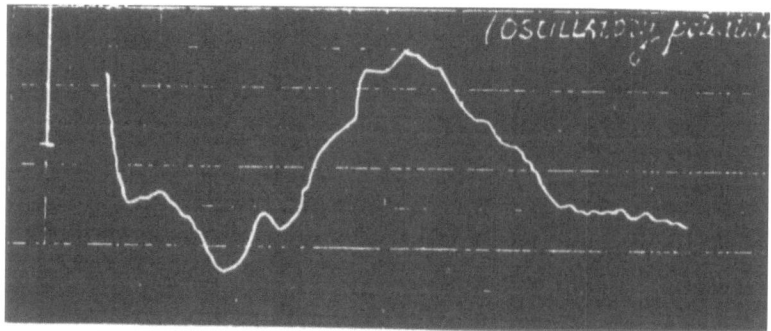

Fig. 4. ERG oscillatory potential of an eye 3 weeks after implantation Zn f.b. in it. Cal. 50 μV.

Two months later, the response of the eyes with Zn and Cu (R 4-5) was just above the base line. The response of the eyes with Cu and ionophoresis with Zn was, similarly, very near the base line.

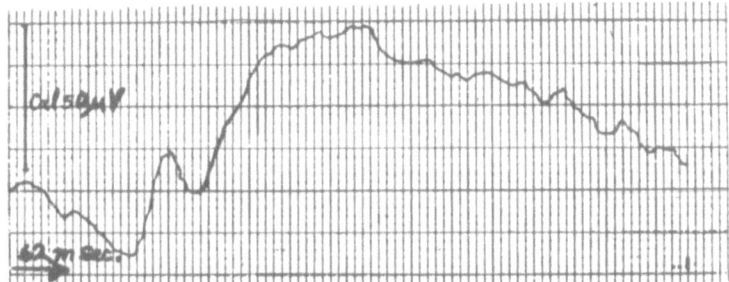

Fig. 5. ERG oscillatory potential of an eye 2 months after implantation of Cu f.b. and iontophoresis with Zn.

The experiment with Intraocular Cu and iontophoresis with Zn was started only 2 months ago; and no additional results are currently available. The oscillary response of the eyes with Cu particle and no treatment had further deteriorated. At nine months the response of the eyes with Cu and Zn was still at the base line and the oscillations were very good.

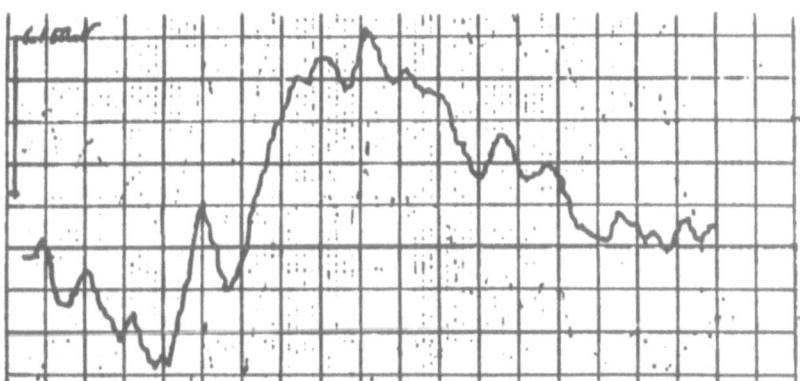

Fig. 6. ERG oscillatory potential of an eye 9 months after implantation of Cu-Zn f.b. in it.

At nine months the response of the eye with Cu and without any treatment was minimal and the oscillation almost completely extinquished.

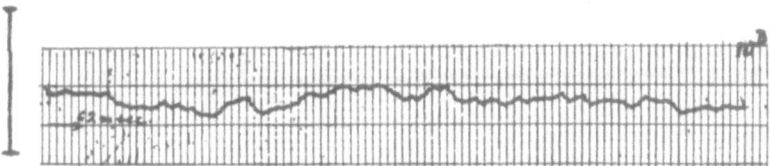

Fig. 7. ERG oscillatory potential of an eye 9 months after implantation Cu f.b. in it. Cal. 50 μV.

COMMENT

1. The increase of the ERG response b-wave of the left eyes with foreign bodies (Cu or Zn, Cu and Zn, or Cu plus iontophoresis with Zn), after the first three days of insertion of these in the eye, of all experimental animals is a remarkable phenomenon. It could be related to the exaltation phase discovered by Wedensky (quoted by Bykov, 1960) in his neuromuscular preparation to which he applied stimulation of different grade, at different lengths of time.

2. Preliminary results indicated that there is some protective action by zinc on an eye which has a copper particle in it. Whether this is similar to the effect described by Itoi in the case of iron, or whether there are additional protective effect on vital enzymes is still to be determined.

3. The obtained results shows that the oscillatory potential is also protected by zinc.

REFERENCES

Bastek, J., J. Bogden, A. Cinotti, W. TenHove, F. Stephens, M. Markopoulos & J. Charles. Trace metals in a family with sex-linked Retinitis Pigmentosa. Proc. ARVO Symp., Durham, N.C., 1975, Retinitis Pigmentosa – Clinical implication of current research, p. 43. Plenum Press, New York (1977).

Bykov, K.M. The refractory and exaltation phase. Textbook of Physiology, p. 509. Foreign Languages Publ. House, Moscow (1960).

Dambit, G.R. The use of tiosulfate of sodium by copper's intraocular foreign bodies. *Oftal. Zh.* 15: *3* (1960).

Delbeque, Ph., J. Sourdille & S. Delthil. Communication sut les Corps Etrangers Intraoculaires. Traitement de la chalcose oculaire d'origine traumatique par la penicillamine. *Bull. Mem. Soc. franç. Ophtal.* 79: *275* (1966).

Habig, J.M., A. Lumen & J. Snacker. Essai de chemiotherapie de cuivre intraoculaire. *Bull. Soc. belge Ophtal.* 98: *287* (1951).

Hogan, M.J. & L.E. Zimmerman. Foreign bodies. p. 159, in: Ophthalmic pathology. Sanders (1962).

Knave, B. Electroretinography in eyes with intraocular metallic foreign bodies. A clinical study. *Acta Ophtal.* Suppl. 100: *5* (1969).

Knave, B. The electroretinographic and ophthalmological changes in experimental metallosis in rabbits. Effect of steel, copper and aluminum particles. *Acta Ophthal.* 48: *159* (1970).

Lawwill, T. Practical rabbit electroretinography. *Am. J. Ophtal.* 74: *135* (1972). Rouher, M.T. Chalcose du cristallin, effets du BAL. *Bull. Soc. Ophthal. France* 1: *19* (1958).

Schmidt, J.G.H., A. Stute & E. Weber. Electroretinographische und Ophthalmoscopische Befunde by Intraocularen Metalfremdkorpern der Rate. *Ber. Dtsch. Ophthal. Ges.* 71: *391* (1971).

Spivey, B.E. & J.T. Pearlman. Day to day variation in ERG of human and rabbit. *Am. J. Ophthal.* 55: *1013* (1963).

Valee, B. Zinc biochemistry, a perspective. Trend in Biochemical Sciences, Vol. 1 (4), p. 88. Elsevier, Amsterdam (1976).

Wald, G. Molecular basis in visual excitation science. 162 (3850): 230 (1969).

Authors' address:
New Jersey Medical School
Eye Institue of New Jersey
15 South 9th Street
Newark, N.J. 07107
USA

Docum. Ophthal. Proc. Series, Vol. 15

CHANGES OF THE ERG IN RABBITS INTRAVITREALLY TREATED WITH BLOOD*

J. RÖVER, H. THEOPOLD, G. SCHAUBELE,
B. OLIVIER & J. FAULBORN
(Freiburg, Br., W. Germany)

Ironions destroy the retinal pigment epithelium and, consequently, the photoreceptors. They may originate from general siderosis, erosion of foreign intraocular bodies, or from haemolysing erythrocytes. Since Karpe's investigation (1948), we know that the destruction of the retina by ironions, deriving from intraocular splinters, has a slow progression. Thus, the function of the retina may easily be controlled by subjective tests and infrequent ERG-recordings.

Far more difficult is a prognostic evaluation when anticipating retinal impairment by ironions, deriving from haemolysis after intravitreal bleeding, as the amount of blood in the vitreous is difficult to judge by inspection. Under these circumstances the ERG becomes the all-deciding test for retinal function. Nowadays it will be even more important, as it has no longer a merely decriptive task but should indicate the necessity and the moment for removing the opacities by vitrectomy. To us it seems necessary to perform vitrectomy dependent upon the ERG-development, as in many cases we observed a spontaneous resorption of the intraocular bleeding and a restitution of good visual function even when an ophthalmoscopic inspection of the fundus proved to be impossible for some months. As vitrectomy bears numerous risks, it should be considered cautiously. Therefore, we investigated the time course of retinal damage in relation to the amount of blood accumulated in the vitreous.

We performed the following test series with rabbits, well aware that the results may not be generally applicable to the situation in human eyes after intraocular bleeding. Nevertheless we hope to contribute some parameters giving hints to the judgement of ERG changes recorded from human diseased eyes. We recorded the ERG with a small corneal electrode as described by Burian and Allan, fitted with a 1oo dptr front lens. We used Maxwellian illumination. The light was provided by a xenon vapour lamp; timing was done by an electronic shutter giving a flash of 16 ms duration, and the intensity varied with neutral density filters. The corneo-fundal potential was recorded with an ink ejection plotter.

First the lens of all rabbits' eyes was extracted, and one week later blood quantities of o.3 to o.8 ml were injected into the vitreous. For control pur-

* Supported by Deutsche Forschungsgemeinschaft SFB 7o.

pose the same amount of sodium chloride was applied to rabbits in a second test series. Removal of the lens was necessary to gain space for the injections, as without these preparations, ruptures of the eyeball of the sutures were observed. The surgery was performed each time with pentobarbiturate anaesthesia and with microsurgery equipment to reduce the traumatic effect on the eye. All the rabbits were recorded after the removal of the lens.

In these preparative studies we encountered a very great difference in amplitude when recording the same animal at different hours of the day as well as between two individuals when recorded under identical conditions. This finding urged us to accept a reliability of 30% variation when interpreting the values recorded after the injection. Our results were favorably comparable to the values published by Ronchi et al.

After the injection the ERG was recorded daily for one week with intensities of 5, 50, 500, 5,000 and 50,000 cd/m^2, then we controlled the ERG the voltage of the ERG-recordings is indicated on the abscissa and the third

In Fig. 1, the time after the removal of the lens is plotted on the ordinate, the voltage of the ERG-recordings is indicated on the abcissa and the third axis gives the intensities of illumination. The a-wave is represented by a dotted line, the b-wave by a continuous line. The amount of blood, applied after the first recording, is indicated by the figure beside the little arrow.

Fig. 2 shows the same graphic display for blood quantities of o.5 ml. It is easy to see, that blood quantities of 0.3 and 0.5 ml have no significant premanent effect on the amplitude of the ERG, equally the ERG recorded from those eyes, treated with sodium chloride solution showed no alteration. However, there is a very significant reduction of the a- and b-wave amplitude with blood quantities of o.8 ml, as shown in Fig. 3. A very drastic effect can be seen between the measurements of the second and third days. This rapid deterioration of the ERG is surprising at first glance, as from the

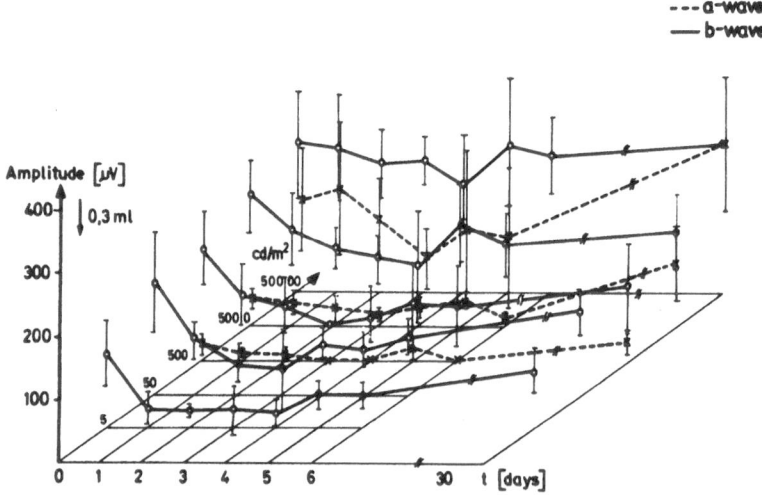

Fig. 1. Time course of the ERG amplitude following the injection of o.3 ml blood into the vitreous of rabbits.

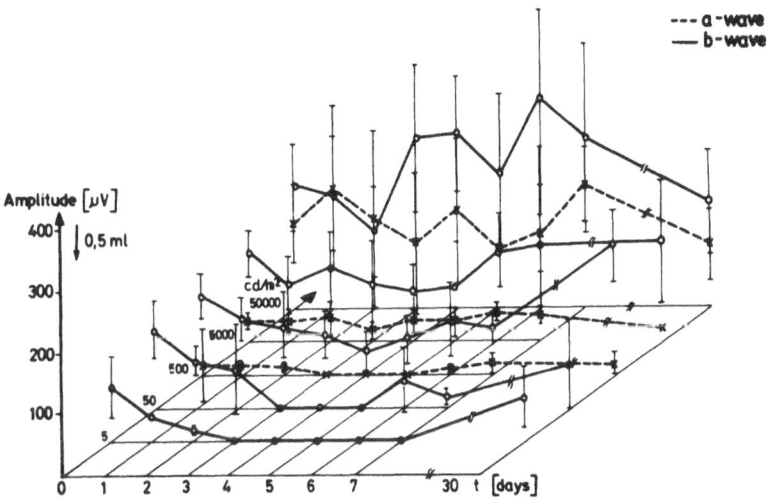

Fig. 2. cf. Fig. 1, injected amount of blood was o.5 ml.

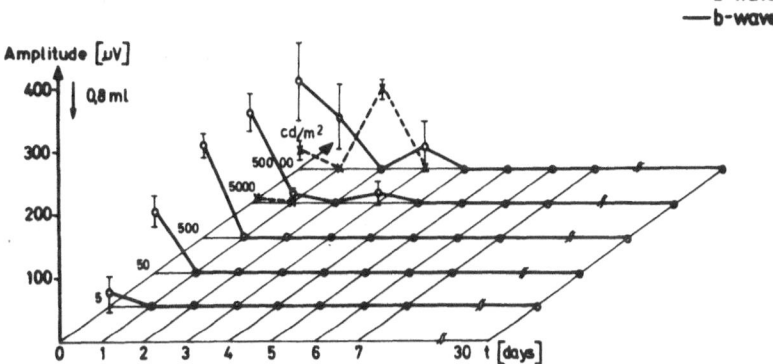

Fig. 3. cf. Fig. 1 and 2, injected amount of blood was o.8 ml.

investigations concerning intraocular splinters we know that the progressive damage of the retina is slow, and there is plenty of time to ponder over therapeutic decisions.

The reason of this rapid diminishing of the ERG could be the very fine and simultaneous release of ironions during haemolysis that cannot be immediately eliminated.

We checked the visual function of those rabbits showing no ERG changes as far as we could by means of electrophysiology. We implanted two electrodes submeningeal above the occipital lobe of the cortex and recorded the VEP with alternating checkerboard pattern. The rabbits showed a typical VEP recording, that did not change, however, with glasses, as shown in Fig. 4.

Our conclusion from our tests is the need for a very frequent control of patients with intraocular haemorrhages by ERG recordings. This is essential

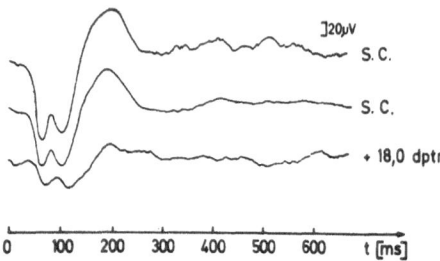

Fig. 4. VEP of a rabbit after removal of the lens and injectionof o.5 ml sodium chloride solution into the vitreous. Recording during checkerboard stimulation with intracerebral electrodes. No alteration of the VEP shape and amplitude visible.

during the first week in order not to miss the moment when surgical intervention becomes necessary.

REFERENCES

Karpe, G. Early diagnosis of siderosis retinae by the use of electroretinography. *Docum. Ophthal.* 2: *277–296* (1948).
Spivey, B.E. & J.T. Pearlman. Day-to-day variation in the ERG of humans and rabbits. *Am. J. Ophthal.* 55: *1013–1020* (1963).
Sugar, H.S., S.D. Kobernick & J.E. Weingarten. Haematogenous ocular siderosis of local cause. *Am. J. Ophthal.* 64: *749–756* (1967).

Authors' address:
Universitäts–Augenklinik
Killianstrasse 21
D7800 Freiburg i.Br.
West Germany

SURFACE AREA SIZES OF INTRAVITREAL COPPER PARTICLES: THEIR EFFECTS ON THE ERG OF RABBITS AND RATS*.

J.G.H. SCHMIDT, V. MIĆOVIĆ & A. STUTE

(Cologne, W. Germany)

It has been clinically and experimentally proven that intraocular copper particles are especially toxic. Single observations, however, have shown that sometimes the effects of particles containing copper are very limited and appear very slowly. In such cases, the cause can very often be found in the fact that copper has been alloyed with other metals, thus changing its toxicity (Schmidt, Blettenberg & Vogelsang, 1975). Another influencing factor is the localization of the foreign body (Schmidt, 1977), since the concentration of oxygen as the main oxidizer in the ocular region varies greatly.

Little quantitative data about foreign particles has been collected thus far. In addition to the effect of various iron particle quantities, Knave has shown on two rabbits the effect of intravitreal copper particles, varying in size, on the ERG. In this study we investigated the effects of surface area sizes of intravitreal copper particles on the ERG of rabbits and rats.

METHODS

Seventeen pigmented rabbits, ranging in weight between 1.7 and 2.6 kg, and 22 albino rats (Wistar), ranging in weight between 140 and 220 g, were used. Electroretinographic recording, anesthesia and the application of copper and contaminating trace metals have been reported previously (Schmidt & Stute, 1972; Stute, Schmidt & Weber, 1977; Stute, 1978).

RESULTS

Rabbits

Fig. 1 shows the mean values of the b-waves of rabbits influenced by intravitreal copper wires of varying size. With very large particles (12.7 mm^2 surface area; 6 eyes), the b-wave is extinguished after seven days, on the average, and the a-wave after ten days. Reducing the surface area of the foreign body drastically changes the speed of intoxication. With copper wire particles ha-

* This research was supported by Deutsche Forschungsgemeinschaft, Bonn/Bad Godesberg.

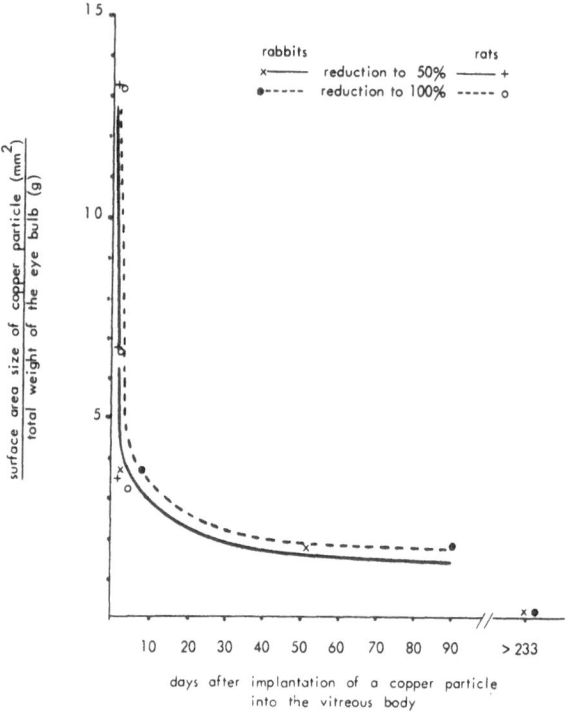

Fig. 1. Surface area size of intravitreal copper particles: their effects on the ERG (amplitude of the b-wave) of rabbits and rats.

ving a surface area between 5.2 and 7.8 mm² (3 eyes), the b-wave is not extinguished for two or three months. Copper splinters with a surface area of o.46 mm² had no influence on the a- or b-wave amplitudes during an observation period of more than 100 days (4 eyes) resp. 233 days (2 eyes). Furthermore, the shapes of the ERG of the implantation eye and the control eye nearly coincided (Fig. 2).

We could discern a clear encapsulation only with the largest foreign particles (12,7 mm² surface area). This developed within the first ten days, then remained, for the most part, constant. Some particles changed their position within the capsule; they slid partly out of the capsule, then a new, thin encapsulation began forming. A change in the surface of the foreign body was not seen ophthalmoscopically until the 191st day.

Rats

The results have been presented previously (Schmidt, Stute & Weber, 1971; Stute, 1978).

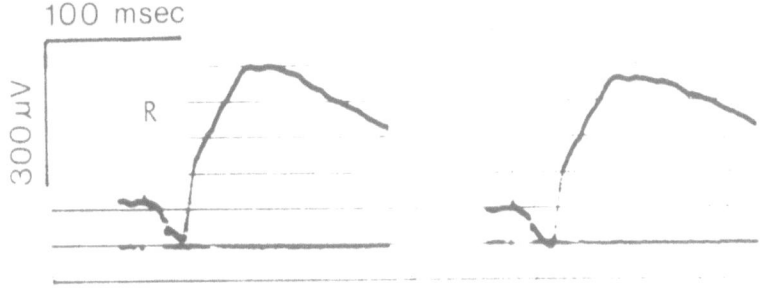

Fig. 2. ERG of rabbit eye (R) with intravitreal copper particle (o.65 mm^2) 233 days after implantation (left) and uninjured fellow eye during same session (right).

Weights of the eye balls of rabbits and rats

For the evaluation of the total ball weights the ocular adnexa were removed as thoroughly as possible.
Eyes of 6 rabbits: $\bar{x} = 3.4$ g; s = 0.296.
Eyes of 10 rats:　$\bar{x} = 99$ mg; s = 5.99.
Ratio of mean values of the two species: 34.3.

DISCUSSION

In earlier experiments (Schmidt, Stute & Weber, 1971; Stute, 1978); we implanted copper splinters into the vitreous body of rats eyes, ranging in size from 0.3 mm^2 (10 eyes) to 0.65 mm^2 (5 eyes) and to 1.3 mm^2 (17 eyes). Even the smallest of the particles destroyed the ERG within a few days. In order to investigate the effect of still smaller particles, we implanted them into the vitreous body of rabbits' eyes. As a basis for comparison, we took the size of the foreign body in relation to the total size of the eye ball, disregarding the anatomical and physiological differences between the eyes of the two species. Within the range of overlapping values of this index figure there was surprisingly good agreement for the corresponding toxicity of copper in the two for the corresponding toxicity of copper in the two species (Fig. 1). The values of the rabbits (6 eyes) and the rats (10 eyes) coincided, for the most part, between 3 and 4 mm^2/g bulbus weight. Impairment of the ERG occurred very quickly with intravitreal particles of more than 3 mm^2/g bulbus weight. A decisive change in the speed of intoxication could be discerned with particles between 3 and 2 mm^2/g bulbus weight. Particles smaller than 1 mm^2/g bulbus weight effected the ERG potentials very slowly, if at all. As the example of animal No. 17 on the 233rd day shows, no change in the shapes of the ERG could be found when comparing the control eye with the implantation-eye (0.14 mm^2/g bulb weight). Ophthalmoscopic investigations did not reveal any changes in the surface of the implant, which could be clearly recognized until the 191st day. Thus, the

65

stability of the ERG potentials in the case of very small foreign particles is not due to encapsulation nor to elimination of the particles.

In the rabbits eyes, the larger particles were localized in the middle of the vitreous body, while the smaller ones were mostly midway between the visual axis and the ciliary body. The values given for the rats' eyes refer to copper particles implanted into the posterior vitrious body region.

Although previous experiments showed an influence of the localization of the foreign body (Schmidt, 1977), the range of changes with varied positions but constant size of the splinter was much smaller than that for varied surface areas reported here. This means that, in clinical cases, the difference in foreign body surface areas is of higher significance than the different localizations of the particles within the vitreous body.

If we convert the values of Knaves's experiments we get a reduction of the b-wave to 50% (resp. to 100%) by one rabbit (3 mm^2 surface area/g weight of the eye ball) within 2 (resp. 60) days, and for another animal (1.4 mm^2/g) values of more than 450 (resp. 450) days. These results are in good accordance with our findings.

Among 280 cases with non-magnetic intraocular foreign bodies (247 intravitreal splinters; 178 containing copper; Neubauer, 1976) of the University Eye Clinic of Cologne only a few large particles of more than 3 mm^2/g bulb weight were removed. As the slope of the curve changes drastically below 3 mm^2/g, this size appears to be of critical importance in patients with copper splinters, assuming that we may transfer the present data on the human eye. Further experiments are necessary to follow up the slope below 3 mm^2/g bulb weight in detail for longer observation time.

During the rabbit experiments with observation periods of up to 233 days, the electric potentials of the control eye remained unchanged. During that time the animals were anesthetized nine times with a mixture of Halothane®-N$_2$O-oxygen for exploratory purposes. In earlier experiments with Wistar rats, there was no recognizable ERG change up to the seventh Halothane® narcosis within twenty-five days. After this, a- and b-waves changes occurred following further periods of anestheses. However, the slightly reduzed amplitudes returned to normal by the 197th day of observation – probably due to longer intervals between anestheses (Stute, Schmidt & Weber, 1977).

SUMMARY

The electroretinogram was investigated in 16 rabbits implanted with intravitreal copper particles ranging in size between 0.65 and 12.7 mm^2 for a period of up to 233 days. Considering also results obtained by the same methods on Wistar rats, we found that the ERG was extinguished after one week, if the surface area of the copper particles exceeded 3 mm^2/g bulbus weight. A surface area half this size impairs the ERG only after two to three months. With very tiny copper splinters (0.14 mm^2/g bulbus weight), no reduction of the electric potentials could be discerned, even after more than 233 days.

Under the given conditions, no effect of Halothane®-laughing gas-oxygen mixture was discerned on the ERG of the control eye.

We are grateful to Miss Christa Schabio and Miss Annegret Weege for their technical assistance.

REFERENCES

Knave, B. The ERG and ophthalmological changes in experimental metallosis in the rabbit. I. Effects on iron particles. *Acta Ophthal. (Kbh)* 48: *136–158* (1970).

Knave, B. The ERG and ophthalmological changes in experimental metallosis in the rabbit. II. Effects of steel, copper and aluminium particles. *Acta Ophthal. (Kbh)* 48: *159–173* (1970).

Neubauer, H. Der nichtmagnetische Fremdkörper. In: H. Neubauer, Intraokularer Fremdkörper und Metallose. Bergmann-Verlag, München (1977).

Schmidt, J.G.H., M. Blettenberg & M.-Chr. Vogelsang. On the recovery of the electroretinogram after the removal of intravitreal copper splinters. Assn of Res. in Vision and Ophthal. (ARVO), Sarasota, Florida (1975).

Schmidt, J.G.H. & V. Micovic. Tierexperimentalle Untersuchungen über die Wirkung intraocularer Fremdkörper auf das ERG. In: H. Neubauer, Intraocularer Fremdkörper und Metallose. Bergmann-Verlag, München (1977).

Schmidt, J.G.H. & A. Stute. Electroretinogram and ophthalmoscopic findings in intra-vitreous iron, copper and lead particles. Proceedings XIth ISCERG Symposium, Los Angeles, 1972. Junk, The Hague (1973).

Schmidt, J.G.H., A. Stute & E. Weber. Elektroretinographische und ophthalmoskopische Befunde bei intraocularen Metallfremdkörpern der Ratte. *Ber. Dtsch. Ophthal. Ges.* 71: *391–396* (1972).

Schmidt, J.G.H. & E. Weber. The effect of intra-ocular copper alloys on the ERG of human and rat retinas. Proceedings VIIIth ISCERG Symposium, Pisa (1970).

Stute, A. Thesis, Cologne (1978).

Stute, A., J.G.H. Schmidt & E. Weber. On the effect of Urethane and Halothane on the ERG of rats. Proceedings 15th ISCEV Symposium, Ghent 1977. Junk, The Hague (1978).

Authors' address:
Universitats-Augenklinik Köln
5000 Cologne 41
West Germany

ELECTROPHYSIOLOGY IN EXPERIMENTAL SIDEROSIS:
A FOLLOW–UP STUDY AFTER REMOVAL OF INTRAOCULAR
FOREIGN BODY*

SONJA S. DECLERCQ & PHILLIP C.A. MEREDITH

(Stanford, Cal., USA)

ABSTRACT

An iron foreign body was placed intravitreously in 19 rabbits. In 11 animals the foreign body was surgically removed after approximately 13 weeks and in 8 animals the extraction was performed after about 2 weeks.

Postoperative complications were encountered in 7 animals. The ERG changes of the remaining 12 animals were recorded over a 56 week period after foreign body removal.

All experiments used one eye as the experimental eye and the fellow eye as the control. The a- and b-wave amplitudes of the experimental eye were expressed in % of the control eye.

The results show that removal of the foreign body does not improve the ERG nor prevent its further deterioration.

INTRODUCTION

We all know and agree that siderosis is a toxic event and that the therapy consists of FB removal (Grant, 1976). However, the prognosis of the eye after removal of an iron FB remains uncertain and controversial (Duke-Elder & MacFaul, 1972). Serial electrophysiological studies in patients in whom an intraocular FB has been removed are considered an objective measure of retinal function (Potts, 1972). The primary objective of this study was to investigate the electroretinographic changes in experimental siderosis after the removal of the intravitreal iron FB.

METHODS AND MATERIAL

Nineteen male albino rabbits weighing about 3 kgs were used in this study. The ERG was recorded using our technique described in detail in a previous publication (Declercq et al., 1977).

ERG sequence: In each recording we used three different stimuli: A photopic ERG was performed using white light intensity 8 (W_8p) on a Grass

---

*This work was supported by Training Grant EY–00051 from the National Eye Institute, National Institutes of Health.
** In the text FB stands for foreign body and IOFB for intraocular foreign body.

photostimulator. After fifteen minutes of dark adaptation, a scotopic ERG was obtained using a white light intensity I reduced by a neutral density filter of 1.0 log unit (W_1ND) and white light intensity 8 (W_8S). All experiments used one eye as the experimental eye and the fellow eye as the control. The a- and b-wave of the experimental eye were expressed as a percent of the intact fellow eye.

Using the above described testing conditions, the a- and b-wave were recorded and studied in nineteen rabbits divided into two groups:

1) In Group 1, consisting of eight animals, a foreign body was placed intravitreously and removed after approximately two weeks.
2) In Group 2 consisting of eleven animals, the foreign body was removed ten to fifteen weeks later.

Implantation technique: this was identical to our technique described in detail in a previous publication (Declercq et al., 1977). A 3 mm long piece of pure iron wire was placed intravitreously, using a lumbar puncture needle, in the lumen of which the iron particle was inserted. The iron FB was released by pushing the stylet of the needle.

Removal technique: Sterile operating conditions were observed. The intraocular FB was removed through the pars plana in eleven cases and through the direct transretinal route in eight cases depending on the FB location. In all cases, the IOFB could be visualized preoperatively. The IOFB was extracted with a foreign body forceps, because very often the magnet could not dislodge the iron particle bound to the retina by fibrous adhesions.

RESULTS

Group 1

The ERG changes occurring after implantation and after removal of the FB are shown in Figure 1.

The a- and b-wave of all eight animals were decreased by approximately 40% at one week after implantation and these values correspond to our previously published results (Declercq et al., 1977). The remaining five were followed up to forty-two weeks after FB removal. At that time, the a-wave of the experimental eye had not changed and remained at 60% of the normal control eye; the b-wave had increased about 15%.

Group 2

The a- and b-wave changes occurring after implantation and removal of the FB are shown in Figure 2. By the seventh week after FB implantation, the a-wave was down to 50% and the b-wave to 60% of the normal fellow eye. The FB was removed and four animals developed a post-operative complication which consisted of a vitreal hemorrhage with or without retinal detachment, these were excluded from the follow-up study.

70

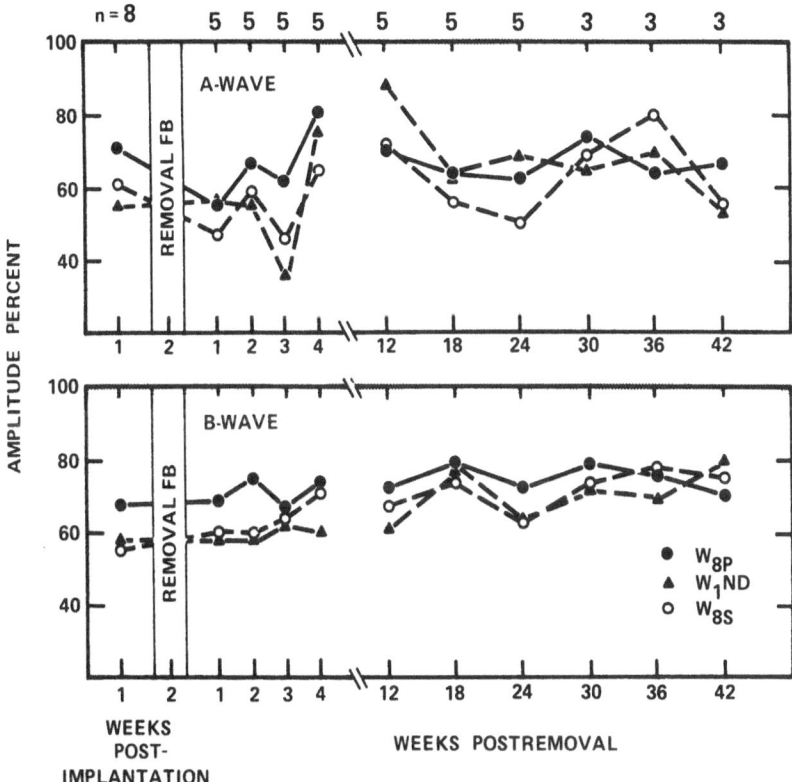

Fig. 1. The a- and b-wave amplitudes, expressed in per cent of the intact fellow eye, of iron implanted eyes in which the FB was removed ten to fifteen days later. Each value represents the mean of n rabbits tested at the given time. ERGs using three different testing conditions were performed weekly during the first four weeks postremoval of the FB and every six weeks thereafter.

The remaining seven animals were studied for a period up to fifty-four weeks following FB extraction. Both a- and b-waves fluctuated in relation to time and relation to stimulus. At the fifty-fourth week after removal, the a- and b-wave values were approximately 50% of the fellow eye.

DISCUSSION

From the results we can say that the IOFB removal does not alter the ERG drastically nor prevent its continued deterioration. If removal is performed early (before two weeks) the electroretinographic values show a very slow improvement, with a b-wave increase of 15%, forty-two weeks later. If removal is performed late, there is no improvement, but after one year a slight decrease in b-wave is present.

The FB extraction per se carries a 36% surgical risk. This corresponds to the latest study done by Percival on 153 human cases (Percival, 1972).

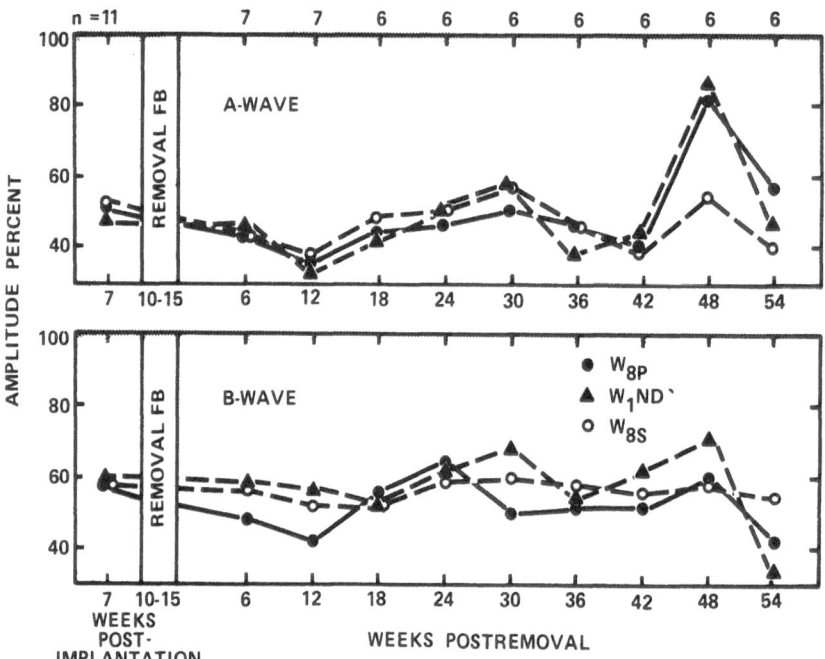

Fig. 2. The a- and b-wave amplitudes, expressed in per cent of the intact fellow eye, of iron implanted eyes, in which the FB was removed between ten and fifteen weeks after implantation. Each value represents the mean of n rabbits tested at the given time. ERGs using three different testing conditions were performed every six weeks after removal.

From our previous studies we know that most of the siderotic electrophysiological damage occurs within one week (Declercq et al., 1977). The values of a- and b-wave after one week are down to 60% and after four months are down to 55% . This agrees with the findings presented in this paper which indicate that FB removal after one week does not result in normalization of the ERG.

REFERENCES

Declercq, S., P.C. Meredith & A.R. Rosenthal. Experimental siderosis in the rabbit. *Arch. Ophthal.* 95: *1051–1058* (1977).

Duke-Elder, S. & P.A. MacFaul. Injuries. Part 1. Mechanical injuries. pp. 525–544 in: Duke-Elder, S., System of Ophthalmology. Mosby, St Louis (1972).

Grant, W.M. Toxicology of the eye. 2nd ed., Chales C. Thomas, Springfield, Ill., pp. 594–604 (1976).

Percival, S.P.B. Late complications from posterior segment intraocular foreign bodies. *Br. J. Ophthal.* 56: *462–468* (1972).

Potts, A.M. Electrophysiological measurements. pp. 187–206, in: Potts, A.M., The assessment of visual function. Mosvy, St Louis (1972).

Authors' address:
Division of Ophthalmology
Stanford University Medical Center
Stanford, California 94305
USA

EXPERIMENTAL STUDY OF SIDEROSIS

P. FRANÇOIS & J.Cl. HACHE

(Lille, France)

The purpose of this work was to find the localization of iron accumulation in relation to the foreign body site. At the same time, the iron rate in aqueous humour and the ERG were studied.

METHOD

Fifteen rabbits were used. Foreign bodies were included either in the lens or in the vitreous close to the retina. For the main elements, the foreign body composition was:

Fe   96%
Cu   2%
Mn   0.06%
Zn   0.03%

The weight of the foreign body was 3 mg for lens foreign bodies and 5 mg for vitreo-retinal foreign bodies.

The ERG was studied with a Henkes contact lens. We used, in photopic condition, a white stimulus of two hundred lux on cornea and a red stimulus. During the darkness, a white stimulus was used. The ERG were studied each month.

Only the results of the first and the last ERG are shown. The puncture for the determination of iron rate in aqueous humour was done just before enucleation. The dosage was realized by atomic absorption spectrophotometry. The normal rate does not overcome 0.11 ppm. The enucleation was done after variable durations, generally when the clinical and electrical signs of siderosis were present. Histologic examinations were realized with optical and electronic methods. Slides were coloured by Perls coloration or Turnbull blue to show the iron depositions. All tissues were studied: cornea, iris, lens, ciliary body, retina, choroid. The siderosis intensity was estimated with the scale 0 to +++ in function of coloration. Only ciliary body and retina are shown.

RESULTS

Lens foreign bodies

It was observed that the lens wound was quickly closed and only a local cataract was developed. The delay of beginning of siderosis is very variable. A marked siderosis happened in thirty-seven days for one rabbit. For another rabbit, the eye with lens foreign body had no siderosis five months after inclusion, but the fellow eye with a vitreo-retinal foreign body developed a siderosis. Iron rate is always increased, but not much. There is no direct relation between iron rate and ERG alterations. ERG alteration was found with reduction of a-wave and b-wave. Histologic alterations are mainly on the ciliary body, lens and iris. There is a marked impregnation with iron in the lens anterior epithelium and above all in pigmented structure of the ciliary body. In the retina, alterations are rather less severe.

Vitreo-retinal foreign bodies

The delay for beginning of the alterations is also variable, but rather earlier than the delay for the lens foreign bodies. However, in one rabbit, there was no siderosis after seven months. The iron rate is more increased than in cases of lens alteration, perhaps because the lens foreign bodies are less heavy than the vitreo-retinal foreign bodies. ERG glterations are slightly more marked and earlier than ERG alterations of lens foreign bodies. In the main phase, a-wave and b-wave are decreased without modification of the latencies. b1 and b2 waves are similarly decreased. In the early phase, b1 wave and response to red stimulus seem slightly decreased. Ferric depositions are yet mainly in the ciliary body but also on the retina. The retina is more impaired and earlier affected than is in cases of lens foreign bodies.

It is noted that iron depositions are in the internal limiting membrane and in the pigmentary epithelium. In inner layers of the retina, there is no pigment, or very little. It seems that iron pigments can cross the retina since there is no 'zonula occludens' in the retina. So, iron pigments can be phagocytosed by pigmentary epithelium.

Table 1. Lens foreign bodies

| Rabbit no. | ERG (μV) | | | | delay | siderosis | | iron rate |
| | before | | after | | | | | |
	a	b	a	b	days	ciliary	retina	ppm
3	45	270	30	180	195	++	+	0.22
5	40	240	30	150	160	+	0	0.12
6	40	300	10	150	37	+++	+	0.18
8	40	200	20	180	250	++	+	0.20
10	50	270	30	250	150	0	0	0.20

Table 2. Retino vitreous foreign bodies

| Rabbit no. | ERG (μV) | | | | delay | siderosis | | iron rate |
| | before | | after | | | | | |
	a	b	a	b	days	ciliary	retina	ppm
1	40	260	20	220	180	+++	+++	0.5
1	50	270	30	200	180	++	++	0.4
2	30	220	10	110	160	++	++	0.35
2	30	230	20	160	160	+	+	0.30
3	50	250	40	200	195	++	+	0.26
4	50	300	20	160	195	+++	++	0.17
4	40	250	10	80	195	0	+++	0.28
5	50	260	30	200	160	+	0	0.28
6	30	210	10	80	37	+++	+++	0.30
7	40	220	15	90	67	++	0	0.17
8	30	190	10	180	250	0	0	0.10
10	50	200	10	160	150	+	+	0.15
12	40	250	20	90	210	+	0	0.30
12	20	250	10	130	210	+	0	0.16
13	40	260	20	200	120	+	0	0.12
13	40	250	20	150	120	+	0	0.10
15	50	250	50	220	210	0	0	0.13
15	50	220	30	200	210	0	0	0.10

DISCUSSION

Ocular siderosis consecutive to lens foreign bodies is not very different from siderosis consecutive to vitreo-retinal foreign bodies. We remark that the retina alteration is slightly less early in the former cases.

In both cases:
— the beginning delay is very variable and we cannot explain this variability;
— there is no hypernormal ERG;
— the impairment of b1 wave and of the response to red stimulus seem to be earlier, but it is possible that the traumatism can be the cause of it.

When the siderosis is more severè, the a-wave and the b-wave of the two systems are equally decreased. The most probable hypothesis is that the b-wave alteration is not due to a primitive siderosis of the inner layers of the retina, but secondary to photoreceptors and the a-wave alteration.

Clinical implications

These results on the rabbit siderosis are slightly contradictory to clinical results. The human ocular siderosis progresses much more quickly than rabbit siderosis and the iron rate is more increased (over 0.5 ppm). The circulation of aqueous humour of the rabbit is probably slightly different from the human circulation of the aqueous humour. This difference explains perhaps the differences of ERG alterations, since J. François, de

Rouck & Golan have found that the earliest alteration was on the scotopic components.

However, we have found in the human iris of siderotic eyes the same affinity of the ferritine for pigmented tissues and melanic structure. On the slides of the electronic microscope of a human iris, iron pigments are seen in the macula or in the cytoplasma near melanin grains. When the intoxication by the iron is so severe, it is very probable that cellular impairments are irreversible.

This affinity of iron for pigmented structures is similar for man and for rabbit. In spite of the difference of evolution, it is probable that, as for the rabbit, the human pigmentary epithelium is the most impaired retinal structure. This is probably the explanation of the early alteration of the EOG and perhaps also of the alteration of the photoreceptors and, consequently, of the ERG.

Authors' address:
Clinique Ophtalmologique
59 Lille
France

EXTENDING RETINAL IMPAIRMENT FOLLOWING IRON INTRAOCULAR FOREIGN BODY

F.A. ABRAHAM

(Jerusalem, Israel)

INTRODUCTION

The specific clinico-pathologic changes of the eye structures caused by the iron contents of intraocular foreign bodies described by von Graefe (1860) were termed siderosis bulbi by Bunge (1890). Since then, the fast industrialization process and the arms used in the last wars highly increased the incidence of iron intraocular foreign bodies, supplying wide clinico-pathologic material (Mayou, 1926; Gulliver, 1942; Loewenstein & Foster, 1947; Roper-Hall, 1954; Hoefle, 1968, Hollwich, 1976). Additional experimental electron microscopic (Barber et al., 1971; Masciulli et al., 1972; Yoo, 1976) and histochemical studies (Matsuo & Hasegawa, 1964; Hasegawa, 1964; Hasegawa, 1966) disclosed specific retinal changes in siderosis. However, the pathogenesis of the retinal disease is still far from being clear. The standard ERG, while cardinal for early diagnosis of siderosis and for prognostic evaluation (Karpe, 1957; Schmöger, 1957; Straub, 1961; Kozousek, 1965; Gorgone, 1966; Knave, 1969), provides only partial information regarding the complex retinal impairment. The purpose of the present study is to analyze and correlate the clinical and visual field changes with the results of fluorescein angiography as well as the electroretinogram (ERG) and electrooculogram (EOG) results in a patient with iron-containing magnetic foreign body on the retina of his single eye. The patient was followed for three years before and seven years after the foreign body was extracted.

METHODS

In addition to the clinical eye examinations the color vision, visual field, fluorescein angiography, psychophysical dark adaptation were examined, and the EOG, ERG and flash visual evoked potential (VEP) were recorded using techniques described in previous studies (Abraham, 1975; Abraham et al., 1976). Under our conditions, the normal ERG elicited by single light flash stimuli of medium intensity (Grass I−2) reaches negative amplitudes of 120−200 μV and positive amplitudes of 430−550 μV after 30 minutes in the dark. For the EOG the criteria of Arden et al. (1962) were used and the lowest normal limit taken as 185%.

An 18 year old soldier was injured by a mine explosion in October 1967 and lost his left eye immediately. The right eye suffered a perforating wound of the sclera at 5 o'clock, 5 mm behind the limbus. The vitreous was full of blood and x-ray revealed a small foreign body at the posterior pole of the eye. An attempt to extract the foreign body was unsuccessful and the wound was sutured primarily. Three months later, when the ocular media had cleared up and vision had returned to 6/6, a glistening, partially incapsulated metallic foreign body of about 0.4 mm diameter could be seen at 5 mm below the optic disk. During three years of observation the eye remained quiet. However, scotopic function became progressively impaired and the visual field decreased concentrically (Fig. 1). Repeated ERG recordings from 1968 to 1970 revealed normal a-wave amplitudes but photopically and mainly scotopically impaired b-waves of moderately subnormal amplitudes (Fig. 2). The EOG was slightly subnormal, reaching only 170%. The VEPs elicited by light flash stimuli were of normal pattern and latency but of subnormal amplitude.

In view of the electrophysiologically impaired retinal function and progressive visual field constriction, extraction of the foreign body became obligatory despite the high risk of the operation. In June 1970 the foreign body

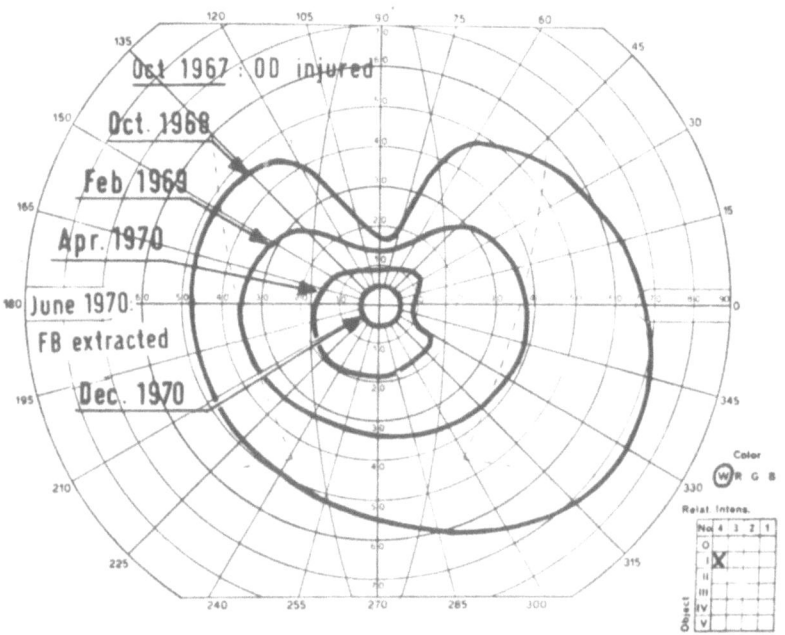

Fig. 1. Follow up of the peripheral visual field tested by I–4 target of the Goldmann perimeter.

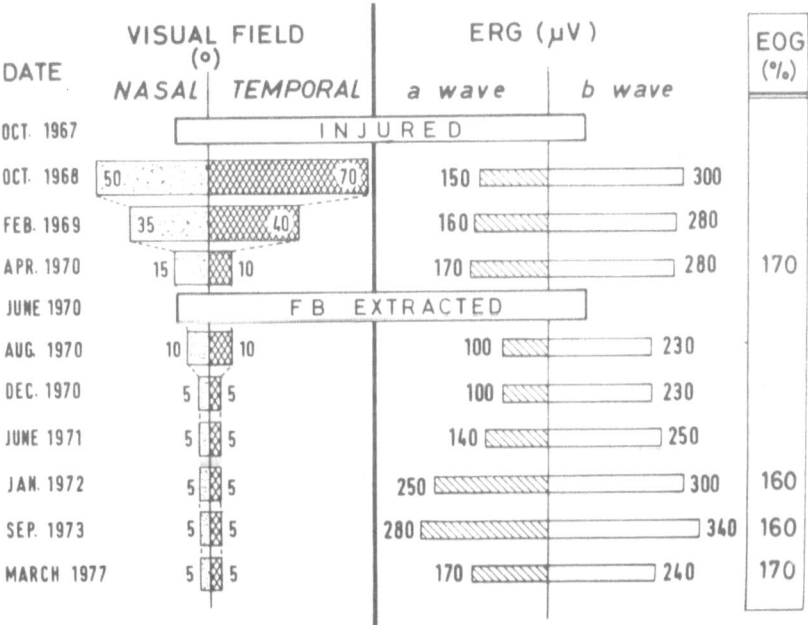

Fig. 2. Follow up of the visual fields horizontal diameter, ERG amplitudes after 30 min. of dark adaptation and EOG values.

was extracted uneventfully by magnet, leaving only a small retinal scar. Postoperatively, the visual field decreased further to 10 degrees diameter (Fig. 1) and remained there according to repeated comprehensive tests. During seven years after operation the eye remained quiet, with normal co- lor vision and a visual acuity of 6/9 due to a small posterior subcapsular lens opacity. Fundoscopy revealed normal appearance of the optic disk, macula, and peripheral retina except the chorio-retinal scar at the lower midperiphe- ry, caused by the injury and surgery. The ERG positive and negative ampli- tudes decreased after operation (Fig. 2), recovered to even higher amplitu- des two years later, but remained photopically and mainly scotopically im- paired. The EOG remained slightly subnormal (160–170%) and the VEPs did not change. Psychophysical measurement of dark adaptation at 4 de- grees above the fovea revealed a photopic plateau at about 2 log threshold higher than normal and missing scotopic function (Fig. 3). Fluorescein an- giography of the posterior pole (Fig. 4), as well as of the midretinal periphe- ry, disclosed normal pigment epithelial structure and retinal circulation.

DISCUSSION

Despite the large number of cases of iron-containing intraocular foreign bo- dies followed clinically and by ERG tests, the progression of the retinal im- pairment and especially the sequence of the retinal layers involvement has

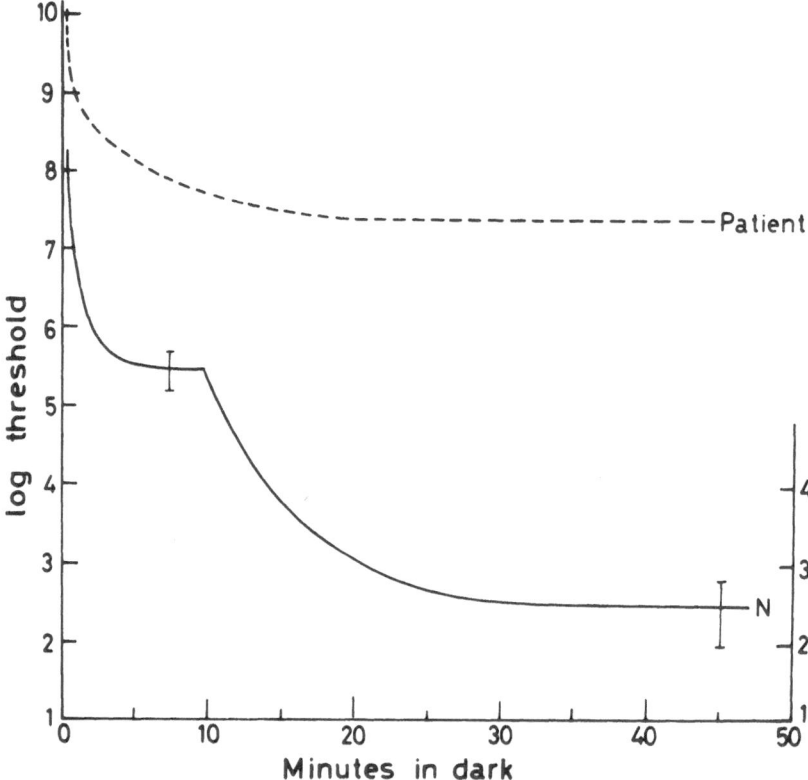

Fig. 3. Dark adaptation curve obtained by psychophisical measurement at 4° above the fovea. N- normal curve measured at 6° above the fovea.

been only partially studied (Karpe, 1957; Schmöger, 1957; Straub, 1961; Kozousek, 1965; Gorgone, 1966; Knave, 1969). The ERG changes were proven to be sufficiently sensitive for an early detection of the retinal iron intoxication process by revealing progressive deterioration of the b-wave followed later on by a decrease of the a-wave amplitude. These ERG changes imply an early affection of the mid-retinal layer followed by the impairment of the photoreceptors (Brown, 1969; Miller & Dowling, 1970). The process seems to progress from the retinal periphery toward the posterior pole (Duke-Elder, 1972). However, to our knowledge, the sequence of the functional impairments was not thoroughly studied by repeated electrophysiological tests. Our patient was unusual in that he enabled us to follow and correlate the functional defects with the electrophysiological results collected over three years before and seven years after the foreign body had been extracted.

It was remarkable that the visual field constriction was not accompanied by progressive changes of the ERG, EOG and VEP. Furthermore, the normal fluorescein angiographic feature of the pigment epithelium and only slightly subnormal EOG, as well as the preserved late receptor potential with

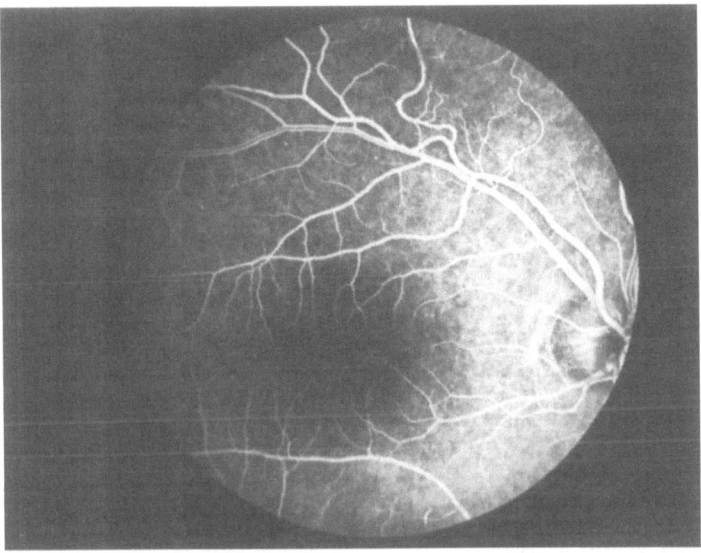

Fig. 4. Arterio-venous phase of the fluorescein angiography.

a just moderately impaired ERG photopic potential, seem to show that in this case the impairment of the outer retinal layers is insufficient for explaining the severe visual field defect (Armington, 1968). On the other hand, the subnormal amplitude but normal pattern of the VEPs and the normal fundoscopic appearance of the retinal nerve fibers and optic disk, do not explain as well the patient's progressive and irreversible visual field constriction (Frisen & Hoyt, 1974; Jakobsen et al., 1968; Holliday et al., 1972). It is therefore tempting to assume that retinal structures located beneath the nerve fibers could be related or responsible for the progressive functional deterioration, and if so, the recording of the ERG oscillatory potentials (Genest, 1964; Algvere & Wachmeister, 1972) may be useful to follow the process of retinal siderosis.

SUMMARY

The retinal function of a young patient with an iron containing foreign body on the retina of his single eye was followed by clinical and electrophysiological tests during three years before and seven years after the foreign body has been extracted. The EOG, ERG, and VEP results while revealing an impaired retinal function, did not follow and did not completely explain the severe and irreversible constriction of the visual field of this patient. In view of the results of the electrophysiological tests and the normal fluorescein angiographic and fundoscopic appearance, an impairment of the retinal structures located beneath the nerve fiber layer were suggested to be related or responsible for the visual field defect.

Abraham, F.A. Sector retinitis pigmentosa. Electrophysiological and psychophysical study of the visual system. *Docum. Ophthal.* 39: *13–28* (1975).

Abraham, F.A. Sector retinitis pigmentosa: a fluorescein angiographic study. *Ophthalmologica* 172: *287–297* (1976).

Algvere, P & L. Wachmeister. On the oscillatory potentials of the human electroretinogram in light and dark adaptation. Part II. *Acta Ophthal.* 50: *837–862* (1972).

Arden, G.B., A. Barrada & J.H. Kelsey. New clinical test of retinal function based upon the standing potential of the eye. *Br. J. Ophthal.* 46: *449–467* (1962).

Armington, J.C. The electroretinogram, the visual evoked potential and the area-luminance relation. *Vision Res.* 8: *263–276* (1968).

Barber, A.N., C. Catsulis & R.J. Cangelosi. Studies on experimental retinitis. Light and electron microscopy. *Br. J. Ophthal.* 55: *91–105* (1971).

Brown, K.T. The electroretinogram: its components and their origins. *Vision Res.* 8: *633 677* (1968).

Bunge. Über Siderosis bulbi. X Int. Cong. Med., Berlin. 4: 151 (1890).

Duke-Elder, S. System of Ophthalmology. Vol. XIV Injuries. Part I. Henry Kimpton, London. p. 533 (1972).

Frisen, L. & W.F. Hoyt. Insidious atrophy of retinal nerve fibers in multiple sclerosis. Fundoscopic identification in patients with and without visual complaints. *Arch. Ophthal.* 92: *91–97* (1974).

Genest, A. Oscillatory potentials in the ERG of the normal human eye. *Vision Res.* 4: *595–604* (1964).

Gorgone, G. Importanza clinica dell' ERG nella siderosis e calcosi oculare. *Boll. Ocul.* 45: *638–645* (1966).

von Graefe, A. Cataracta traumatic und chronishe Chorioditis durch einen fremden Korper in der Linse bedingt. *von Graefes Arch. Ophthal.* 6: *134–139* (1860).

Gulliver, F.D. Particles of steel within the globe of the eye. *Arch. Ophthal.* 28: *896–903* (1942).

Hasegawa, H. Histochemical studies on lactic dehydrogenase in the experimental siderotic retina. *Folia Ophthal. Japan* 15: *494–498* (1964).

Hasegawa, E. Histochemical studies on glucose-6-phosphate dehydrogenase in experimental siderosis of the retina. *Folia Ophthal. Japan* 17: *189–294* (1966).

Hoefle, F.B. Initial treatment of eye injuries. *Arch. Ophthal.* 79: *33–35* (1968).

Holliday, A.M., W.I. McDonald & J. Mushim. Delayed visual evoked response in optic neuritis. *Lancet* 1: *982–985* (1972).

Hollwich, F., E. Damaske & H. Liermann. Misdiagnosis of intraocular iron foreign bodies. *Klin. Mbl. Augenheilk.* 169: *481–488* (1976).

Karpe, G. Das Electroretinogram bei Siderosis bulbi. *Bibl. Ophthal.* 48: *182–193* (1957).

Knave, B. Electroretinography in eyes with retained intraocular metallic foreign bodies. A clinical study. *Acta. Ophthal. Suppl.* 100: *5–63* (1969).

Kozousek, V. Electroretinographic et microscopie electronique dans les metalloses. *Ann. Oculistique* 198: *694–702* (1965).

Loewenstein, A. & J.F. Foster. A contribution to the knowledge of ocular siderosis and posterior degenerative pannus. *Am. J. Ophthal.* 30: *275–288* (1947).

Masciulli, L., D.R. Anderson & S. Charles. Experimental ocular siderosis in the squirrel monkey. *Am. J. Ophthal.* 74: *638–661* (1972).

Matsuo, N. & E. Hasegawa. Histochemical and electron microscopical studies on retinal siderosis. *Acta. Soc. Opthal. Japan* 68: *1702–1717* (1964).

Mayou, M.S. Siderosis. *Trans. Ophthal. Soc. U.K.* 46: *167–180* (1926).

Miller, R.F. & J.E. Dowling. A relationship between Müller cell slow potentials and the ERG b-wave. Intern. Soc. Clin. Electroretinography Symp., Pisa, pp. 85–100 (1970).

Roper-Hall, M.J. Review of 555 cases of intraocular foreign body with special reference to prognosis. *Br. J. Ophthal.* 38: *65–99* (1954).

Schmoger, E. Electroretinographie bei Siderosis und Chalcosis. *Klin. Mbl. Augenheilk.* 128: *158–166* (1956).

Straub, W. Das Electroretinogramm. Bücherei des Augenarztes, Ferdinand Enke Verlag, Stuttgart (1961).

Yoo, J.H. Responses of Müller cells of rabbit retina in experimental siderosis. *Japan J. Ophthal.* 20: *149–158* (1976).

Author's address:
Vision Research Laboratory
Hadassah University Hospital and Medical School
Jerusalem
Israel

Docum. Ophthal. Proc. Series, Vol. 15

THRESHOLD ERG STUDY OF EXPERIMENTALLY
INDUCED METALLOSIS
(A preliminary report)*

J.R. BRUNETTE, S. WAGDI & G. LAFOND

(Sherbrooke, Que., Canada)

The complex decision making process which occurs in the presence of a retained metal or possibly metallic foreign body in the eye is a frequent and almost intractable feature of ophthalmic practice in populations of workers exposed to such industrial hazards. Any technique that could possibly detect metallosis or metallosis arrest in time, or help differentiate eye lesions due to trauma itself as opposed to the toxic effects of metallosis would certainly be welcome. The examination of extensive series of threshold ERGs (Brunette, 1973) has allowed us to propose a possible differentiation of degenerative processes in the retina, as in tapetoretinal degenerations, from destructive lesions, as in traumatic retinal detachment or extensive scarring. Models of these two types of electrophysiological responses are currently under study. It is the purpose of this paper to clarify the electrophysiopathological process induced by metallosis and determine whether it is of the degenerative or destructive type.

Induced metallosis in rabbits using iron and copper particles, will be reported here. This presentation will be limited to the mode of alteration of the ERG produced by these controlled ocular intoxications. No effort will be made to cover the factors governing the severity of the affection, the nature and the usefulness of the inflammatory reaction which follows implantation. These aspects shall be discussed in a future presentation.

MATERIAL AND METHODS

Forty-nine healthy adult Albino rabbit eyes were used, for over 190 ERG sessions. Ten eyes served for surgery controls and ERG preliminary studies. Surgical procedure alone did not induce ERG changes in controls. Eyes which presented evidence of post-operative complications such as retinal detachment, or hemorrhage were discarded. We have had no post-operative infections.

Surgical protocol

Particles of commercial iron and copper wire were cut into small pieces of an approximate surface area of 1.125 mm² (0.15 diam. x 2.5 long). One,

* This work was done under a research grant of the Canadian Medical Research Council.

three or six of these were introduced into the eye through as aseptic scleral flap at the pars plana, under direct visualization through a corneal contact lens. Particles were localized in the vitreous at varying distances from the retina. Eyes were examined and medicated daily, photographed, and complete follow-up records maintained.

ERG protocol

Subjects were light pre-adapted for two minutes with a background intensity of five footcandles. Cone threshold was then determined by adjusting the intensity of stimulation (in 0.1 log unit increments) to obtain a 50 μv criterion response (threshold ERG). A dark adaptation period of 20 minutes followed, during which threshold ERGs were recorded at one minute intervals. At the end of this period, the rod threshold was found. Then, the intensity of stimulation was increased by 0.5 log units increments to the full intensity of stimulation.

Technical data

The stimulator used a 300 watt Sylvania concentrated arc lamp, Type K-300, light source collimated to a Uniblitz shutter, with a time duration of 100 ms. Neutral density filters were mounted on discs, electromechanically controlled through drived Slow Syn motors, One disc supports neutral density Wratten filters calibrated from 1 to 9 log units, and a second disc, filters from 0.1 to 0.9 log units. The same possibilities exist for the background source, a DYS 600 watt Sylvania Tungsten Lamp. Light from the background and the stimulator source are each focused in a 1/4 inch fiber optic light guide, which divided in two 1/8 inch fiber bundles. These four sources are directed on a flat back plate mounted on a ping-pong ball one third of which has been cut out. This produces a reflected light into the diffusing sphere, or a ganzfeld effect. The back plate bears a 1 cm hole. The light sources are not directly visible to the eye under evaluation. The full intensity of the stimulus was evaluated at 1.8 lumens sec./pi^2 and that of the background at 2.1 lumens sec./pi^2.

Responses were amplified 1000x on Tektronix low-level pre-amplifier type RM 122, using a band pass of 0.8 to 50 cycle/sec. They were amplified and monitored on a Tektronix type 3A 74, model 564, four trace oscilloscope and photographed for later use. Animals were maintained in a head holder, in a shielded cage, under light Pentothal anesthesia. Pupils were maximally dilated.

RESULTS

We have now followed 29 eyes. These eyes were sequentially studied by ERG until extinction of the response. At the time of extinction the eyes were enucleated for eventual histologic studies. Many eyes are still under long term follow up. Thirteen have been studied with copper implantations and fourteen with iron implantations of 1, 3 and 6 particles. Follow-ups range from 1 to 145 days in the more chronic cases, 1 to 3 particles; and from 10 to 168 hours in the more acute cases of six particles implantations. The actual report is based on 150 ERG recording sessions as described in protocol done on 29 eyes. ERG evolution varies from total extinction to still normal responses with 'in between' possibilities of continuing decrease of response.

ERG evolution of two typical cases of acute and chronic copper metallosis will be presented as examples. Rod and cone threshold and peak times responses of an acute intoxication are shown. Evolution ranges from normal response at outset, to extinction over a period of 164 hours. Figure 1, upper part, presents in graph form progressive threshold increase and, lower, pro-

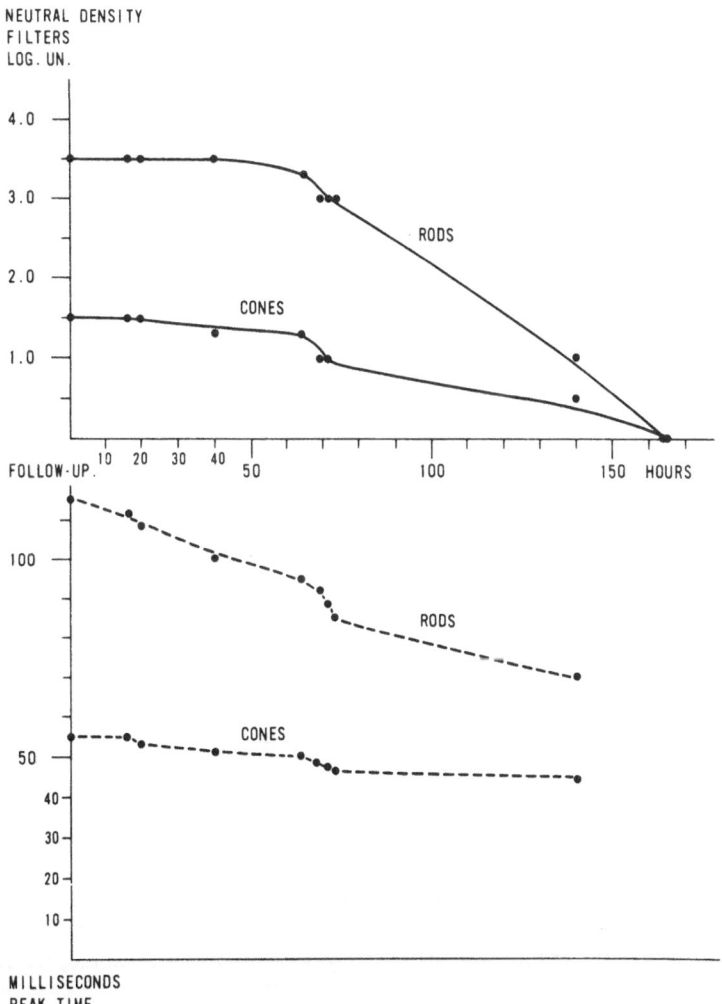

Fig. 1. Upper graphs: Rod and cone threshold measured in log units of neutral density filtering during an acute metallosis produced by the introduction of 6 particles of copper in the eye. Lower graphs: Rod and cone implicit time (peak time) of response in the same case.

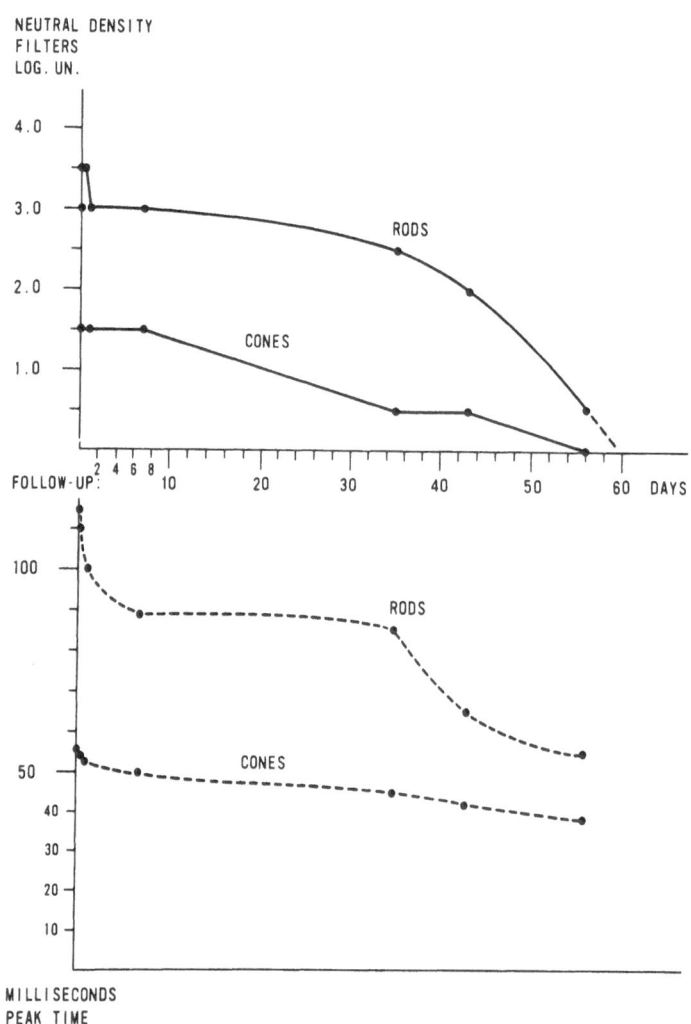

Fig. 2. Upper graphs: Rod and cone threshold measured in log units of neutral density filtering during a chronic metallosis produced by the introduction of one particle of copper in the eye. Lower graphs: Rod and cone implicit time (peak time) of response in the same case.

gressive peak time values over that same period of time. Figure 2 shows the same values in a case of more chronic copper metallosis over a period of 60 days.

Rapidity and severity of ERG evidence of metallosis is generally proportional to the quantity of metal introduced in the eye. All variations observed during the progressive ERG deteriorations in all cases are, without exception, along the same lines. These are, progressive threshold elevations and decrease in peak time values.

Results are still incomplete. The first series were of copper cases. There is less extensive follow-up in the iron implantation series. These results are currently being followed on a chronic basis for completion.

DISCUSSION

Again, we would like to stress the point that no effort is being made to draw conclusions on the clinical evolution or the differences encountered between cases or series. It is our aim to limit our discussion to the time parameter of the ERG response. All time modifications of the responses met in all cases and both series are consistent and of the same pattern.

That the ERG would become rapidly 'extinct' with the experimental introduction of a number of metallic particles in eyes is certainly not surprising or new. The same is evidently applicable to the progressive elevation of threshold.

The clear cut conclusions that stem out from the results in relation with ERG deterioration patterns are threefold. Directly related to the progression of the metallosis the threshold raises or, in other words, sensitivity decreases. This may be due to a decreasing number of firing receptors, or, alternately or simultaneously to a general decrease in sensitivity of all/or affected receptors. The second point is that the peak time value decreases progressively. Responses come earlier as metallosis progresses. That peak time decreases while intensity increased to maintain a constant criterion response could be related to the undergoing pathological process. But it must not be forgotten that peak time of response is directely related to intensity of stimulation, increasing intensity producing earlier responses (Brunette & Lafond). It is our belief that in the present cases, this anticipation of the response is intensity related. Conclusive clinical material in this regard is currently being published (Brunette & Lafond, in press). Finally, the third observation is that there is no rod-cone difference in the pattern of ERG alteration, pointing rather to a diffuse pathological process.

The pathological ERG pattern of these induced metallosis is interesting to compare with the tapeto-retinal degenerative pattern (Brunette, 1973). This delayed response in retinal degenerations is a current observation in our laboratory as well as in the literature. It is currently under study, here, in experimental hereditary retinal degenerations in rats. On the other hand we have clinical material pointing to the fact that simple destruction of parts of the retina produce elevated thresholds without peak time value increase. Rather, peak times values decrease in direct proportion to the elevation of the intensity of stimulation needed to obtain the threshold response. Lesions producing such changes are long standing partial post-traumatic retinal detachments and extensive chorioretinal scars. For these reasons these two types of threshold ERG response have been termed tentatively the 'degenerative pattern' and the 'destructive pattern'. The ERG modifications induced by metallosis being an elevated threshold and decreased peak time values, these suggest that the electrophysiopathological process should be classified in the 'destructive pattern'.

Although the changes caused by the toxic process of metallosis can not be differentiated from the traumatic lesion itself. There is one clear cut conclusion that can be drawn from this material. There are at least two patterns of retinal lesions that can be monitored by ERG. Both have elevated thresholds but differ by the peak time values of the responses. This therefore warrants the importance of evaluating the time parameter in clinical electroretinography.

REFERENCES

Brunette, J.R. A standardizable method for separating rod and cone responses in clinical electroretinography. *Am. J. Ophthal.* 75: *833–45* (1973).

Brunette, J.R. & G. Lafond. Intensity of stimulation and rods and cones evaluation in clinical ERG. Submitted for publication, *Can. J. Ophthal.* 13: *27–31* (1978).

Brunette, J.R. & G. Lafond. The time parameter of the threshold ERG response as intensity rather than dark adaptation related. *Can J. Neurol. Sci.* (in press).

Authors' address:
Département d'Ophtalmologie
Centre Hospitalier Universitaire de Sherbrooke
Sherbrooke, Québec
Canada J1H 5N4

Reprint requests to Dr Brunette at the above address.

THIORIDAZINE (MELLARIL^R) OCULAR TOXICITY

J. COHEN, J. WELLS & R. BORDA

(Houston, Texas, USA)

Thioridazine retinopathy has been well documented in patients receiving in excess of the recommended maximal daily dosage of 800 mg (Siddall, 1968). Clinical signs and symptoms of toxicity include decreased visual acuity, visual field defects and retinal pigment epithelial disturbances. Marked suppression of the ERG and diminished reactivity of the EOG are characteristic of advanced toxicity with this drug. The pathogenesis of this disorder is thought to be selective uptake of thioridazine in pigmented uveal tissue and the retinal pigment epithelium with resultant local toxicity. The present report concerns a schizophrenic patient who developed ocular symptoms of thioridazine toxicity after self-regulating her medication dose. After thioridazine was discontinued, visual acuity returned to normal, but even six months following cessation of the medication the ERG and EOG were still abnormal.

CASE REPORT

The patient is a 50 year-old schizophrenic black female with previously documented vision of 20/20 in each eye, despite many years of Thorazine® therapy and resultant tardive dyskinesia. Due to lack of control of her psychiatric symptoms, her medication was changed to thioridazine at a dosage of 200 mg daily. Two weeks later, the patient reported that she had increased her daily dosage to 800 mg. She was warned of possible ocular complications with thioridazine and was instructed to use only 600 mg daily. A two-month supply of medication was prescribed, but she exhausted this supply (36 grams) in the next 23 days. Five days later she complained of blurred vision. An ophthalmologic consultation was requested.

At that time, her best corrected visual acuity was noted to have decreased to 20/40 in each eye without obvious explanation. No detectable pigment-ary changes were present in either fundus. Visual field testing was attempted but was not reliable. An ERG was obtained and found to be severely suppressed in all parameters (Fig. 1). Thioridazine was discontinued and two weeks later the patient's vision had improved to 20/25 in the right eye and 20/30 in the left eye; the fundi still appeared normal. After another two weeks, however, definite pigment mottling was evident in both fundi, the

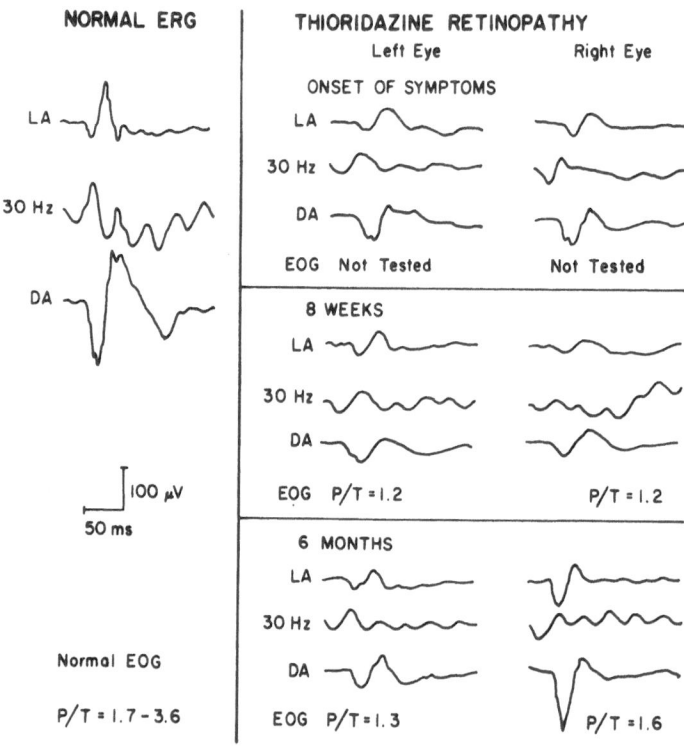

Fig. 1. ERG and EOG findings following onset of ocular toxicity during thioridazine administration. On the left are normal tracings for comparison: LA = light-adapted (room illumination approximately 540 lux), 30 Hz = flicker response to flash train at 30/sec, DA = dark-adapted ten minutes. The patient was tested at the onset of visual symptoms, then at 8 weeks and 6 months following cessation of thioridazine therapy. All recordings were obtained with a Life-Tech Instruments Recorder, Model 7102, Stimulator, Model 7310, with Parabolic Reflector for ERG, Model 7310M, and Signal Averager, Model 7402. Flash intensities for LA, 30 Hz, and DA ERG were approximately 5×10^{-3} lum. secs/cm^2. For the EOG, the patient was adapted to room illumination of 540 lux, dark adapted for 12 minutes, then re-adapted to a background light of 40 lux for 12 minutes.

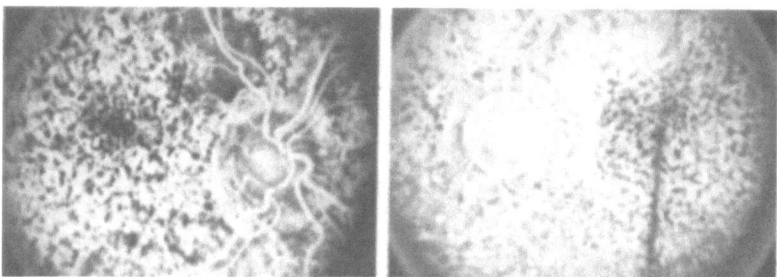

Fig. 2. Fluorescein angiograms obtained four weeks after thioridazine therapy had been discontinued.

abnormalities being particularly noticeable with fluorescein angiography (Fig. 2).

Eight weeks after thioridazine was discontinued the visual acuity had improved to 20/20 in each eye but there was little improvement in the ERG. The EOG also continued to be markedly below normal in the peak/trough ratio (Fig. 1).

Six months following cessation of thioridazine therapy the vision remained normal but electrophysiologic testing revealed persistent ERG and EOG abnormalities. The ERG had increased in amplitude slightly in the right eye, while the ERG in the left eye was still grossly abnormal. The EOG evidenced increased reactivity to dark and light adaptation in the right eye, but the left showed no significant improvement (Fig. 1). At this time pigmentary mottling was more pronounced in the fundi of both eyes, as was seen by ophthalmoscopy and with fluorescein angiography.

DISCUSSION

In 1960, Weekley et al. reported 4 cases of 'pigmentary retinopathy' in patients using thioridazine. They postulated that the toxic effects were due to a high local concentration of the drug in the uvea and that possibly there was a moderate enzyme inhibiting action of the drug.

Later experiments demonstrated that thioridazine has an affinity for melanin granules and tends to accumulate in close association with uveal pigment, especially in the choroid. Increasing drug levels in the choroid may lead to damage of the choriocapillaris which, in turn, results in damage to the pigment epithelium. Drug accumulation in melanin granules of pigment epithelial cells may also contribute to the damage of these pigment epithelial cells. The metabolic products of some phenothiazines have been found to produce alterations in the enzyme systems of the Müller cells and photoreceptors in experimental animals (Meier-Ruge & Cerletti, 1966), and these alterations, added to the drug's direct effect on the choriocapillaris and pigment epithelium, presumably result in abnormal nutrition to the rods and cones and altered retinal function.

ERG and EOG abnormalities appear early in thioridazine toxicity and, thus, these tests are especially helpful in confirming this diagnosis before pigmentation changes are visible. Alterations in photoreceptor nutrition, Müller cell enzymes, and pigment epithelial function all have cumulative effects on the ERG. As the drug level decreases, the ERG slowly recovers. Enough damage may occur, however, to permanently alter the ERG. Davidorf (1973) has reported an abnormal macular ERG six years after cessation of thioridazine treatment, while the full field ERG was normal. Similarly, the EOG usually returns to normal, but with acute toxicity also can be permanently altered.

Thioridazine ocular toxicity is interesting because blurring of vision usually occurs days to weeks before any observable retinal pigment changes. Due to the accumulation of drug in the uvea, fundus changes occur even after the discontinuation of the drug. The early stages of the retinopathy typically are characterized by coarse black pigmentary stippling mostly in the central portion of the fundus. After cessation of the drug therapy, visual acuity generally returns to normal over periods ranging from weeks to months, while the pigmentation either remains unchanged or forms large plaques.

Our present case report illustrates the possible consequences of patients altering their medication dosage when the toxicity level is not much higher than the therapeutic level. At present, it is recommended that a daily dose of 300 mg of thioridazine be exceeded *only* in severe conditions, and doses of greater than 800 mg/day are not recommended.

Clearly, electrophysiological measures of retinal function can be especially valuable in following non-institutionalized patients who are being treated with thioridazine. Since toxic side effects may occur fairly rapidly when dosages exceed 800 mg/day, high-risk patients should probably have ERG and EOG recordings performed once every two or three weeks when feasible.

REFERENCES

Davidorf, F.H. Thioridazine pigmentary retinopahty. *Arch. Ophthalmol.* 90: *255* (1973).

Meier-Ruge, W. & A. Cerletti. Zur experimentellen pathologie der phenothiazin-retinopathie. *Ophthalmologica* 151: *512–533* (1966).

Siddall, J.R. Ocular complications related to phenothiazines. *Dis. Nerv. Syst.* 29 (Suppl. 3): *10–13* (1968).

Weekley, R.D., A.M. Potts, J. Reboton & R.H. May. Pigmentary retinopathy in patients receiving high doses of a new phenothiazine. *Arch. Ophthalmol.* 64: *65–76* (1960).

Authors' address:
Neurophysiology Department
Methodist Hospital
6516 Bertner Blvd.
Houston, Texas 77030
USA

THE ERG OF CHLOROQUINE INDUCED RETINOPATHY: THE PROGNOSTIC SIGNIFICANCE OF ABNORMALITIES ON THE ERG

YASUO KUBOTA, SCHUKUKO KOBOTA & KAORU ASANIGI

(Chiba, Japan)

As is well known, the fundus changes of chloroquine retinopathy often progress to severe degeneration even after discontinuation of the drug. However, in some cases the fundus changes remain stationary.

Fifteen cases of chloroquine retinopathy were followed for a prolonged period in our clinic. Electroretinographic evaluations were made on these cases and the prognostic significance of the abnormalities were studied.

CASE REPORTS

Case 1

A 27 year old woman was admitted to our clinic in February, 1964. She had been taking chloroquine for systemic lupus erythematosis. The period of chloroquine administration was 3 years, and the total dosage was 510 gm.

The visual acuity of both eyes was 0.9. Ophthalmoscopic examination revealed a ring-shaped discoloration at the parafoveal region of the retina. Visual field examination confirmed the presence of a small ring scotoma.

The ERG of the patient revealed the following: the amplitudes of a- and b-wave were normal. The peak time of the b-wave was slightly prolonged. Oscillatory potentials disappeared. (Later, the amplitudes of a- and b-wave were reduced.) (Fig. 1)

The diagnosis of chloroquine retinopathy was made, and the administration of chloroquine was stopped. Although chloroquine was discontinued at an early stage of retinopathy, the degeneration progressed. The ring-shaped discoloration at the macula changed to the so-called Bull's eye conformation. Furthermore, almost all of the posterior region of the retina had degenerated. The visual acuity became gradually impaired (Fig. 2, 3).

Case 2

A 64 year old man had been taking chloroquine for over 7 years for nephritis. The total dose administered was 900 gm. He complained of impaired vision and visited our clinic in November, 1966.

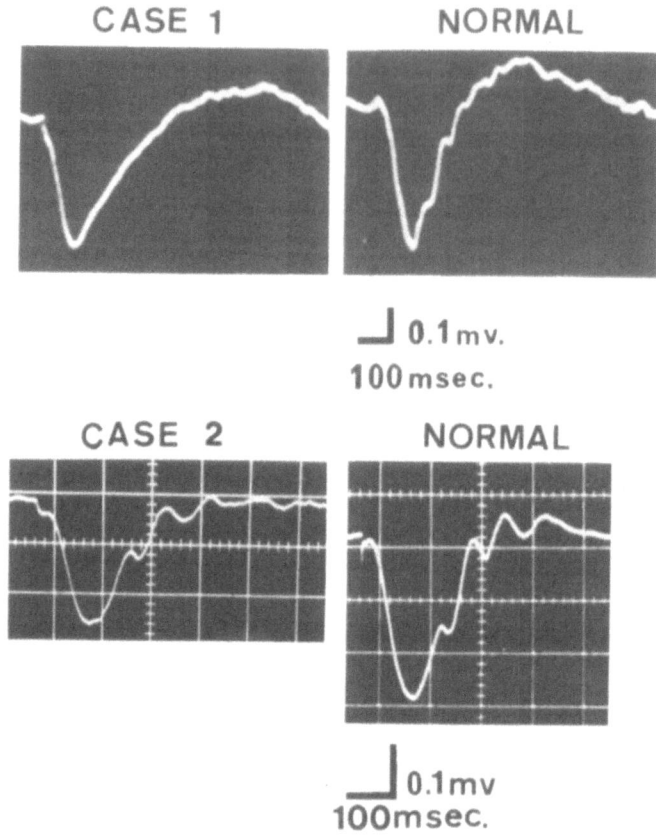

Fig. 1. The ERG of case 1 (upper) and case 2 (lower).

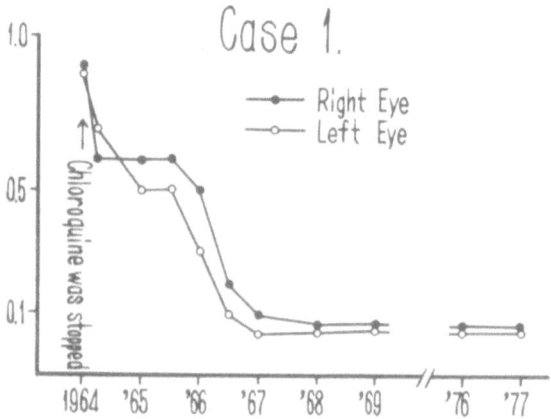

Fig. 2. Visual acuity of case 1 after stopping chloroquine (progressive).

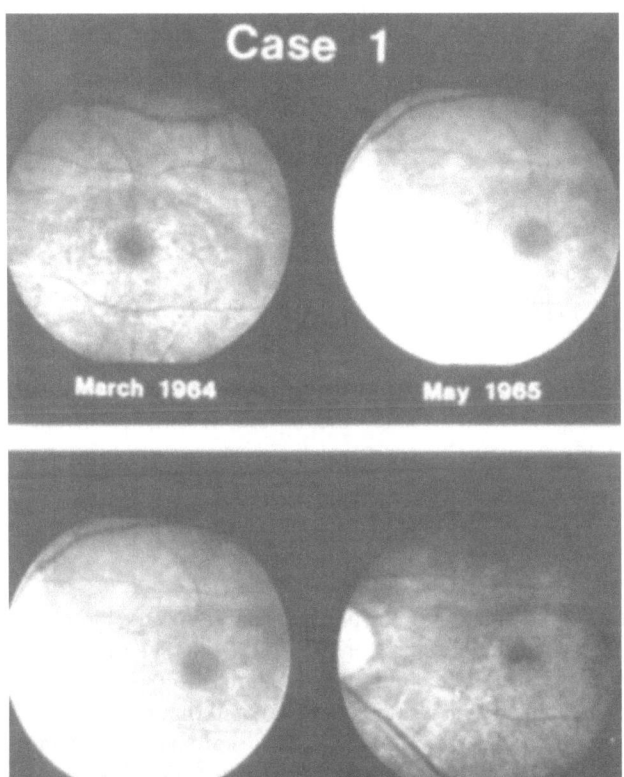

Fig. 3. The fundus changes of case 1. Slight discoloration around the macula changed to so-called Bull's eye. Furthermore, the retinopathy progressed to severe retinal degeneration.

The visual acuity of both eyes was 0.6. The visual field examination showed a small central ring scotoma. On the retina, in the parafoveal region, a ring-shaped discoloration was observed.

The ERG of this case was almost normal. However, the amplitudes of the a- and b-wave were slightly reduced. A diagnosis of chloroquine retinopathy was established, and the chloroquine discontinued.

After stopping the chloroquine, the visual field, visual acuity and the fundus changes remained nearly the same. The size of the ring-shaped discoloration of the retina slightly enlarged; however, the degeneration was still limited to parafoveal region (Fig. 4).

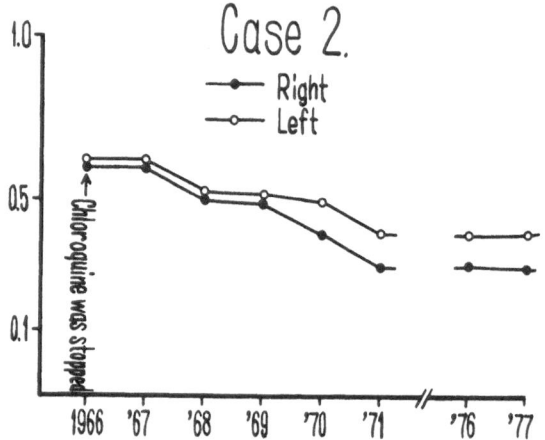

Fig. 4. Visual acuity of case 2 after stopping chloroquine (almost stationary).

Case 3

A 28 year old woman with nephritis, had received chloroquine for 14 months. The total dose administered was 255 gm. She complained of visual impairment when she visited our clinic in March, 1973.

The visual acuity of the right eye was 0.6, and that of the left 0.4. The visual field examination revealed a small ring scotoma. Ophthalmoscopically, the so-called Bull's eye pattern was seen on the retina. Electroretinographic examination showed charateristic abnormalities. The amplitudes of the a- and b-waves were reduced. The peak time of the b-wave was prolonged. The oscillatory potentials were clearly recognized. The ERG of this case resembled that of Case 2.

After stopping the chloroquine, the fundus picture, visual acuity and the visual field remained unchanged.

Case 4

A 9 year old boy received chloroquine for epilepsy. The period of drug administration was 2 years and the total dose administered was estimated to be 400 gm. He complained of dimness of vision when visiting our clinic in December 1967.

At the time of the first visit, the retinal degeneration was already far advanced. Although the visual acuity of his right eye was 0.5, and that of the left 0.3, the visual fields were extremely constricted.

The ERG was non-recordable. Ophthalmoscopic examination revealed widespread retinal degeneration involving almost the entire retina. Only the localized foveal region remained unimpaired.

After discontinuation of chloroquine, the degeneration progressed further. The central macular region was also impaired. The constricted visual field vanished, and the visual acuity took a turn for the worse.

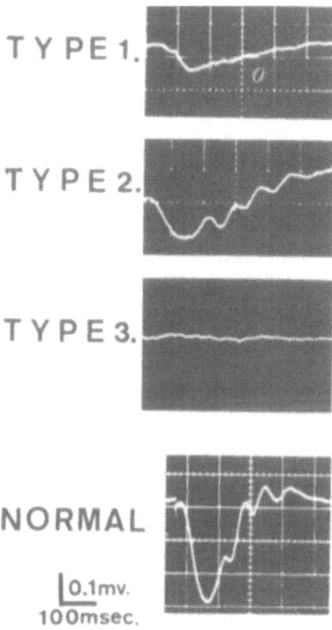

Fig. 5. The ERGs of chloroquine retinopathy were classified into three types.

Four representative cases of chloroquine retinopathy were described above. The ERGs are classified into the following three types (Fig. 5):

1.The amplitudes of the a- and b-waves were reduced. The peak time of the b-wave was extended. Oscillatory potentials disappeared. The abnormalities were seen in 8 cases.

2. The a-wave was normal or slightly decreased. The amplitude of b-wave was reduced. Oscillatory potentials were clearly recognized. These abnormalities were observed in 4 cases.

3. Extinguished ERG (non-recordable). These were seen in 3 far advanced cases.

DISCUSSION

Long-term follow up examinations were done on cases of chloroquine retinopathy and electroretinographic evaluations were made. Many studies have been made on the ERG of this disease (Okun et al., 1963; Henkind et al., 1964; Carr et al., 1966; Krill et al., 1971). However, these were concerned mainly with the diagnostic significance of the ERG abnormalities.

In our clinic, not only cases at an early stage, but also those of intermediate stages were examined. Generally, intermediate stages progressed to severe retinal degeneration after discontinuation of chloroquine. Some cases in early stages, however, progressed to widespread degeneration after stopping the chloroquine. The relationship between the ERG abnormalities and degenerative progression was studied.

The prognosis of cases with a 'Type 2' ERG were generally good, and the retinopathy was stationary. The degeneration of cases with 'Type 1' ERG, but poor in others. This may be related to the fact that, in the cases where there is relatively extensive intoxication of the retinal epithelium, there already exists a severe degeneration, even if only slight changes are ophthalmoscopically found; and the prognosis in such cases is poor.

Extinguished ERG (Type 3) was seen in the far advanced cases. Understandably, the prognosis was poor in these cases.

SUMMARY

Electroretinographic evaluations were made on cases of chloroquine retinopathy. The prognostic significance of the ERG abnormalities was discussed. It is concluded that from the ERG abnormalities the prognosis of these cases could be estimated.

REFERENCES

Carr, R., P. Gouras & R. Gunkel. *Arch. Ophthal.* 75: *171* (1966).
Henkind, P., R. Carr & I. Siegel. *Arch. Ophthal.* 71: *157* (1964).
Krill, A.E., A.M. Potts & C.E. Johanson. *Am. J. Ophthal.* 75: *531* (1971).
Okun, E., P. Gouras, H. Bernstein & von Sallmann. *Arch. Ophthal.* 69: *59* (1963).

Authors' address:
Department of Ophthalmology
Chiba University
Chiba-shi
Japan

FOLLOW-UP IN A CASE OF RETINOPATHY MORE THAN 10 YEARS AFTER STOPPING CHLOROQUINE THERAPY

E. SCHMÖGER, W. MÜLLER & E. HAASE

(Erfurt, German Dem. Republic)

After becoming aware of the irreversible damage to the retina from chloroquine therapy ophthalmologists have been concerned for many years how to determine a safe dose and duration of therapy for this drug. We have found it difficult to determine a borderline of safety in the individual case. Cessation of therapy is not certain to prevent progression of the retinal damage which depends not only on the dosage but also on the melanine content of the choroid and retina which is unknown in the individual case. These problems have been discussed by Zvaifler, Bernstein and Rubin, Potts, François, Meier-Ruge, and others. The subject was also discussed at length at the Amsterdam Congress of the European Society for Ophthalmology in 1968. Since the Amsterdam Congress there have been fewer reports of chloroquine retinopathy. This is probably due to the awareness of physicians of the danger of this treatment. There are few follow-up reports after stopping treatment. We were able to find no reports of a more than 4 years' follow-up (for instance, Carr and co-workers, or mentioned by Bruckner). For this reason we thought that it would be valuable to publish the course of the most severe case seen in our clinic.

The patient, Mrs. Magdalena Z., was 55 years old when she came into our clinic for the first time, and the diagnosis of chloroquine retinopathy was made. In the course of more than 5 years before she had received altogether about 550 g chloroquine. This therapy had been stopped for about 4 months when we first saw her. She still had a good visual acuity but severe defects in the visual fields. Her colour sense was rather defective, examined with Farnsworth 100 hue test and she had subnormal ERG and a nearly flat EOG and the beginning of a so-called bull's eye macula. This was in 1965. We saw her again in 1967, 1968 and 1977. Up to 1968 the visual field became somewhat worse but this did not concern so much the subjective vision, specially not the visual acuity. ERG, EOG and fundus oculi did not change very much.

A noticeable diminution of function followed later than 3 years after cessation of drug therapy. Today the visual field defect has reached the fixation point for usual testmarks, therefore, the visual acuity is reduced, the same as the colour sense with very large errors in Farnsworth tests, now similar to a tritanopia. In the fundus there is a pale degenerative zone around the dark red fovea, a typical bull's eye.

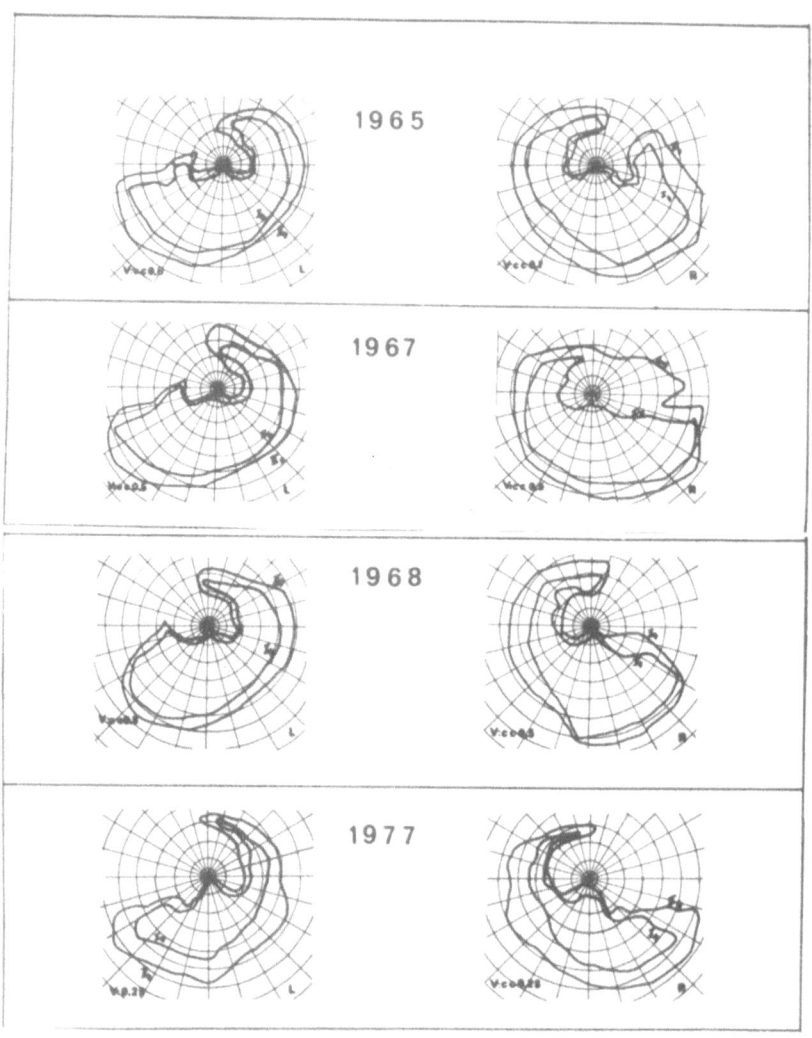

Fig. 1. Visual fields in chloroquine retinopathy, Pat. M.Z., 550 g Chloroquine 1959–1965. Testmarks I_4 and II_4 (Goldmann-Perimeter). Visiual acuity 1965: R = 0,7; L = 0,8; 1977: R = L 0.25

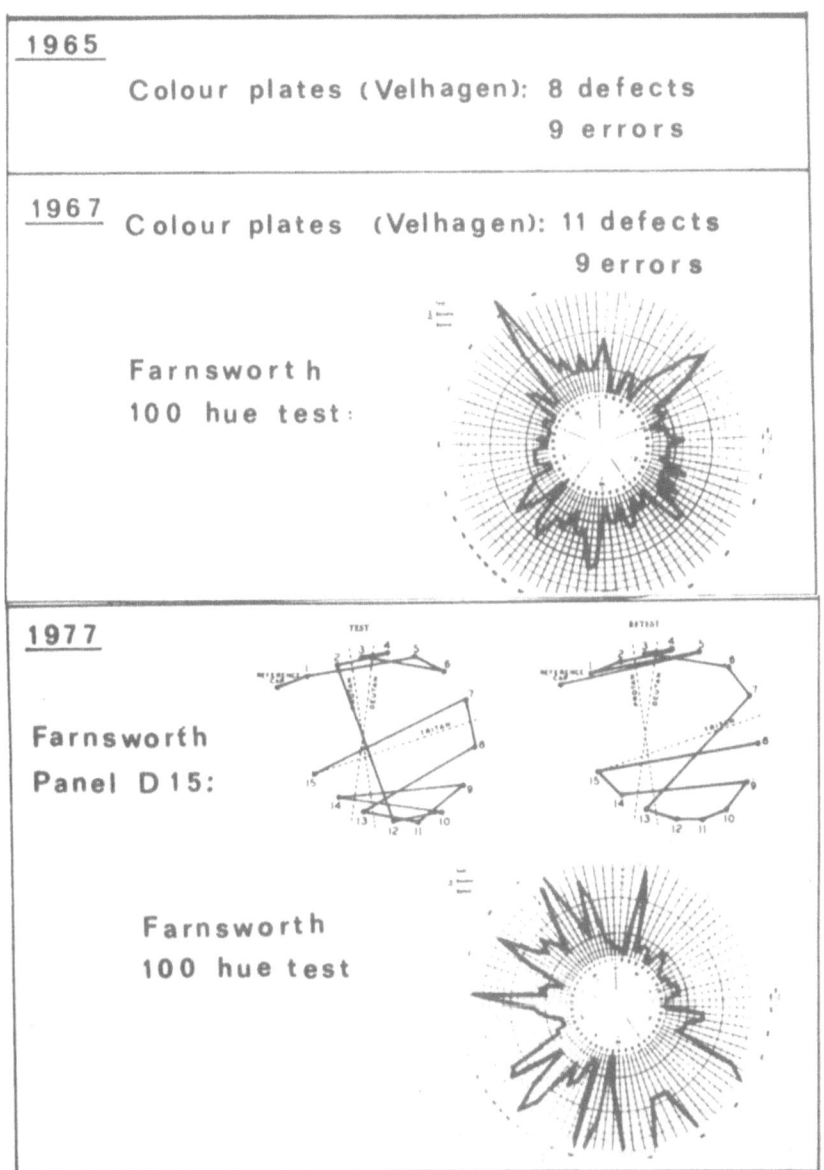

1965

Colour plates (Velhagen): 8 defects
9 errors

1967 Colour plates (Velhagen): 11 defects
9 errors

Farnsworth
100 hue test:

1977

Farnsworth
Panel D 15:

Farnsworth
100 hue test

Fig. 2. Same patient, colour defects.

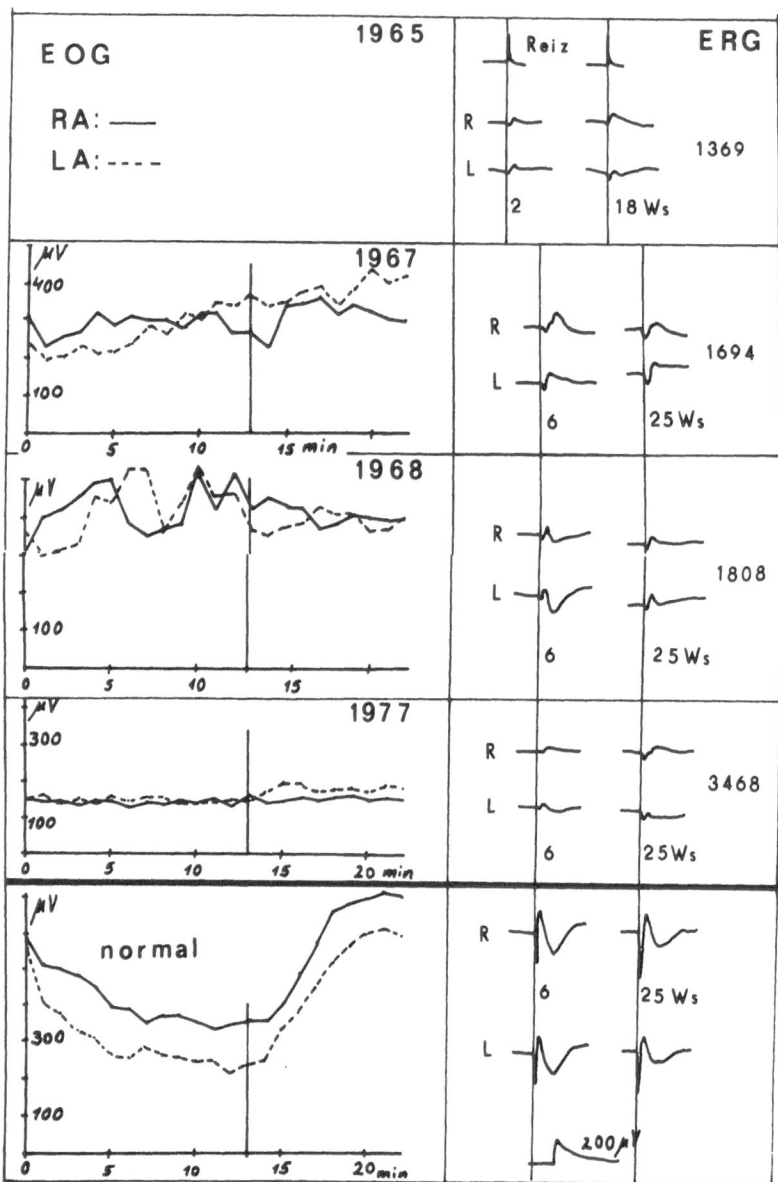

Fig. 3. Same patient, ERG and EOG. In 1965 EOG was not registered and the ERG has a stimulus different from that in later years.

Concerning the ERG, we noticed a scotopic ERG with severely subnormal amplitude, almost no photopic ERG is to be registered, it has a very low amplitude, a_2 seems to be absent, but the time relations are nearly normal. The EOG is now an absolutely flat curve with rather low voltage (Fig. 1-3).

We have also registered the subjective dark adaptation curve; it is reduced, but does not differ much over the years. We also did quantitative perimetry, which showed large defects.

SUMMARY

The reduced function and electrodiagnostic symptoms in a patient of 55 years at the time of stopping chloroquine therapy seemed to cease in severe further detoriation for several years, but later continued in reducing central vision. ERG and EOG became severely reduced in comparision to the status during the first years after cessation of drug therapy.

REFERENCES

Brückner, R. Frühdiagnose medikamentöser Schäden von Netzhaut und Sehnerv. 3. Kongr. europ. Ges. Ophthal., Amsterdam 1968. *Ophthalmologica* 158: *245–272* (1969).

Carr, R.E., P. Henkind, N. Rothfield & I.M. Siegel. Ocular toxicity of antimalarial drugs: long-term follow-up. *Am. J. Ophthal.* 66: *738–744* (1968).

François, J. & M.C. Maudgal. Experimental chloroquine retinopathy. *Ophthalmologica* 148: *442–452* (1964).

Meier-Ruge, W. Die Morphologie der experimentellen Chlorochinretinopathie des Kaninchens. *Ophthalmologica* 150: *127* (1965).

Meier-Ruge, W. Drug induced retinopathy. 3rd Congr. europ. Soc. Ophthal., Amsterdam 1968. *Ophthalmologica* Addit. ad Vol. 158; *561–573* (1969).

Potts (1964): cited by Meier-Ruge.

Zvaifler, Bernstein & Rubin (1962): cited by Meier-Ruge.

Authors' address:
Augenklinik der Medizinischen Akademie
Nordhäuser Str. 74
50 Erfurt
German Dem. Republic

TOXIC RETINOPATHY IN MALARIA TROPICA

BARBARA SCHMIDT

(Berlin, Federal Rep. Germany)

The retina is known to be vulnerable to many toxic agents. For many years antimalarial drugs have been known to exert an apparently selective toxic effect on the eye. The doses used in malaria have relatively few secondary effects.

The ocular manifestations are of two kinds: deposits of chloroquine crystals in the epithelial cell of the cornea and possibly in Bowman's membrane (Pau & Bäumer, 1959) or retinal alterations. If the treatment is discontinued the corneal formations disappear within a few weeks but the fundus degenerations do not. Certain drugs induce morphological alterations in the eye which are histologically and electron-microscopically identical with those found in hereditary lipidoses (Seiler, Thiel & Wassermann, 1977).

Chloroquine seems to have an affinity for melanin (Meier-Ruge, 1967). Accumulation of the toxic substance results in a functional destruction of the pigment epithelium, a destruction which effects the retina secondarily. The experiments of Meier-Ruge have revealed an accumulation of lipids and mucopolysaccharides in the pigment epithelium. For many years we have known that there is a correlation between the duration of treatment and the total dose of the drug administered. I just remember the slide shown at the first session of this society in 1961 (Schmidt, 1962). In patients without eye disturbances it could be demonstrated that there is a decrease of the electric responses, due to doses and time of uptake. It seems probable that advanced age in the patient also favours retinal intoxication.

CASE REPORT:

M., Margaret, a 49 year old white female, is living in Ghana, West-Africa. There is no family history of eye disease. She has never been seriously ill, but living in a region of high incidence of malaria tropica, she needed anti-malaria drugs for prevention, but also for acute attacks. She received about 260 g as preventive medicine, and roughly 180 g for intensive care during attacks, i.e. over 10 years a total dosis of 440 g chloroquine diphosphate had been administered. At times she got camoquine, the total dose is roughly 200 tablets.

She complained of difficulties in night vision, constricted visual fields, and visual deterioration, also of flickering sensations and light sensitivity. The follow-up has been done in several hospitals throughout the years. I will report on my own examinations and those by one eye specialist.

The visual acuity was normal in 1969, and is now reduced to 0.7 in both eyes. The field has become more and more narrow. It started with losses temporally and is now constricted to about $30°$ only.

Dark adaptation thresholds were elevated in 1969, there is now a loss of about 2.5 log units. The electrophysiological findings revealed only small potentials, up to 35 μV in 1969, now the ERG is extinguished. Also, the EOG showed no light peak , and a just slightly visible dark trough: Arden ratio about 100.

In the cornea there had been chloroquine deposits in 1969, now there are none.

The fundus had no well-defined discs, they were slightly prominent, the arteries narrow. In the retinal tissue there seem to be small dots, like capillary ectasias. Now there is heavy pigmentation, the vessels are extremely narrow. So there is the picture of a classical retinopathia pigmentosa.

Discussion

Until now toxic retinopathy due to antimalaria drugs has been reported only in cases of collagen diseases and sarcoidoses. The small doses used in malaria prevention and treatment have relatively few secondary effects.

In collagenoses the daily dose of chloroquine is usually 250 to 500 mg, whereas in prevention of malaria 250 mg are taken once or twice weekly. It is most noticeable that in almost all severe cases of retinopathy the patients have been given the drug in large doses and without interruption for several years. The drug is incorporated for a long time, even after many years there still is some urinary excretion.

There seems to be a correlation between the duration of treatment and the total dose of the drug administered (Babel & Meyer, 1965). It also seems probable that advanced age of the patient favours retinal intoxication. But, apparently, quite a number of questions remain open. Our patient, otherwise of good health, took 440 g chloroquine and camoquine as malaria therapy. She seems to be pre-aged. According to Babel & Meyer, advanced age of the patient favours retinal intoxication.

Chloroquine is excreted from the body very slowly. Urinary excretion never exceeds 10% to 20% of the dose administered (Thorp, 1961, in Franceschetti, Francois & Babel, 1974) and following cessation of the treatment, chloroquine or one of its metabolites may still be found in the urine for months and even 5 years later (Bernstein et al., 1964). Living in a hot and dry tropical region, our patient may have had not enough urinary excretion. How far chloroquine may be excreted by skin perspiration is not known. Chloroquine deposits can also be found in the skin tissue.

Furthermore, our patient belongs to the dark pigmented type. The work of Bernstein et al. has acquainted us with the affinity of chloroquine for melanin. Accumulation of the toxic substance results in a functional destruction of the pigment epithelium, pigmented subjects seem to be more prone to chloroquine retinopathy.

This may altogether have caused a toxic retinopathy. This seems to be the first case suffering from toxic retinopathy by antimalaria drugs taken against malaria.

REFERENCES

Babel, J. & E. Meyer. Fréquence et prevention des lésions rétiniennes dues à la chloroquine. *Schweiz. Med. Wschr.* 95: *1125–1130* (1965).

Bernstein, H. N. & J. Ginsberg. The pathology of chloroquine retinopathy. *Arch. Ophth.* 71: *238–245* (1964).

Franceschetti, A., J. François & J. Babel. Chorioretinal heredo-degenerations. Charles C. Thomas, Publisher, Springfield, Ill. (1974).

Meier-Ruge. W. Experimental investigation of the morphology of chloroquine retinopathy. *Arch. Ophthal.* 73: *540–544* (1965).

Meier-Ruge, W. Medikamentöse Retinopathie. Thieme, Stuttgart (1967).

Nylander, U. Ocular damage in chloroquine therapy. *Acta Ophthal. (Kbh).* 92: *5–71* (1967).

Pau, H. & A. Bäumer. Resochineinlagerung in der Kornea. *Klin. Mbl. Augenheilk.* 135: *363–377* (1959).

Schmidt, B. & W. Müller-Limmroth. Electroretinographic examinations following the application of chloroquine. *Acta Ophthal. (Kbh).* suppl. 70: *245–251* (1962).

Seiler, K.U., H. J. Thiel & O. Wassermann. Die Chloroquinkeratopathie als Beispiel einer arzneimittelinduzierten Phosphalipidosis. *Klin. Mbl. Augenheilk.* 170: *64–73* (1977).

Author's address:
Klinikum Steglitz
Augenklinik
I Berlin 45
Fed. Rep. of Germany.

Docum. Ophthal. Proc. Series, Vol. 15

TOXIC RETINOPATHY INDUCED BY SODIUM IODATE IN RABBITS: CORRELATION BETWEEN ELECTRORETINOGRAPHY, VITAMIN A LEVELS IN BLOOD, ELECTRONMICROSCOPIC HISTOLOGY AND COLOUR FLUORESCEIN ANGIOGRAPHY

PIERRE SOLE, RINALDO ALFIERI, FRANCK BACIN
PIERRE TRONCHE & BERNADETTE KANTELIP
(Clermont-Ferrand, France)

ABSTRACT

Experimentally induced retinoses are useful in that they give the possibility of stu-dying the pathogenesis of human tapeto-retinal degeneration. Intravenous injections of sodium iodate at 20 mg/kg were chosen to intoxicate rabbits of the "Fauve de Bourgogne" variety. At varying times after the injections, the following were carried out:

1. An electroretinography study: this shows the early disappearance of the e-waves, followed by a change in the b_2-wave.
2. A biochemical study: this shows a drop of the vitamin A level in the blood, which happens long after the electroretinographic changes.
3. An electronmicroscopic study: this shows early changes in Bruch's membrane and the pigment epithelium.
4. A colour fluorescein angiographic study: this shows an abnormal distribution of the fluorescein which probably indicates perturbations in the permeability of the pigment epithelium.

The strange chronology (precocious electrical extinction, delayed drop in vitamir level) may be explained by a unitary hypothesis based on the correlations existing be tween these different types of test: sodium iodate reacts first on the enzyme systern which affects vitamin A isomerisation.

INTRODUCTION

Experimental retinoses induced in animals enable a better understanding of tapeto-retinal degeneration in man. Franceschetti, François & Babel (1963) published an overall study. We have personally studied the correlation be-tween the adapto-electroretinogram and the variations in circulating vitamin A levels in rabbits injected with sodium iodate (Alfieri & Solé, 1965; Al-fieri, Solé & Tronche, 1966). Since then, ultrastructural observations, com-bined with electrophysiology, have been made, more especially by Kobaya-shi (1970) and by Imaizumi et al. (1973). Lastly, Shimotori (1971) studied the retinal lesions using fluorescein angiography. Here we have tried to es-tablish a more general correlation by observing concomitantly the electro-physiological, biochemical, ultrastructural and angiographic changes.

PROCEDURE

Retinoses were induced in 20 rabbits of the "Fauve de Bourgogne" variety, by means of one intravenous injection of sodium iodate of 20 mg/kg. The anaesthetic was administered intraperitoneally (Imalgène 500 : 0.5 ml/kg + Vetranquil : 0.1 ml/kg).

Electroretinography

The electroretinograms were obtained by white stimulation; the active corneal electrode is a Worst type suction electrode and the indifferent electrode is a needle stuck in the skin in the middle of the forehead. The recording is made by means of a transient averager (ART 1000 SAIP). The rabbits eye is first adapted to mesopic conditions. After four minutes dazzling at 3,000 lux, an adapto-electroretinogram is recorded every 2 minutes for 30 minutes.

This recording was made at times varying between a few minutes after the injection for early effects and 40 days after for the last recordings.

Biochemistry

Vitamin A dosages were carried out on blood samples taken by intracardial puncture using the colorimetric reaction to antimony trichloride of Carr and Price, adapted to the French Pharmacopeia and the directions of Embree et al. (1957). We would like to point out that under these conditions the vitamin A isomers are measured globally whereas β-carotene does not react.

The blood samples were taken after consideration of the variations in the electroretinogram.

Electron microscopy

The eyes were enucleated 48 hours, 60 hours and 12 days after sodium iodate injection. The retinas were fixed in 1% buffered glutaraldehyde and postfixed in 1% buffered osmic acid. Following dehydration and embedding in TAAB resin, ultrathin sections were prepared, stained with uranyl acetate and lead citrate, and examined in an electron microscope (Philips EM 300).

Fundus photography and fluorescein angiography

We used the technique developed by Shikano & Shimizu (1968) and by Matsui et al. (1969), and which we described at Bad Nauheim (Alfieri, Sole & Rigal, 1974). A half cm^3 of 20% fluorescein was injected in the ear vein; colour photographs were taken everey second after the injection, using a fundus camera (KOWA) covering a field of 45°. The interferential exciter filter used was a Spectrotech Z6 and the interferential barrier filter was a Spectrotech Z7.

RESULTS

Electroretinography

1. *Static electroretinogram.* The most frequently observed phenomenon is that of a decrease in amplitude and even disappearance of the e-waves. This change comes about as from the 17th hour and reaches a peak between the

112

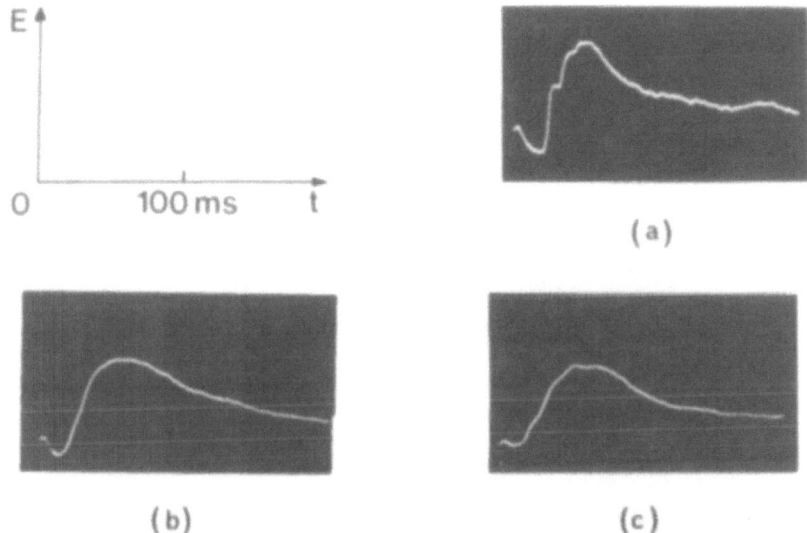

Fig. 1. Static electroretinogram in the rabbit. E: potential; t: time.
(a) Before sodium iodate injection, the e-waves are clearly visible.
(b) 41 hours after injection, the e-waves have disappeared.
(c) 60 hours after injection, the e-waves begin to reappear.

41st and 48th hour (Fig. 1, b). After the 60th hour following the injection of sodium iodate, the e-waves begin to reappear (Fig. 1,c).

2. *Dynamic electroretinogram.* The scotopic b_2-wave decreased slightly between the 2nd and 17th hour following the injection and became practically extinct between the 84th and 96th hours. As from the 12th day a complete recovery of the wave is noted. We must point out that in our earlier work (1965) we observed a change in the b_2-wave over 5 months after the injection.

Biochemistry

The same results were noted as in our earlier works. The level of circulating vitamin A remains constant during the first few days after injection but drops as from the 12th day, from about 2.0 U.I. to 1.5 U.I. per cm^3 of blood.

Electron microscopy

As from the 48th hour signs of damage appear :
a) the pigment epithelium cells present a pycnotic nucleus (Fig. 2 : 1), a vacuolar cytoplasm (Fig. 2 : 2) with few organites and a plasmic membrane which has in general lost its basal and apical invaginations;

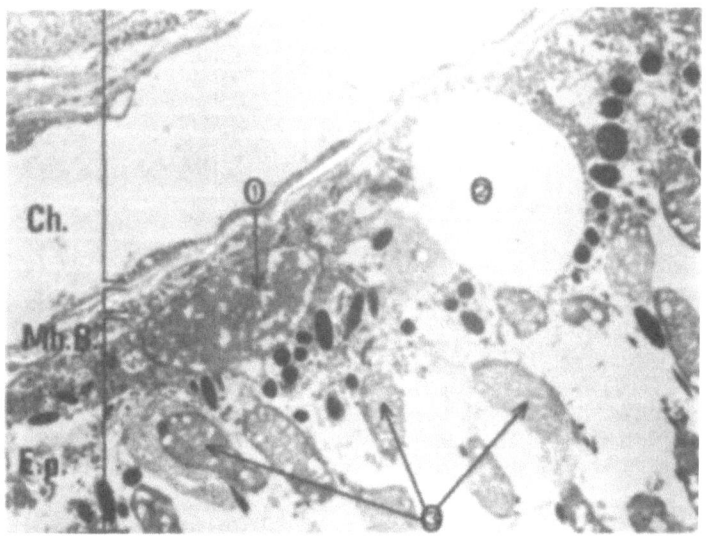

Fig. 2. (x3,200). Electron micrograph of the rabbit choroid and retina, 48 hours after sodium iodate injection. Ch.: choriocapillaris; Mb. B.: Bruch's membrane; E. p.: pigment epithelium. 1: pycnotic nucleus; 2: vacuolar cytoplasm; 3: the regular structure of the photoreceptor discs has disappeared.

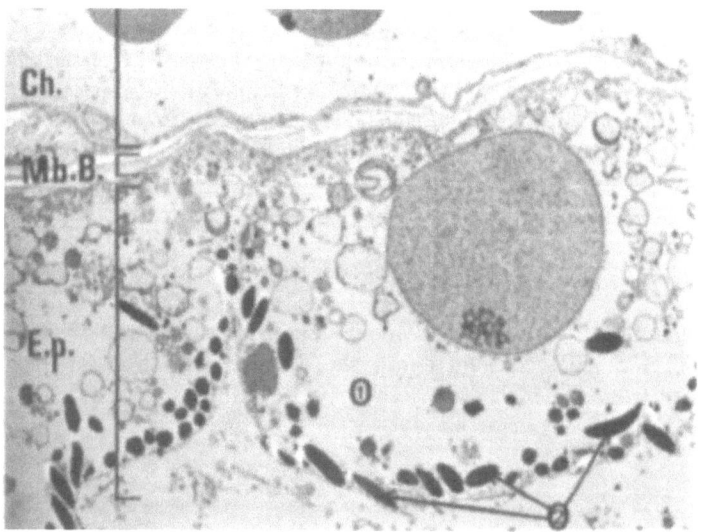

Fig. 3. (x3,200). Electron micrograph of the rabbit choroid and retina, 60 hours after sodium injection. Ch.: choriocapillaris; Mb. B.: Bruch's membrane; E. p.: pigment epithelium. 1: oedema of the cytoplasm; 2: the pigment grains are pushed out to the cellular periphery.

b) the regular structure of the discs in the outer segments of the photo-receptors has become disorganised (Fig. 2 : 3).

At the 60th hour the signs of damage seem to reach a maximum : there is considerable oedema of the cytoplasm in the cells of the pigment epithelium (Fig. 3 : 1), unrecognisable organites and all the pigment grains have been pushed out to the cellular periphery (Fig. 3 : 2).

On the twelfth day, the signs of damage begin to disappear:

a) Bruch's membrane is broken (Fig. 4: 1) which probably explains the presence of cells 'rather difficult to identify' which were observed by Babel et al. (1977) under the basal membrane of the pigment epithelium cells (Fig. 4: 2);

b) the cells of the pigment epithelium present easily identifiable organites: mainly mitochondria (Fig. 4: 3) and endoplasmic reticulum (Fig. 4: 4); the presence should be noted of a large lamellar body (Fig. 4: 5) inside an epithelial cell.

For all samples, no matter at what time they were taken, the capillaries of the choriocapillaris are dilated, Bruch's membrane is abnormal and the cells of the pigment epithelium have become thinner.

Colour fundus photography and colour fluorescein angiography

Colour fundus photography. Compared to a normal fundus (Fig. 5, a), the following may be observed on the 30th day following the injection of sodium iodate:

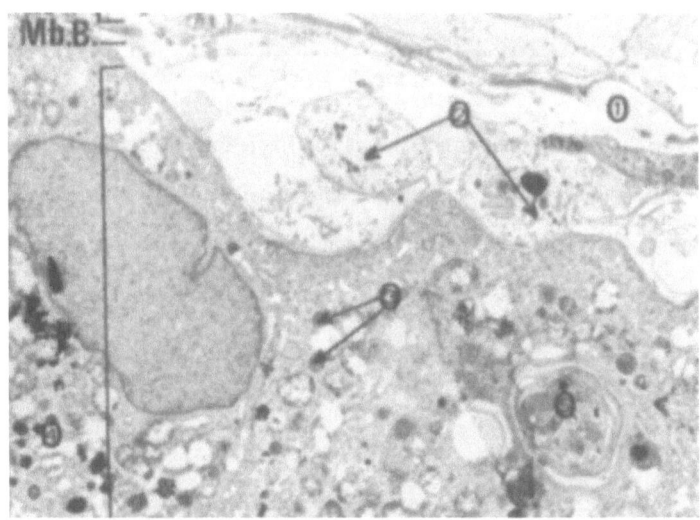

Fig. 4. (x5,600). Electron micrograph of the rabbit choroid and retina, 12 days after sodium iodate injection. Ch.: choriocapillaris; Mb.B.: Bruch's membrane; E. p.: pigment epithelium. 1: Bruch's membrane is broken; 2: cells 'rather difficult to identify' (Babel et al., 1977); 3: mitochondria; 4: endoplasmic reticulum; 5: lamellar bodies.

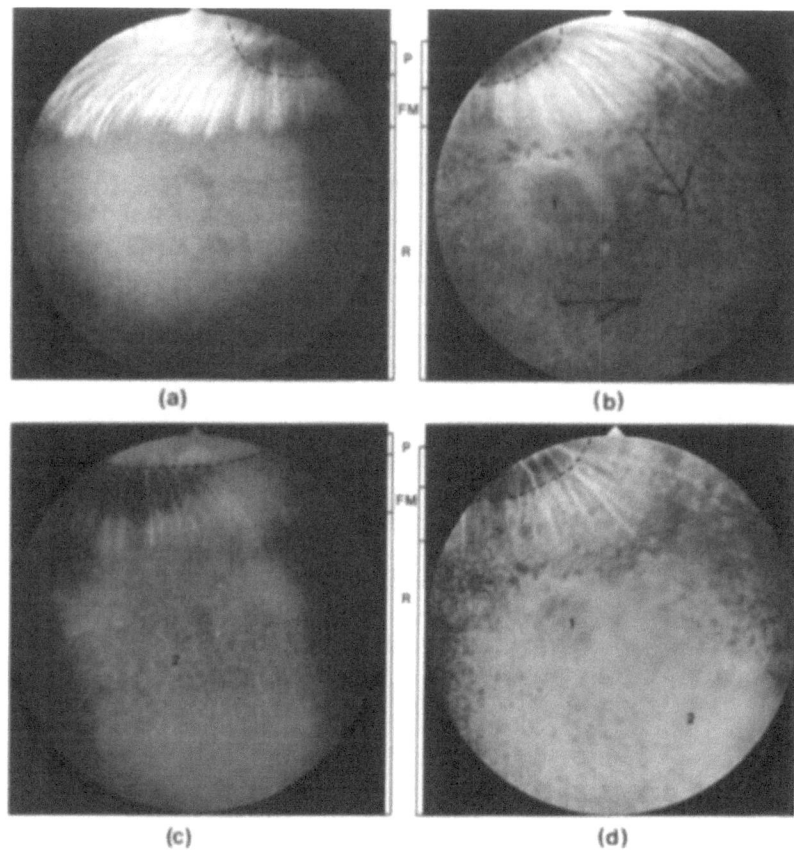

Fig. 5. Colour fundus photograph and colour fluorescein angiograph in the rabbit.
(a) Normal fundus photograph.
(b) Fundus photograph 30 days after sodium iodate injection. 1: rounded lesion;
2: pigment clumping; 3: choroidian vessels.
(c) Normal fluorescein angiograph (20 seconds after fluorescein injection). 1: retinal vessels; 2: 'choroidian mottling'.
(d) Fluorescein angiograph 30 days after sodium iodate injection (20 secondes after fluorescein injection). 1: probable serous detachment; 2: hyperfluorescence.
P: Papilla; F.M.: medullated fibers; R: retina.

a) a rounded lesion (Fig. 5, b, 1), the nature of which will be explained by angiography;

b) widespread hyperpigmentation (Fig. 5, b, 2) with pigment clumping;

c) some choroidal vessels (Fig. 5, b, 3) which appear between the pigmented areas.

Colour fluorescein angiography. The normal photograph, taken after 20 seconds, shows a retinal vascularisation very different to that in man: the retinal vessels remain localised in the medullated fibers area (Fig. 5, c, 1); the rest of the picture however reminds one of the 'choroidal mottling' normally found in man (Fig. 5, c, 2).

On the 30th day following the injection of sodium iodate, the following may be observed:

a) the rounded lesion already seen on the fundus photograph: it shows up as an abnormal distribution of fluorescein (Fig. 5, d, 1) and probably corresponds to a serous detachment of one of the retinal layers; this is in agreement with the electronmicroscopic picture (in the upper part of Figure 4);

b) hyperfluorescence of the remainder of the retina (Fig. 5, d, 2); this disappearance of the 'choroidal mottling' may, in our opinion, result from a dilation of the capillaries of the choriocapillaris and/or from a permeabilisation of the pigment epithelium.

CONCLUSIONS

This work should be considered as only partial since further study, especially in histo-enzymology, should be carried out. However the following points are worth noting:

1. The existence of pluritissular lesions. Even though most of the early stage lesions are found in the pigment epithelium, we observed vascular changes in the choriocapillaris such as vasodilation, exudation and even a serous detachment of the pigment epithelium.

2. The electrophysiological, biochemical and histological results may be separated into several stages:

a) an initial, acute, local attack (first 12 days) which is shown from an electrophysiological point of view by an overall modification of the electroretinogram (photopic: e-waves, and scotopic: b_2-wave), from a biochemical point of view by a constant level of circulating vitamin A which remains normal and from a histological point of view by considerable damage to all the retinal cells;

b) then local repair sets in from the 12th day as can be seen from normal electroretinographic recordings and from the sections where subnormal epithelial cells reappear; the level of circulating vitamin A begins to drop, however;

c) finally, secondary effects are noted, doubtless due to extra-ocular enzymatic changes, probably hepatic (Kalt, 1937), which lower the level of circulating vitamin A by blocking the isomerases systems and alter the b_2-wave in ERG, which shows qualitative or quantitative rhodopsine changes (Grignolo et al., 1970).

ACKNOWLEDGEMENTS

We would like to express our thanks to Misses Force, Laurent, Lenient, Maugein, Oron, Viader and Warren and Messrs. Bastide, Bourges, Danne, Heydel and Tronche for their suggestions and/or technical assistance.

REFERENCES

Alfieri, R. & P. Solé. L'adapto-électrorétinogramme du Lapin au cours des rétinoses expérimentales provoquées par l'iodate de sodium. *C.R. Soc. Biol.* 159: *1511–1516* (1965).

Alfieri, R., P. Solé & D. Rigal. Coupled electrophysiological and colour fluorographic studies as a part of the anatomical diagnosis of retinopathies. In: Docum. Ophthal. Proc. Series, Vol. 4, 11th ISCERG Symp., Bad Nauheim 19–22 Sept. 1973, pp. 409–418. Junk, The Hague (1974).

Alfieri, R., P. Solé & P. Tronche. Rétinose expérimentale induite chez le Lapin par l'iodate de sodium: parallèle entre les modifications électrorétinographiques et les variations du taux sanguin de vitamine A. *C.R. Soc. Biol.* 160: *993–994* (1966).

Babel, J., N. Stangos, S. Korol & M. Spiritus. Ocular electrophysiology, pp. 142–147. Georg Thieme, Stuttgart (1977).

Embree, N.D., S.R. Ames, R.W. Lehman & P.L. Harris. Determination of Vitamin A. In: Glick, D. (ed.). Methods of biochemical analysis, Vol. 4, pp. 78–81. Interscience, New York (1957).

Franceschetti, A., J. François & J. Babel. Les hérédodégénérescences chorio-rétiniennes, Vol. 2, pp. 1578–1623. Masson, Paris (1963).

Grignolo, A., N. Orzalesi & G.A. Calabria. Studies on the fine structure and the rhodopsin cycle of the rabbit retina in experimental degeneration induced by sodium iodate. *Exp. Eye Res.* 5: *86–97* (1966).

Imaizumi, K., Y. Tazawa & H. Kobayashi. Electrophysiological and histopathological studies on the rabbit retina treated with sodium and sodium l-glutamate. In: Docum. Ophthal. Proc. Series, Vol. 2, 10th ISCERG Symp., Los Angeles 20–23 Aug. 1972, pp. 105–118. Junk, The Hague (1973).

Kalt, E. De l'action nocive sur l'épithélium pigmentaire de la rétine des solutions de certains composés iodiques injectés par voie parentérale. *Bull. Soc. Ophtal. Paris* 49: *304–308* (1937).

Kubayashi, H. Electron microscopic observation on the rabbit retina treated with long term daily administration of small dose of sodium iodate or sodium l-glutamate. *Acta Soc. Ophthal. Jap.* 74: *902–908* (1970).

Matsui, K., Y. Oka & T. Matsui. Fluorescein fundus angiography in color. *Acta Soc. Ophthal. Jap.* 73: *653–658* (1969).

Shikano, S. & K. Shimizu. Atlas of fluorescence fundus angiography. Saunders, Philadelphia (1968).

Shimotori, M. Fluorescein angiography of experimental retinal degeneration on rabbits. In: Proc. Int. Symp. Fluorescein Angiography, Albi 9–14 June 1969, pp. 309–311. Karger, Basel (1971).

Authors' addresses:
P. Solé & F. Bacin
Department of Ophthalmology

R. Alfieri
Department of Biomathematics

B. Kantelip
Department of Pathologic Anatomy
of the Faculty of Medicine
P.O. Box 38
63001 Clermont Ferrand CEDEX
France

Pierre Tronche
Department of Chemical Pharmacy
of the Faculty of Pharmacy
P.O. Box 38
63001 Clermont-Ferrand Cedex
France

Docum. Ophthal. Proc. Series, Vol. 15

SLOW OFF-EFFECTS OF THE HUMAN D.C. REGISTERED ERG*

KLAS-OLAV SKOOG, SVEN ERIK G. NILSSON & EVA WELINDER
(Linköping, Sweden)

ABSTRACT

The d.c. registration technique developed in our laboratory in connection with the study of slow on-effects, particularly the c-wave, has now been used to demonstrate equally slow, marked off-effects of the human ERG. The eyes of human volunteers were adapted to various light intensities and then exposed to total darkness. At 'off' the following changes appeared: a very fast positive d-wave, a fast negative change (the f-wave), a slower positive wave with a maximum at 0.9–1.5 sec after 'off' (the g-wave) and a slow negative change with a maximum at 4–6 sec (the h-wave). The amplitudes and implicit times of the g- and h-waves were roughly proportional to the intensity of the preceding adapting light. The behaviour of the h-wave was similar to that of the slow positive on-effect, the c-wave. It thus seems that the h-wave at 'off' represents the reverse of the process underlying the c-wave at 'on'. The h-wave was followed by a positive maximum at about 45 sec after 'off', corresponding to the SP deflection previously shown by us in direct recordings and to the fast EOG peak.

INTRODUCTION

Relatively little work has been devoted to the study of off-effects in the ERG, although fast off-events (d-wave) were reported already by Holmgren (1865) (frog). A slow negative off-effect was found by Noell (1953) (rabbit). Dodt (1952), Bornschein & Schubert (1953) and others described fast off-effects (d-waves) in the human ERG.

There has been very little information concerning the precise potential variations in the human eye in the time interval between the fast ERG d-wave and the potential maximum seen 45 sec after off. The latter peak was indirectly recorded by Täumer, Hennig & Pernice (1974) and others by means of EOG. It was also demonstrated by Skoog (1975) with the aid of a method for long-term (more than 90 min) direct registrations of the standing potential (SP). The direct technique has also been used to study the slow on-effect (the c-wave) in detail (Skoog & Nilsson, 1974a, b; Skoog, 1974; Nilsson & Skoog, 1975). This procedure also permits a study of off-events

* This investigation was supported by grants from the Swedish Medical Research Council (Project No. 12X–734), the Research Committee of the Östergötlands läns landsting and Ollie and Elof Ericsson's Research Foundation.

occurring in the gap between the limits of standard ERG and EOG techniques. There is evidence of slow off-effects in some human c-wave registrations (Skoog & Nilsson, 1974a). In that study the authors aimed at developing a method which could be easily used even with untrained patients. Consequently a 1 sec stimulus was found suitable, although off-effects seemed to cause a slight change of slope of the rising phase of the c-wave. This observation suggested the present investigation, where two new slow off-effects of the human ERG are revealed. The interaction between the c-wave and the slow off-responses has been analysed in another study from our laboratory (Textorius, 1977).

MATERIAL AND METHODS

The present method is presented in more detail elsewhere (Skoog, Welinder & Nilsson, 1977a).

Nine female and five male volunteers (aged 18—30 years) took part in the study. The pupils were dilated. The signals from a scleral contact lens and a reference chamber on the forehead passed through saline-agar bridges to matched calomel half-cells which served as recording and reference electrodes. The contact lens was stabilized on the cornea by means of slight suction. Further stability was obtained by letting the volunteer fixate a very weak deep red light during registrations. A low-drift d.c. amplifier, a signal analyzer and an analogue tape recorder were used.

Adapting light (0.6, 6, 60 or 600 Lux) came from a xenon lamp. Since the surface of the contact lens was slightly opaque, a uniform wide angle illumination of the retina was obtained. The eye was adapted to each intensity for 10 min. The first time after the application of electrodes an adaptation of 30 min was allowed. The light was turned off for 0.2, 10 or 60 sec and off-effects were recorded. The 0.2, 10 and 60 sec registrations were repeated with 20 sec, 1 min and 10 min intervals, respectively. Four 0.2 and 10 sec recordings were averaged. 60 sec registrations were not averaged. A series of registrations consisted of responses with adapting light intensities from 0.6 to 600 Lux. 17 series of 0.2 sec and 10 sec recordings were performed. The 60 sec registrations consisted of 14 series.

It seemed practical for easy identification of the various off-effects to suggest a new nomenclature (see labelling of Fig. 1) in addition to the established a-, b-, c-, d- and e-waves.

RESULTS

In Fig. 1a-c the electrical events after 'off' are illustrated. To save space only three recordings with different time-scales from a typical experiment are shown. Adapting intensity (AI) was 60 Lux in the recording of Fig. 1a, and 6 Lux in the registrations of Figs. 1b-c.

Very soon after 'off' there is a positive d-wave with multiple peaks and then a negative f-wave (Fig. 1a). Multiple d-wave peaks were also seen at

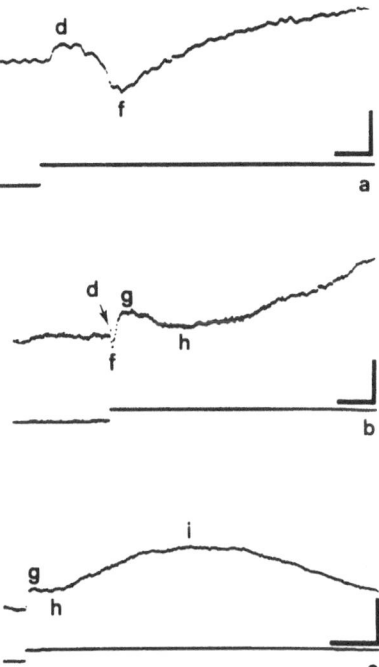

Fig. 1a-c. Fast (d- and f-wave), slow (g- and h-wave) and very slow (i-wave) potential variations after the termination of an adapting light of (a) 60 Lux and (b-c) 6 Lux. Amplitude calibration (a) 50 μV, (b) 100 μV and (c) 200 μV. Time calibration (a) 50 ms, (b) 2 s and (c) 10 s.

600 Lux. After the f-wave there is a slower increase in potential which (as seen in Fig. 1b with its compressed time-scale) builds up a rather slow positive off-effect, the g-wave. The g-wave is considerably larger than the d-wave. It is followed by a through, the h-wave. Then the trace starts climbing very slowly again. In Fig. 1c (with an even more compressed time-scale) it may be seen how a positive peak (the i-wave) is formed about 45 sec after 'off', followed by a steady decrease in potential.

Recordings at the other adapting light intensities were principally similar but amplitudes and implicit times differed as demonstrated in Figs. 2–4. The d, g and i-wave amplitudes were measured from the iso-electric line. The f- and h-wave amplitudes were measured from the peaks of the d- and g-waves, respectively.

In some cases the potential variations were recorded for one hour to confirm that the decrease after the i-wave continued in a damped SP oscillation with a frequency of about 2/h.

The d-wave was barely detectable at AI 0.6 Lux, but its amplitude increased with rising intensities and showed multiple peaks at 60 and 600 Lux. The implicit time (measured from 'off' to the first peak) declined between AI 0.6 and 60 Lux. The f-wave-amplitude increased between AI 0.6 and 600 Lux. Its implicit time was rather constant.

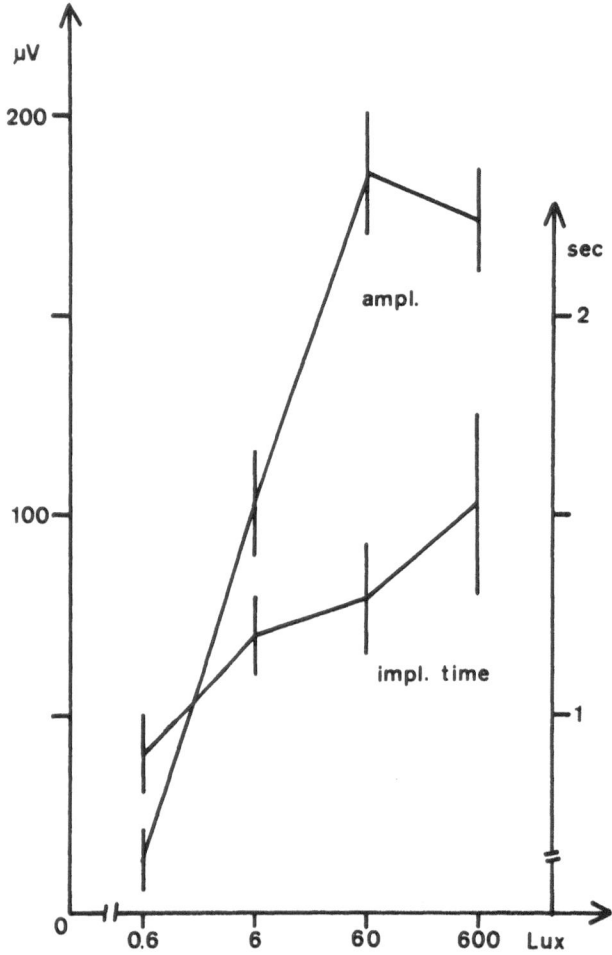

Fig. 2. The relationship between g-wave amplitude (left ordinate), implicit time (right ordinate) and adapting light intensity. Means and standard error of the mean from 17 experiments. (Figs. 2–4 from Skoog, Welinder & Nilsson, 1977a).

Fig. 2 demonstrates that the g-wave amplitude (left ordinate) rose between 0.6 and 60 Lux and then tended to decrease. There was a steady increase in implicit time (left ordinate) between 0.6 and 600 Lux.

As shown in Fig. 3 both the h-wave amplitude (left ordinate) and implicit time (right ordinate) increased with rising AI (abscissa).

In Fig. 4 i-wave amplitude (left ordinate) and implicit time (right ordinate) are plotted against AI (abscissa). Amplitudes increased between 0.6 and 60 Lux while implicit times were more or less constant.

In preliminary experiments no off-effects were detected at AI 0.006 Lux. Off-responses were very weak and consequently difficult to measure at 0.06 Lux. The termination of stronger illuminations than 600 Lux sometimes provoked disturbing eye movements.

122

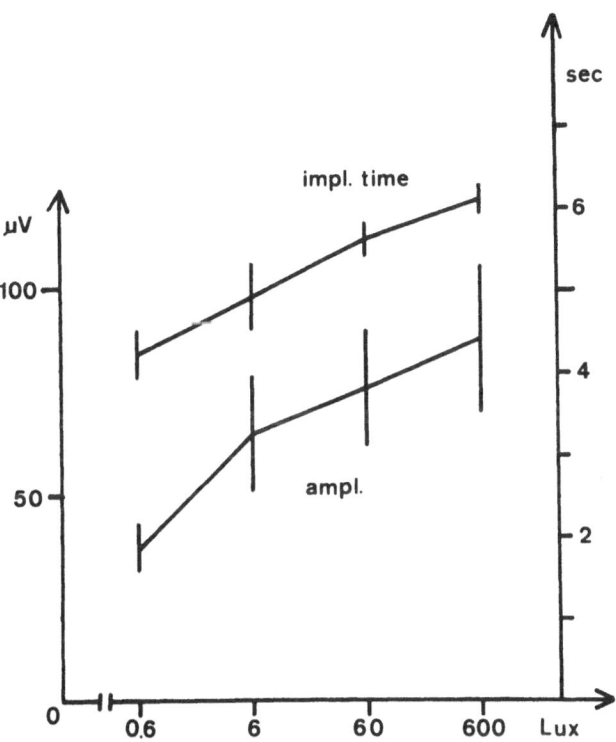

Fig. 3. The relationship between h-wave amplitude (left ordinate), implicit time (right ordinate) and adapting light intensity (abscissa). Means and standard error of the mean from 17 experiments.

DISCUSSION

The characteristics of the d-wave observed in the present study are in accordance with the findings of Best & Bohnen (1955) and others. The f-wave is a constant and reproducible deflection in our recordings. A fast through after the d-wave may be seen also in the paper by Best & Bohnen (1955) and others.

The g- and h-waves of the present study have not been clearly shown in earlier human registrations, since they cannot be demonstrated with ordinary ERG and EOG techniques. Slow off-effects were reported in animal experiments by Noell (1953), Faber (1969) and Hanitzsch (1970). Faber considered the slow negative off-response of the rabbit retina as the result of an interaction between a positive 'slow-PIII-off' and a slow negative 'off-c-wave'. It seems reasonable to the authors to propose that also the g- and h-waves of the human ERG are created by the sum of at least two processes. Tentatively, the rising limb of the g-wave is built up by the beginning of a human counterpart of Faber's 'slow-PIII-off'. The h-wave would then arise when human equivalent of Faber's 'off-c-wave' is superimposed upon 'slow-PIII-off'. In the rabbit the 'off-c-wave' predominates so that the result is a

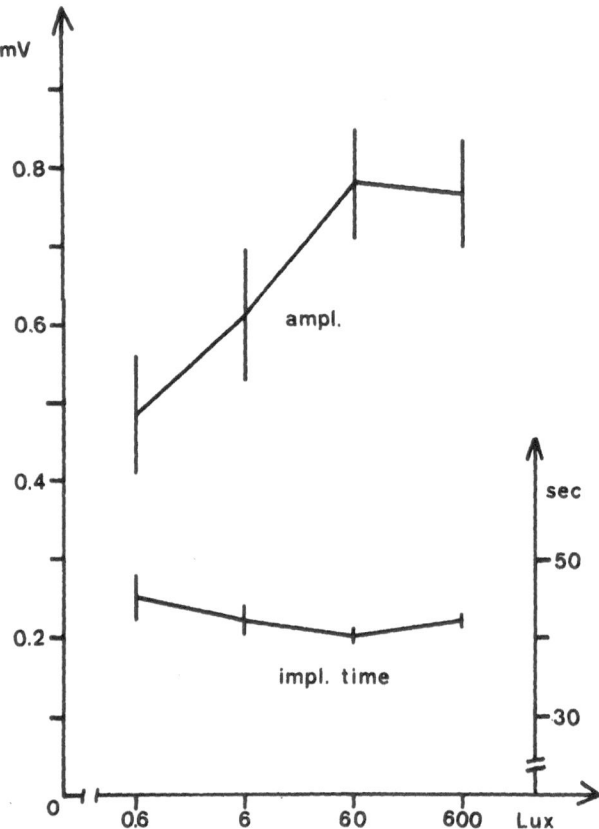

Fig. 4. The relationship between i-wave amplitude (left ordinate), implicit time (right ordinate) and adapting light intensity (abscissa). Means and standard error of the mean from 14 experiments.

negative off-response. In man, the positive component is relatively stronger, so that a positive and a negative off-effect, the g- and h-waves, are produced.

Crescitelli & Sickel (1968) and Crescitelli (1968) described slow e-waves in the frog ERG. Experimental conditions were quite different from those of the present study, so it is somewhat difficult to compare the e-wave with the present g-wave. A relationship cannot be excluded, however.

As to timing, intensity-amplitude relationships, intensity-implicit time relationships and reactions to ethanol the slow on-effect (the c-wave) and the h-wave show considerable similarities (Skoog & Nilsson, 1974a; Skoog, 1974; Skoog, Welinder & Nilsson, 1977a,b). Moreover, both the major positive component of the rabbit c-wave and the major negative part of its slow off-response are eliminated by sodium iodate, which suppresses the pigment epithelium (Noell, 1953, Faber, 1969). The major positive part of the c-wave is generated by the pigment epithelium-receptor complex in response to a decrease in potassium ion concentration around the receptor cells occurring during light stimulation (Steinberg, Schmidt & Brown, 1970;

Oakley & Green, 1976; Oakley, Steinberg, Miller & Nilsson, 1977). It may be speculated that the negative component of the h-wave, seemingly a mirror image of the major positive part of the c-wave, is generated by a reversal of the ion concentration and polarization changes which are related to the c-wave.

REFERENCES

Best, W. & K. Bohnen. Über den 'off-Effekt' im Elektroretinogramm des Menschen. *A. v. Graefes Arch. Ophthal.* 158: *568–577* (1955).

Bornschein, H. & G. Schubert. Das photopische Flimmer-Elektroretinogramm des Menschen. *Z. Biol.* 106: *229–238* (1953).

Crescitelli, F. The e-wave and inhibition in the developing retina of the frog. *Vision Res.* 10: *1077–1091* (1970).

Crescitelli, F. & W. Sickel. Delayed off-responses recorded from the isolated frog retina. *Vision Res.* 8: *801–816* (1970).

Dodt, E. Beiträge zur Elektrophysiologie des Auges. II. Mitteilung. Über Hemmungsvorgänge in der menschlichen Retina. *A. v. Graefes Arch. Ophthal.* 153: *152–162* (1952).

Faber, D.S. Analysis of the slow transretinal potentials in response to light. Thesis. State University of New York at Buffalo (1966).

Hanitzsch, R. Vergleichende Untersuchungen an isolierten, umströmten Warmblüternetzhäuten über das Verhalten intraretinaler langsamer Belichtungspotentiale und das Elektroretinogramms-II. Einfluss der Reizparameter an der helladaptierten Netzhaut. *Vision Res.* 10: *1011–1023* (1970).

Holmgren, F. Method att objectivera effecten af ljusintryck på retina. *Upsala Läk. Fören. Förh.* 1: *184–198* (1865).

Nilsson, S.E.G. & K.-O. Skoog. Covariation of the simultaneously recorded c-wave and standing potential of the human eye. *Acta Ophthal. (Kbh.)* 53: *721–730* (1975).

Noell, W.K. Studies on the electrophysiology and metabolism of the retina. U.S.A.F. School of Aviation Medicine, Randolph Field, Texas (1953).

Oakley II, B. & D.G. Green. Correlation of light-induced changes in retinal extracellular potassium concentration with c-wave of the electroretinogram. *J. Neurophysiol.* 39: *1117–1133* (1976).

Oakley II, B., R.H. Steinberg, S.S. Miller & S.E.G. Nilsson. The in vitro frog pigment epithelial hyperpolarization in response to light. *Invest. Ophthal.* 16: *771–774* (1977).

Skoog, K.-O. The c-wave of the human d.c. registered ERG. III. Effects of ethyl alcohol on the c-wave. *Acta ophthal. (Kbh.)* 52: *913–923* (1974).

Skoog, K.-O. The directly recorded standing potential of the human eye. *Acta ophthal. (Kbh.)* 53: *120–132* (1975).

Skoog, K.-O. & S.E.G. Nilsson. The c-wave of the human d.c. registered ERG. I. A quantitative study of the relationship between c-wave amplitude and stimulus intensity. *Acta Ophthal. (Kbh.)* 52: *759–773* (1974a).

Skoog, K.-O. & S.E.G. Nilsson. The c-wave of the human d.c. registered ERG. II. Cyclic variations of the c-wave amplitude. *Acta ophthal. (Kbh.)* 52: *904–912* (1974b).

Skoog, K.-O., E. Welinder & S.E.G. Nilsson. Off-responses in the human d.c. registered ERG. *Vision Res.* 17: *409–415* (1977a).

Skoog, K.-O., E. Welinder & S.E.G. Nilsson. The influence of ethanol on slow off-responses in the human d.c. registered ERG. *Vision Res.* Accepted for publication (1977b).

Steinberg, R.H., R. Schmidt & K.T. Brown. Intracellular responses to light from cat pigment epithelium: origin of the electroretinogram c-wave. *Nature* (Lond.) 227: *728–730* (1970).

Textorius, O. The influence of stimulus duration on the human d.c. registered c-wave. A quantitative study. *Acta ophthal. (Kbh.).* 55: *561–572* (1977).

Täumer, R., J. Hennig & D. Pernice. The ocular dipole – a damped oscillator stimulated by the speed of change in illumination. *Vision Res.* 14: *637–645* (1974).

Authors' address:
Department of Ophthalmology
University of Linköping
S-581 85 Linköping
Sweden

ETHANOL–INDUCED CHANGES IN A SLOW OFF–EFFECT (THE h-WAVE) OF THE HUMAN D.C. REGISTERED ERG*

SVEN ERIK G. NILSSON, KLAS-OLAV SKOOG & EVA WELINDER

(Linköping, Sweden)

ABSTRACT

Slow off-effects in the human d.c. registered ERG were recently analysed in our laboratory. The fast positive d-wave was followed by a fast negative wave (the f-wave), a slower positive wave (the g-wave) and a slow negative change (the h-wave). The h-wave showed great similarities to the c-wave (a slow on-effect) with respect to time course and the relationship between amplitude and implicit time, on the one hand, and the intensity of the preceding adapting light on the other hand. The present study demonstrates that the h-wave reacted to ethyl alcohol in the same way as the c-wave. A small dose of ethanol given orally to human volunteers provoked a marked increase in amplitude (in a negative direction) of the negative h-wave. The increase reached a maximum after about 12 min and was followed by a very slow oscillation. This finding further supports the hypothesis that the h-wave at 'off' reflects the reverse process represented by the c-wave at 'on'.

INTRODUCTION

Fast and slow off-effects of the human d.c. registered ERG were recently studied by the authors (Skoog, Welinder & Nilsson, 1977 a.b; Skoog, Nilsson & Welinder, 1977). A new nomenclature was suggested in order to facilitate identification and discussion of the various off-effects (see labelling of Fig. 1). The fast positive d-wave and the fast negative f-wave were followed by a slow positive g-wave (0.9 − 1.5 s after 'off') and then a slow negative h-wave (4−6 s after 'off'). These slow off-variations in the human ERG may be compared to those of the rabbit, where there is only a slow negative response after 'off' (Noell, 1953; Faber, 1969). Noell and Faber regarded the slow off-response of the rabbit as the result of an interaction between a negative 'off-c-wave' and a positive 'slow PIII-off' (Faber's nomenclature). The present authors (Skoog, Welinder & Nilsson, 1977 a,b; Skoog, Nilsson & Welinder, 1977) suggested that there are human counterparts of the two off-components: the rising part of the g-wave being generated by the human 'slow PIII-off'. The h-wave would be produced by the depression in the slow PIII-off' caused by the human 'off-c-wave'. The great similarities be-

*This investigation was supported by grants from the Swedish Medical Research Council (Project No. 12X−734), the Research Committee of the Östergötlands läns landsting and Ollie and Elof Ericsson's Research Foundation.

tween the c-wave at 'on' and the h-wave at 'off' were also pointed out. It was speculated that the negative component of the h-wave (which behaves more or less like a mirror image of the major positive component of the c-wave) is generated by a reversal of ion concentration and polarization changes connected to the c-wave. The latter were recently studied by Oakley & Green (1976) and Oakley, Steinberg, Miller & Nilsson (1977).

In the present study a further similarity between the c- and h-waves was sought. It is known that a small oral dose of ethyl alcohol provokes a large increase in c-wave amplitude (Knave, Persson & Nilsson, 1974; Skoog, 1974). The present authors found an equally dramatic increase of the h-wave amplitude in response to ethanol.

MATERIAL AND METHODS

A more detailed description of the method may be found elsewhere (Skoog, Welinder & Nilsson, 1977a,b).

Registrations were performed on two male and two female volunteers, aged 20—26 years and weighing 55—85 kg. The pupils were dilated. The recording system consisted of a suction contact lens on the cornea and a reference chamber on the forehead, saline-agar bridges leading to calomel half-cells and a low-drift d.c. amplifier. The signals from the amplifier were led to a signal analyzer and an analogue tape recorder. During recordings the volunteer fixated a very weak deep red light with his free eye.

The eye was adapted to a uniform wide angle illumination of 60 Lux for 30 min. Then it was suddenly subjected to total darkness and off-responses were registered. Each 'dark flash' lasted 10 sec. The stimulus interval was 1 min.

After 30 min of repeated recordings, the volunteer was given an oral dose of 0.4 g ethanol/kg body weight between two registrations. Electrodes were kept in place. Then another 30—40 min of registrations were carried out at one min intervals.

The volunteers had not eaten for 3 hours before the experiment. Before that they had only a very light meal. There was no influence from ethanol or drugs prior to the experiment. Alcohol was taken in the form of brandy with added pure ethanol to make 50 vol%. The Department of Clinical Chemistry performed blood alcohol analyses (gas chromatography).

Four experiments were performed. The g-wave was measured from the iso-electric line. The h-wave was measured between the g-wave maximum and the h-wave trough.

RESULTS

In Fig. 1a one can see normal slow off-effects of the human d.c. registered ERG. Ethanol has a prominent effect on the h-wave, which becomes very deep (Fig. 1b). Both registrations are taken from the experiment illustrated in Fig. 2.

During the 30 min before ethanol was given there were only slight and

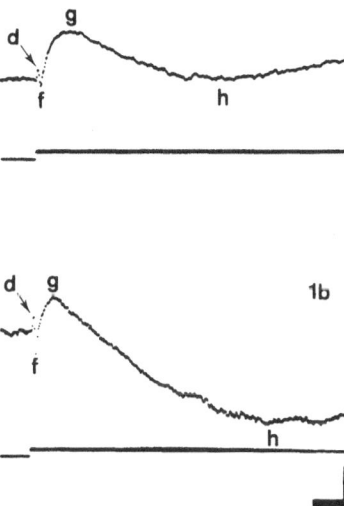

Fig. 1. D.c recordings of fast (d- and f-waves) and slow (g- and h-waves) off-effects after the termination of an illumination of 60 Lux. Photographs taken from the experiment illustrated in Fig. 2.
1 a: An average of two recordings before ethanol.
1 b: An average of two registrations with a pronounced alcohol effect.
Amplitude calibration 100 μV. Time calibration 1 s. 'Off' is indicated on the line below each recording. (Figs. 1–3 from Skoog, Welinder & Nilsson, 1977b).

seemingly random changes in the g- and h-wave amplitudes. In two experiments the variations might be interpreted as 2/h amplitude oscillations of the h-wave. However, the authors are not yet fully convinced that there are cyclic variations of the h-wave amplitude in response to repeated 'dark flashes'. The recordings were more or less constant after 20 min.

The h-wave changes in a typical experiment are illustrated in Fig. 2. The first 20 min are not plotted. The h-wave amplitude had been rather stable for 13 min, when at 0 min (arrow) o.4 g ethanol/kg body weight was administered orally. A small minimum of the h-wave amplitude appeared after 5 min, soon followed by a dramatic increase leading to a peak at 10 min. The variation continued with a minimum at 24 min followed by another increase. Initial h-wave amplitudes were almost reached at 30 min. Ethanol seems to have provoked a cyclic change of the h-wave amplitude. The g-wave amplitudes varied like a less pronounced oscillation, which was a mirror image of that of the h-wave. Both the d- and the f-waves remained more or less stable during the experiment.

Sometimes it was difficult to detect the small h-wave minimum 5 min after ethanol. In other respects the other experiments fully substantiated the above findings. An average of all four experiments is plotted in Fig. 3. The average standard error of the mean of the -9-0 min, 1-10 min, 11-20 min and 21-30 min intervals was 30 μV, 41 μV, 36 μV and 32 μV, respectively.

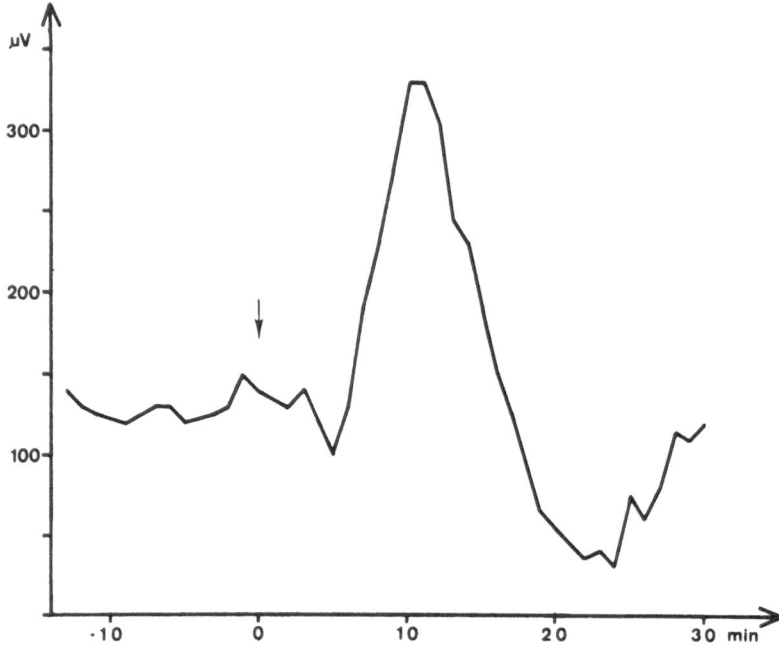

Fig. 2. A typical experiment where repeated registrations of the h-wave amplitude (measured from the peak of the g-wave) were performed before and after the oral administration (arrow) of 0.4 g ethanol/kg body weight. Stimulus interval 1 min. Adapting light intensity 60 Lux.

DISCUSSION

The present experiments support the hypothesis that there exists a close similarity between the slow positive on-effect (the c-wave) and the slow negative off-effect (the h-wave). Both the former (Skoog, 1974) and the latter ERG component react with slow amplitude oscillations after small oral doses of ethanol.

On repeated registrations the c-wave amplitude varies like a damped oscillation (Calissendorff, Knave & Persson, 1974; Skoog & Nilsson, 1974). This cyclic change is probably caused by the average increase in illumination of the eye after the beginning of registrations (Nilsson & Skoog, 1975). In the present study there were possibly faint indications of a 2/h oscillation of the h-wave in response to repeated 'dark flashes'. We do not consider such cyclic changes of the h-wave demonstrated beyond doubt, since the variation was blurred by apparently random amplitude changes. At the time when ethanol was administered the h-wave amplitude was more or less constant, so that the following changes must be considered true ethyl alcohol effects.

It is not yet possible to decide in what way ethanol influences the h-wave. Knutsson (1961) and others showed that ethanol influences cell membrane potentials. Knave, Persson & Nilsson (1974) suggested an effect on both the neuroretina and the pigment epithelium. From the work of Noell (1953) and Faber (1969), it seems probable that these structures are related to the 'slow PIII-off' and 'off-c-wave', respectively.

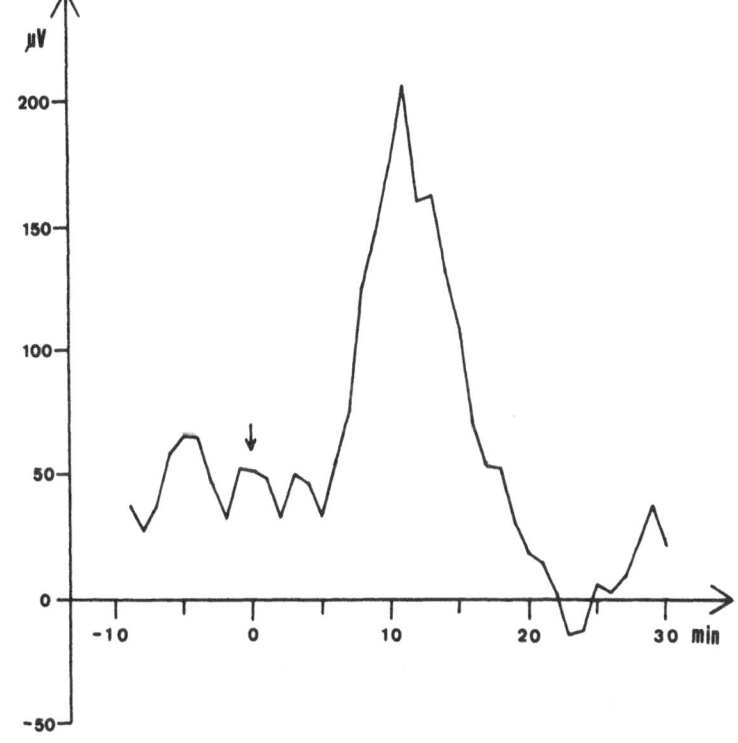

Fig. 3. The average of 4 experiments where repeated registrations of the h-wave amplitude (measured from the peak of the g-wave) were performed before and after the oral administration (arrow) of 0.4 g ethanol/kg body weight. Stimulus interval 1 min. Adapting light intensity 60 Lux.

REFERENCES

Calissendorff, B., B. Knave & H. E. Persson. Cyclic variations in the c-wave amplitude of the sheep ERG. *Vision Res.* 14: *1141–1145*, (1974).

Faber, D. S. Analysis of the slow transretinal potentials in response to light. Thesis. State University of New York at Buffalo. (1969).

Knave, B., H. E. Persson & S. E. G. Nilsson. A comparative study on the effects of barbiturate and ethyl alcohol on retinal functions with special reference to the c-wave of the electroretinogram and the standing potential of the sheep eye. *Acta ophthal. (Kbh.)* 52: *254–259*, (1974).

Knutsson, E. Effects of ethanol on the membrane potential and membrane resistance of frog muscle fibres. *Acta physiol. scand.* 52: *242–253*, (1961).

Noell, W.K. Studies on the electrophysiology and metabolism of the retina. U.S.A.F. School of Aviation Medicine, Randolph Field, Texas, (1953).

Oakley II, B & D.G. Green. Correlation of light-induced changes in retinal extracellular potassium concentration with c-wave of the electroretinogram. *J. Neurophysiol.* 39: *1117–1133*. (1976).

Oakley II, B., R.H. Steinberg, S.S. Miller & S.E.G. Nilsson. The in vitro frog pigment epithelial cell hyperpolarization in response to light. *Invest. Ophthal.* 16: *771–774* (1977).

Skoog, K.-O. The c-wave of the human d.c. registered ERG. III. Effects of ethyl alcohol on the c-wave. *Acta ophthal. (Kbh.)* 52: *913–923,* (1974).

Skoog, K.-O. & S. E. G. Nilsson. The c-wave of the human s.c. registered ERG. II. Cyclic variations of the c-wave amplitude. *Acta ophthal. (Kbh.)* 52: *904–912.* (1974).

Skoog, K.-O., S. E. G. Nilsson & E. Welinder. Slow off-effects in the human d.c. registered ERG. Proceedings 15th ISCEV Symposium, Ghent, 1977. Junk, The Hague (1978).

Skoog, K.-O., E. Welinder & S. E. G. Nilsson. Off-responses in the human d.c. registered electroretinogram. *Vision Res.* 17: *409–415,* (1977a).

Skoog, K.-O., E. Welinder & S. E. G. Nilsson. The influence of ethanol on slow-responses in the human d.c. registrered ERG. *Vision Res.* Accepted for publ. (1977b).

Authors' address:
Departement of Ophthalmology
University of Linköping
S-581 85 Linköping
Sweden

THE INFLUENCE OF ETHANOL
ON RETINAL OSCILLATORY POTENTIALS*

J. LEVETT & F. MORINI
(Chicago, Ill., USA)

ABSTRACT

This study confirms the already reported electroretinographic effects of alcohol. It furthermore demonstrates that the e-wave, or first positive component of the oscillatory potential subsequent to the b-wave, is selectively attenuated following ethanol injection. In the chronic situation the e-wave is completely extinguished. Subsequent to the removal of ethanol the ERG is transiently increased, becomes faster and then diminishes somewhat to a new steady-state. The e-wave reappears after several days.

INTRODUCTION

The studies reported in this paper deal with the application of both the acute and chronic ethanol state in the frog. The critical parameter of interest is the frog electroretinogram. Of particular interest is a little explored minor component designated the e-wave that follows the major b-wave component in the light-adapted state. The e-wave, which is the first positive potential subsequent to the b-wave and can be followed by further damped oscillations, can be found in several other species as well. In the human it appears to be cone mediated (Auerbach, 1967; Brunette, 1973). Subsequent to the application of intraperitoneal (IP) alcohol in the frog, both the b-wave and the e-wave change. The e-wave completely disappears but return after several hours. Chronic ethanol through daily immersions produces extinction of the e-wave. Subsequent to removal from ethanol the ERG rebounds and slightly overshoots pre-alcohol amplitudes before assuming its new and faster steady state. Over this period of several days the e-wave returns and the ERG is essentially the same as for the normal. All frogs were treated with a solution of antibacterial agents for 24 hours upon arrival from supplier. Both large (*Rana catesbeiana*) and small frogs. (*Rana pipiens*) have been used. They were periodically fed meal worms.

More than 20 acute experiments have been conducted on intact frogs. Ethanol was administered via the intreperitoneal (IP) cavity. IP injections

---

* Supported by a grant from NIAAA #IROI AA02156-01 and The Regenstein Fund, Department of Ophthalmology, Rush-Presbyterian-St. Luke's Medical Center.

were given in saline solutions in strengths of 5–40% ethanol. Corneal recordings of ERGs were taken before and subsequent to the injection. Three populations of frogs were started on daily immersions of 2% ethanol for periods of 20 minutes. This dose was arrived at by observing that immersion in a 10% solution for 10 minutes produced deep anesthesia. Blood samples obtained from frogs subsequent to immersion in a 2% solution for 20 minutes showed blood alcohol levels of about 0.2% rising to roughly 0.3% 10–20 minutes later. Upon removal of the frogs from 2% ethanol their righting reflexes are impaired and this can last up to one hour. Electroretinography was performed periodically. From the original populations only two frogs survived for more than two months. These frogs were removed from alcohol and electroretinography was performed during the period of withdrawal. Subsequently they were returned to daily ethanol immersions.

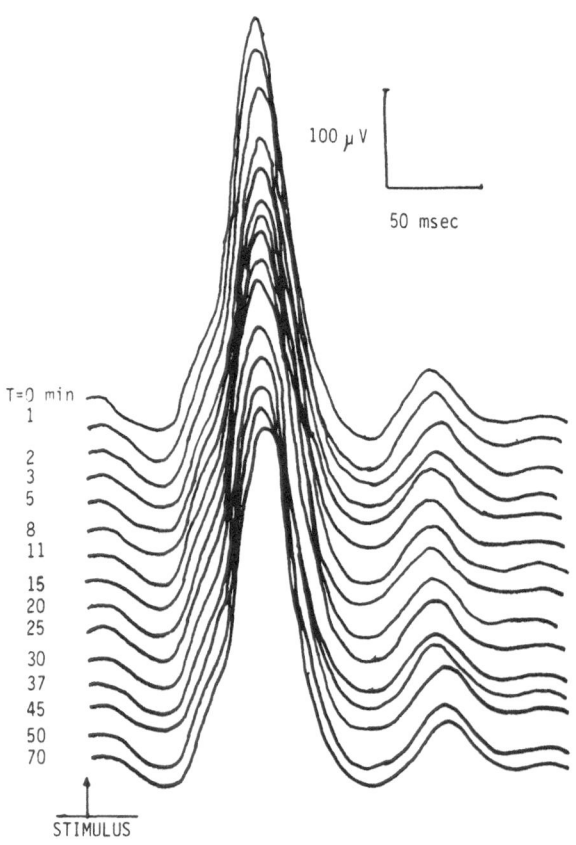

Fig. 1. At T=0 an injection of 10cc (0% Alcohol) saline solution was administered IP. The ERG was followed for 70 min.

134

Typical results are shown in Figures 1, 2 and 3, for the acute ethanol state. This data demonstrates the way in which the e-wave is affected. Figure 4 is a plot of amplitude ratios subsequent to ethanol. In the chronic condition the e-wave is absent and the ERG generally depressed. Subsequent to ethanol withdrawal the amplitudes rebound and the e-wave reappears. This sequence of events is shown in Figure 5. Figure 6 indicates various amplitudes displayed graphically subsequent to withdrawal.

DISCUSSION

The results presented in this paper demonstrate that the retinal response to light subsequent to ethanol ingestion are markedly changed and those changes are dose related for acute situations. Such findings are not new since Ikeda (1963) reported changes in the human, and more recently Sasovetz (1974) has reported similar results for rats. The results reported here are the first quantitative studies for a poikilotherm that we know of and these findings extend our knowledge of ETOH effect on retinal response in vertebrates. One important result is a differential effect of a minor compenent of the ERG, designated the e-wave.

Chronic frogs show a generally depressed, retarded ERG with an absent e-wave. Withdrawing the animals from ethanol provokes a gradual increase in amplitude, a faster response and the return of the e-wave. A transient amplitude overshoot also occurs before the response settles back to a new

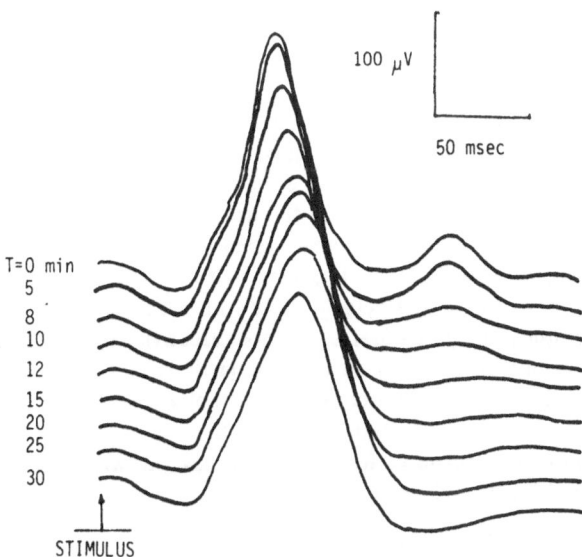

Fig. 2. At T=0 an injection of 10cc (10% Alcohol) saline solution was administered IP. The ERG was followed until the e-wave disappeared.

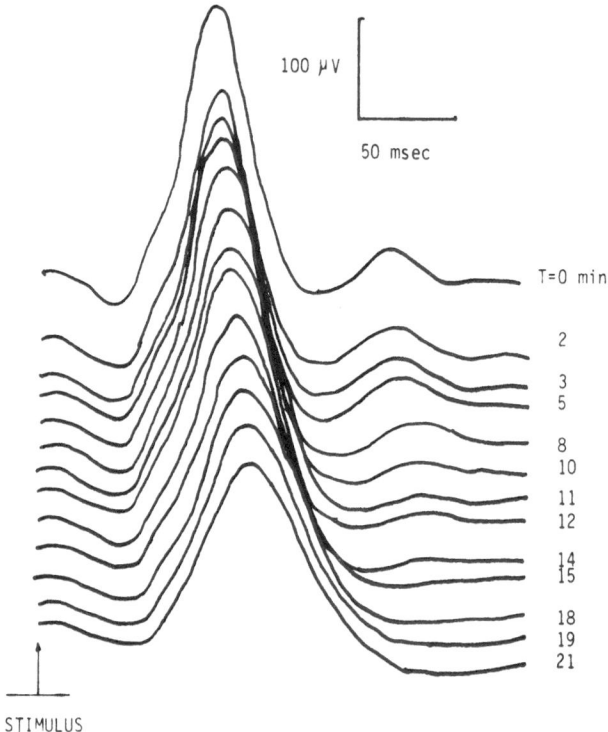

100 μV

50 msec

T=0 min

2

3
5

8
10

11
12

14
15

18
19
21

STIMULUS

Fig. 3. At T=0 an injection of 10 cc (30% Alcohol) saline solution was administered IP. The ERG was followed until the e-wave disappeared.

steady state that is qualitatively normal. For animals that have received ethanol for about two months, return to the normal steady-state required approximately 4–5 days. Since only two frogs survived from the original three populations, we have insufficient data to be quantitative. Nevertheless, qualitatively the described pattern of events is present.

Our preliminary studies encourage the use of the frog as model for ETOH effects on the CNS and for objective evaluations of both acute and chronic alcohol in man.* Our ERG findings lead us to conclude that a frog ETOH model will show us CNS effects. While we have ensured that all drugs and solutions employed by themselves do not affect the ERG, (see Fig. 7) we can not rule out entirely a possible synergistic relationship between them and alcohol. However, such a consideration appears unlikely. Furthermore, we have no way of relating our results to the nutritional state of the frog. While attemps were made to feed them, we have no way of telling whether all their nutritional needs were accounted for.

* Patient data presented by Van Lith (this symposium) appears to confirm these findings in man.

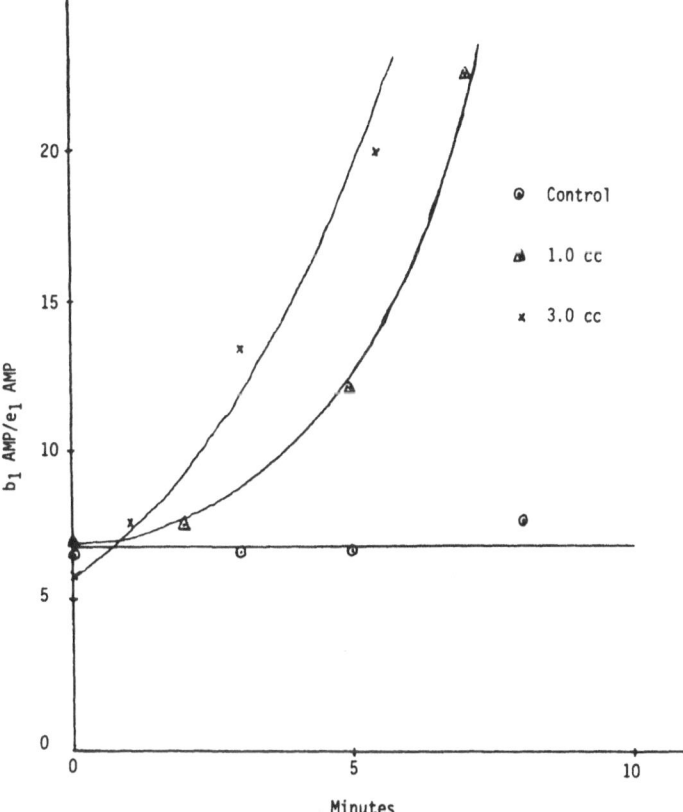

Fig. 4. The absolute magnitude of the ERG varies with each preparation. To minimize the effect of this variability on the analysis of the data the ratios of b-wave amplitude/ e-wave amplitude is plotted against time for three different dosages in the acute situation.

The Müller cell membrane behaves as a K^+ specific ion-exchange membrane (Miller & Dowling, 1970; Miller, 1973). Assuming that this membrane is also capable of oscillatory behaviour (McAvinn, 1976) then both the b-wave of the ERG and the subsequent wavelets can be assumed to stem from the same underlying mechanisms. Under appropriate conditions the work of Teorell (1960) provides an actual physical membrane model which will act as an oscillator. Subsequent to chronic alcohol, swelling of Müller cell membranes may result in a diminished penetration of K+ through the membrane and a reduction on the light-adapted oscillatory potential.

137

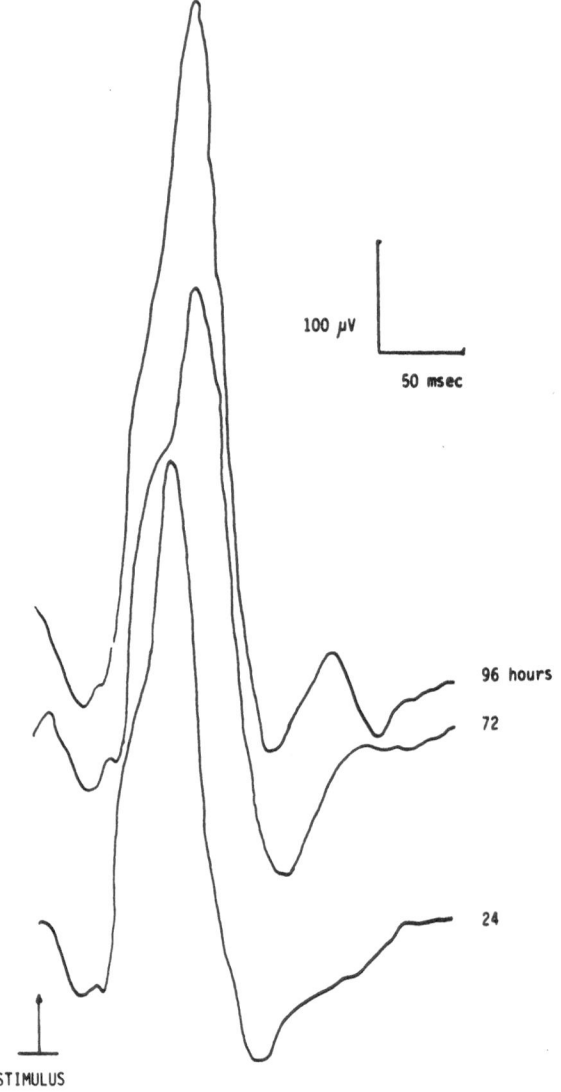

100 μV

50 msec

96 hours

72

24

STIMULUS

Fig. 5. Frog C was given 13 twenty minute baths in a 2% alcohol solution over an 11 day period. Baths were discontinued and on the 12th day the ERG showed no e-wave. On the 14th day, 72 hours after the last bath, the ERG showed signs of e-wave revocery. On 15th day, 96 hours after the last bath, there was a complete return of the e-wave.

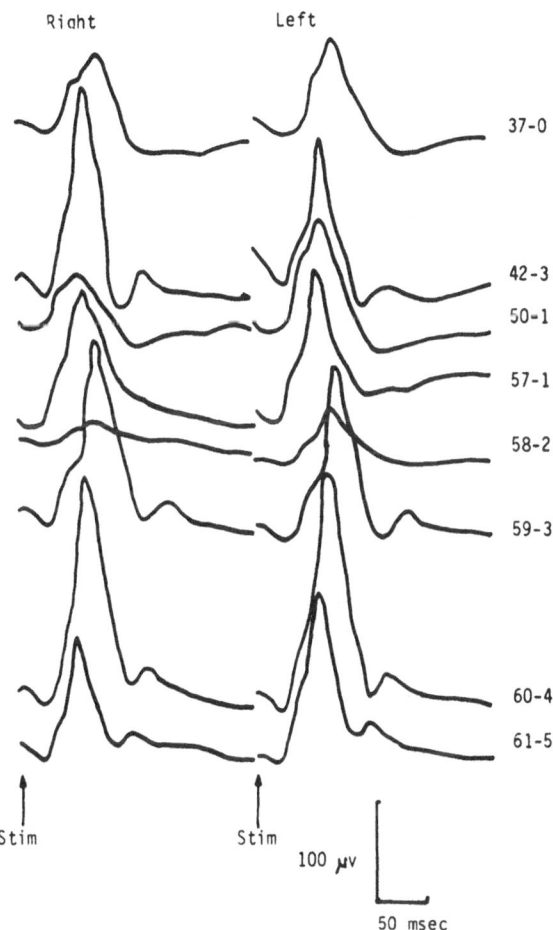

Fig. 6. At T=0 (days) frogs began receiving daily 20 minutes baths in 2% alcohol solution. On three occasions during the course of the experiment frogs were allowed to 'dry out' for periods of 3 to 5 days and the ERG's followed daily. The numbers to the right of the tracings mark the number of days into the experiment and the number of days since the last alcohol bath, i.e. ERG no. 37–0 was recorded on the 37th day of the experiment while the animal was still on alcohol and ERG no. 59–3 was recorded on the 59th day of the experiment while the frog was in the 3rd day of no alcohol. The recordings show the e-wave is extinguished by alcohol and requires 3 to 5 days to recover in the chronic case.

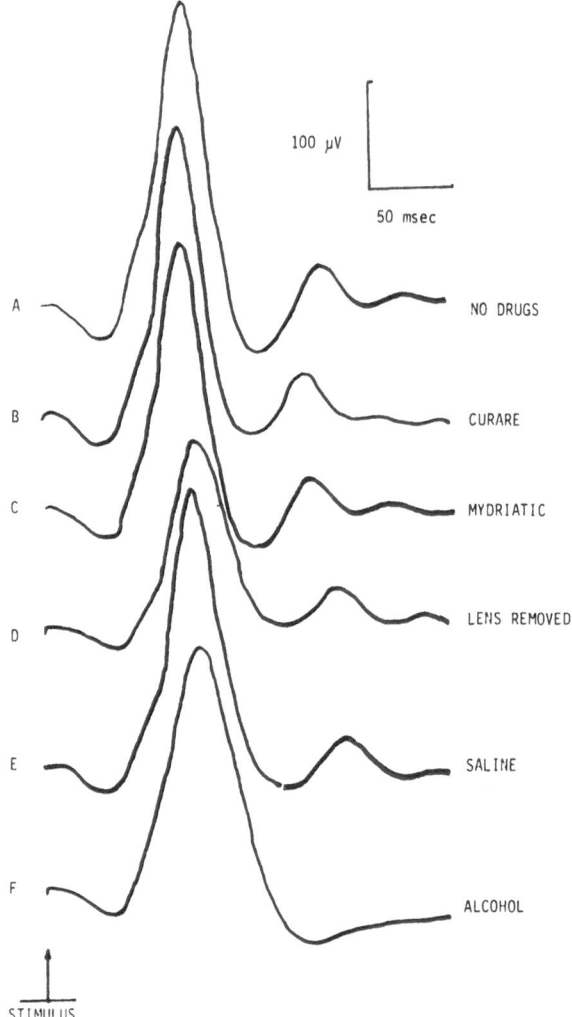

Fig. 7. ERG's of frogs which received: a) no drugs or anesthetics b) tubocurarine chloride injection IP, 0.01 mg/gram frog weight. ERG followed for two hours c) a mydriatic agent: Neo-synephrine, two drops/eye. ERG followed for 30 min: d) curare and had lens removed as a possible source of contamination e) curare, Neo-synephrine and a 10cc injection of (0% Alcohol) saline solution. ERG followed for two hours: f) curare, Neo-synephrine and a 10cc IP injection of (40% Alcohol) saline solution. ERG followed for 35 min.

140

REFERENCES

Auerbach, E. The human electroretinogram in the light and during dark adaptation. *Docum. Ophthal.* 22: *1* (1967).

Brunette, J. R. Standardizable method for separating rod and cone responses in clinical electroretinography. *Am. J. Ophthal.* 75: *833* (1973).

Ikeda, H. Effects of ethyl alcohol on the evoked potentials of the human eye. *Vision Res.* 3: *155–159* (1963).

McAvinn, J. D. The effects of neural adaptation on the b-wave and oscillatory potential of the frog electroretinogram. Master's Thesis, Univ. of Illinois, Chicago (1976).

Miller, R.F. Role of K+ in generation of b-wave of electroretinogram. *J. Neurophysiol.* 36: *28* (1973).

Miller, R. F. & J. E. Dowling (1970). A relationschip between Müller cell slow potentials and the ERG b-wave; pp. 85–100, in: Proceedings of the ISCERG Symposium, Pisa (1970).

Sasovetz, D. The electroretinographic response to alcohol of the rat retinal under various light adapted states. *Ann. Ophthal.:* *797–802* (1974).

Teorell, T. Application of the voltage clamp to the electrohydraulic nerve analog. *Acta Soc. Med. Uppsala* 65: *231* (1960).

Authors' address:
Rush Presbyterian St Luke's Medical Center
Department of Physiology
Chicago, Ill. 60612
USA

CHANGES INDUCED BY GANGLIOSIDES ON THE
C-WAVE IN THE RABBIT

G. CAVALLACCI, G. TOTA & A. WIRTH

(Pisa, Italy)

Gangliosides represent a group of glycolipids like N-acetilneuroaminic acid (NANA), sphingosine, fatty acids, N-acetilglycoseamine, glycose and galactose. Their molecular structure has been sharply defined by DeRobertis et al. (1960). It is shown in Figure 1.

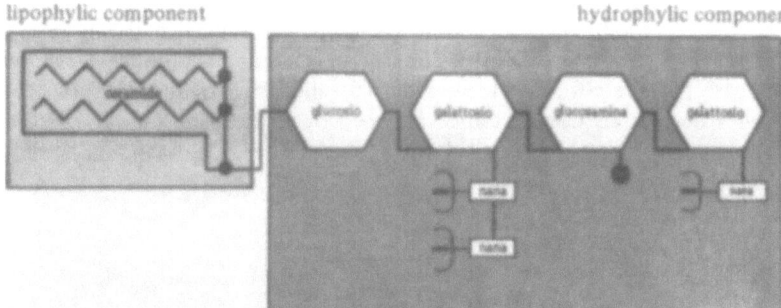

Fig. 1. Schematic view of a ganglioside molecule

Since gangliosides are mainly localized in the membrane of the nervous terminals, in dendrites and axons, they are of primary importance at the synaptic level, for they contribute to the determination of the membrane receptive properties.

We felt it would be of interest to study the effect, if any, of these substances on the slow components of the ERG in the rabbit, primarily on the c-wave and, consequently, on the properties of the pigment epithelium (Noell, 1953).

MATERIAL AND METHOD

Experiments have been performed on 22 pigmented male and female rabbits, weighing 1500–2000 g, and between 3–5 months of age. The basal c-wave was recorded under general anesthesia (Valium 5 mg/kg + Ketalar 10 mg/kg) in full dark adaptation: the gangliosides were injected intravenously at a dose of 5 mg/kg. Changes of the c-wave were followed, as a rule, for 1 hour; in some cases the tracings were checked from the first hour until 8 days after.

The recording technique was the routine one of our laboratory: a small Ag-AcCl ring electrode was kept in contact with the cornea mounted on a plexiglass blepharostat; the indifferent electrode being a needle inserted in the skin of the ear. Leads were taken through a FET small box to a high impedence (up to 50 MΩ) differential amplifier having a time constant of 10 sec with a band-pass at high frequencies up to 8 Hz, connected with the DC input of a Tektronix 502A oscillograph.

The sweep was synchronized with the aid of a photodiode, so that the onset of the stimulus coincided with the onset of the sweep of $\simeq$ 5 sec duration. Tracings were recorded on stationary paper. The light stimulus, set at 1 sec duration, was provided by a Philips 8 volt/50 watt, type 131/3 c/04 bulb, brought to focus on the cornea by a fiber optics bundle. Measurements at the cornea at the standard distance of 1 cm with a conventional luxmeter gave a value of 1150 lux.

RESULTS AND DISCUSSION

The results of our experiments are synthetised in Figure 2: it can be seen that gangliosides injected intravenously in the rabbit produce a marked decrease of the c-wave, which, after 10 minutes, is of the order of 30%. Such a decrease is transient and vanishes slowly within 8 hours. Statistical treatment of the results revealed a high significance at the Student t-test (P = 0.01).

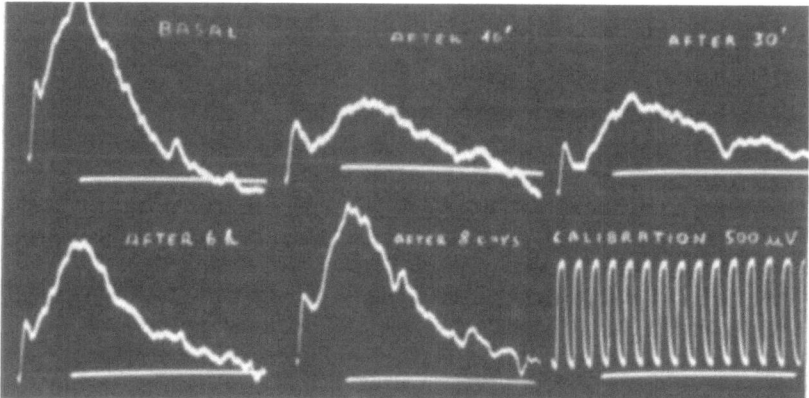

Fig. 2.

On the basis of the results obtained so far, it is rather difficult to explain the mechanism by which gangliosides decrease the c-wave. However, one can suggest that gangliosides interfere at the level of the pigment epithelium with the properties of the cell membrane. It is known that the c-wave is the result of an active transport of ions across the pigment epithelium (Noell, 1953) and that the cells of this layer are of main importance in the processes of nutrition and regeneration of photoreceptors and in the synthesis of photopigments (Hubbard & Wald, 1951). The pigment epithelium serves as a barrier between two compartments of quite different structure, like the choroid and the neuroretina. Such a barrier is of major importance in the vertebrate, insofar as it represents the way across for the exchange of electrolytes and other molecules. It is interesting to recall that a common component of the ganglioside molecule, viz. N-acetilneuraminic acid (NANA), contributes with its carboxyl groups to maintain a negative charge at the external surface of the cell. Chemical analysis of the plasma membrane (Albers & Koval, 1962; Gammack, 1963) showed that gangliosides, like phospholipids, have a hydrophobic and a hydrophylic component as well, the latter containing NANA, and that when this is removed by hydrolysis in presence of a neuroamidase the negative charge external to the cell is diminished (Berkaloff er al., 1967).

We can summarize the topic as follows: the fundamental structure of the cell membrane, including the pigment epithelium, is composed of a lipid bilayer, which acts as a barrier such that the small hydrophilic molecules can cross only with the help of a carrier, especially when there is a unidirectional flow. A process like this, insofar as it means work, requires energy available from cell metabolism. If we admit that gangliosides have a facilitating action on the permeability of the cell membrane of the pigment epithelium, one can suppose a change in the energy consumption with quick exhaustion of the recoverability of electrochemical equilibrium, needed for maintaining a steady-state c-wave voltage.

SUMMARY

Gangliosides injected intravenously into the rabbit at a dose of 5 mg/kg decrease the c-wave amplitude of 30% after 10 minutes. The effect vanishes slowly within 8 hours. It is suggested that gangliosides have a facilitating action on the permeability of the cell membrane of the pigment epithelium, therefore inducing a change in the energy consumption with a quick exhaustion of the recoverability of electrochemical equilibrium, which is needed to maintain the steady-state c-wave voltage.

REFERENCES

Alberts, R.W. & G.J. Koval. The interaction of gangliosides with cationic molecules. *Biochim. Biophys. Acta* 60: *359* (1962).

Berkaloff, A., J. Bourguet, P. Fauard & M. Guinnebauet. Biologie et physiologie cellulaire. Hermann, Paris (1967).

Gammack, D.B. Physiochemical properties of ox-brain gangliosides. *Biochem. J.* 88: *373* (1963).

Hubbard, R. & G. Wald. The mechanism of rhodopsin synthesis. *Proc. Nat. Acad. Sci.* 37: *69* (1951).

Noell, W.K. Studies on the electrophysiology and the metabolism of the retina. US School of aviation medicine, Rep. 1. Randolph Field, Texas, p. 122 (1953).

Authors' address:
Clinica Oculistica Università
Pisa
Italy

Docum. Ophthal. Proc. Series, Vol. 15

CLINICAL ELECTRO-OCULOGRAPHY:
OPTIMUM ILLUMINATION LEVELS FOR THE
LIGHT-ADAPTATION PHASE

R.P. BORDA

(Houston, Texas, USA)

A review of the literature on the clinical applications of the EOG reveals a wide range of illumination levels being utilized for the light adaptation phase in different laboratories. Most, however, approximate the 20,000 trolands reported by Arden et al. (1962); a commonly used light source for EOG seems to be a fluorescent tube X-ray view box.

After the typical dark-adaptation period of 12 minutes, most normal individuals experience considerable discomfort when required to view a light of this intensity. Patients with photophobia can experience fairly profound discomfort. While their discomfort is usually not of long duration, the tearing and blinking typically accompanying the sudden re-adaptation can disrupt the recording procedure for several minutes. While this would be acceptable if it were essential to the diagnostic procedure, the question arises as to whether re-adaptation levels of this magnitude are truly necessary, or whether they have been adopted only out of tradition.

There have been few studies of the effect of illumination level on EOG parameters. One well-designed study by Gouras & Gunkel (1963) reported data which showed that typical EOG dark-trough and light-peak parameters could be elicited by illumination levels over a range of 1–1000 ft. lamberts. The testing procedure used by Gouras & Gunkel required that the subject pre-adapt to a background illumination of 9 ft. lamberts, then the EOG was recorded for 11–12 minutes in darkness, followed by an additional 15 minutes of re-adaptation to light of varying intensities. They noted that in a single subject, the peak-to-trough ratio (P/T), suggested by Arden et al. as the clinically significant parameter of the EOG, increased as the re-adapting illumination was increased in log steps over the range of 1–1000 ft. lamberts. This was in agreement with the observations of Arden & Kelsey (1962). Gouras & Gunkel reported an additional finding of potential importance to clinical electro-oculography: as re-adapting levels of illumination are increased, the range of normal P/T values (or their variability) increases. These authors suggest, for this reason, that re-adaptation levels should be near 1000 trolands.

These findings were considered when constructing a new test facility for routine visual electrodiagnosis. A system was designed using incandescent bulbs for re-adaptation illumination with levels 1–3 log units lower than those commonly reported in the literature. In its present form, the system provides a re-adaptation illumination level of 3.5×10^{-3} lum/cm^2 (35 lux). Our standard test procedure requires that the patient pre-adapt to room levels of illumination of approximately 540 lux. The room lights are extinguished and the EOG sampled once every minute during 12 minutes of dark adaptation. The background illumination of 35 lux is then switched on and the EOG recorded for an additional 12 minutes.

In a retrospective study of 376 normal eyes, the mean P/T with this system was found to be 2.28 with a standard deviation of 0.39. The range of values found in this series was 1.7–3.6, a range which compares favorably with those reported by other laboratories.

Without direct comparisons of our system and one utilizing higher levels of re-adapting illumination, it would be impossible to determine which would be superior in diagnostic accuracy. In our experience, however, our system yields results which are identical to those reported for various pigmentary retinopathies. In the recessively inherited form of retinitis pigmentosa, for example, P/Ts of 1.0–1.2 are found, and in vitelliform macular degeneration slightly higher P/Ts ranging to 1.5 are seen. From the results of studies by Gouras & Gunkel and Arden & Kelsey it might be expected that a system such as that described here would tend to yield more 'false positive' EOGs, i.e., P/Ts which are artificially low. In a series of family members (N = 5) with 'sector-like' pigmentary changes, EOG P/Ts were found which had a mean value of 2.0, clearly within the range of normal variation. Similarly, in a family with a 'pseudo-vitelliform' degeneration (N = 10), the mean P/T was 2.2.

In our experience, then, the lower levels of re-adapting illumination provided by the system used in this new laboratory produce results comparable to those obtained with the higher levels commonly used elsewhere. Patient tolerance of these lower levels is much greater, however, and it would appear from the low variability of P/Ts found in normal eyes that the lower levels may be superior for routine clinical evaluation.

REFERENCES

Arden, G.B. & J.H. Kelsey. Some observations on the relationship between the standing potential of the human eye and the bleaching and regeneration of visual purple. *J. Physiol.* 161: *205–226* (1962).

Arden, G.B., A. Varrada & J.H. Kelsey. New clinical test of retinal function based upon the standing potential of the eye. *Br. J. Ophthal.* 46: *449–464* (1962).

Gouras, P. & R.D. Gunkel. The EOG in chloroquine and other retinopathies. *Arch. Ophthal.* 70: *629–639* (1963).

Author's address:
Neurophysiology Department
Methodist Hospital
6516 Bertner Blvd.
Houston, Texas 77030
USA

THE INITIAL PHASE OF THE EOG-OSCILLATION*

P. HEILIG, A. THALER & V. SCHEIBER

(Vienna, Austria)

The first minutes in the course of the electrooculogram are dominated by the 'fast oscillation of the corneoretinal potential' (Kolder & Brecher, 1966). The potential reaches its peak within approximately 45 seconds. Light stimulation elicits a potential of corneonegative polarity. Transition from light to darkness causes a corneopositive deflection.

METHODS

Nine EOG recordings of one male subject (37 years, emmetropic) were obtained on different days. No other volunteers were included in the study, hence interindividual variation was ruled out. Examination under steady state conditions guaranteed the recording of potentials uninfluenced by preceding oscillations (Thaler et al., 1978). The amplitudes were measured at the peak of the fast oscillation and from that point every minute up to the fifth one.

RESULTS

The peak amplitude of the light induced fast oscillation was found to be higher than that in darkness (Tab. 1). Analysis of variance revealed additional differences between the time course of both potentials. The response to light differs from that to darkness in linear trend ($p < 0.001$) as well as in curvature ($p < 0.001$) (Fig. 1).

Table 1. Mean values (x) and standard deviations (s) of EOG-amplitudes. Responses to light (L) and to darkness (D). n = 9.

minutes		1	2	3	4	5
L	x	84.6	91.9	99.2	111.6	128.0
	s	3.8	3.1	4.8	5.1	9.3
D	x	110.3	101.8	96.3	93.2	90.2
	s	1.7	4.7	2.8	3.8	4.3

* Supported by 'Fonds zur Förderung der wissenschaftlichen Forschung' Grant nr. 2455 and by 'Jubiläumsfonds der Österreichischen Nationalbank' Grant nr. 1151.

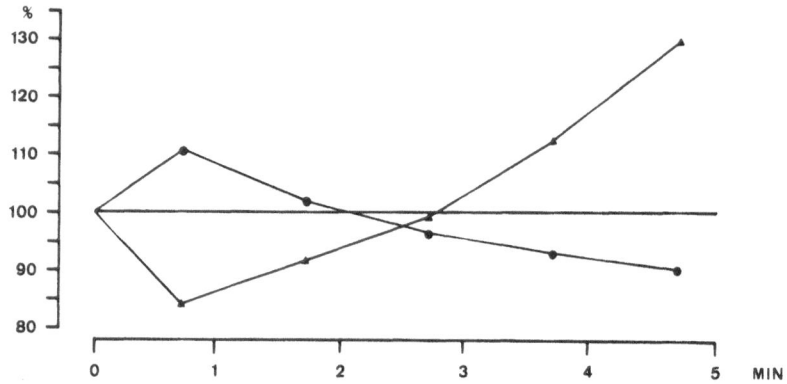

Fig. 1. Mean values of EOG amplitudes. ▲ = response to light. ● = response to darkness. n = 9.

DISCUSSION

The difference in amplitude of light and dark response indicates that these
potentials do not reflect merely the reversion of one process.

No sequential fast oscillation was observed under these experimental conditions. This impression was corroborated by the results of EOG examinations in patients with ischemic retinopathy. This lesion annihilates the
influence of the slow EOG-oscillation, thus displaying the isolated fast oscillation (Thaler & Heilig, 1977). Considering the recordings in normal eyes
and in eyes with ischemic retinopathy two conclusions can be drawn:
1. The peak amplitudes of the fast oscillations of the corneoretinal potential are reflecting the processes generating the fast oscillations exclusively.
2. The course of the EOG following the peak of the fast oscillations is
shaped by a combined activity of both the fast and slow oscillations. With
elapsing time the slow oscillation is gaining more influence on the course of
the EOG curve. No exact point of transition can be determined. Nevertheless, the dominating influence of the slow oscillation takes place almost immediately after the peak of the fast oscillation. Consequently the main
differences in linear trend and curvature have to be attributed to the generators of the slow oscillation.

REFERENCES

Kolder, H. & G.A. Brecher. Fast oscillation of the corneo-retinal potential in man.
    Arch. Ophthal. 75: 232–237 (1966).
Thaler, A. & P. Heilig. EOG and ERG components in ischemic retinopathy. *Ophthal.
    Res. 9: 38–46* (1977).
Thaler, A., P. Heilig, V. Scheiber. Fast oscillation of the corneoretinal potential in
    ischemic retinopathy. *Ophthal. Res. 9: 324–328* (1978).

Authors' address:
II. Augenklinik der Universität
4 Alserstrasse
Vienna A-1090
Austria

THE INITIAL PHASE OF THE EOG-OSCILLATION IN ISCHEMIC RETINOPATHY*

A. THALER, P. HEILIG & V. SCHEIBER
(Vienna, Austria)

In normal eyes the fast EOG-oscillation is influenced by the slow oscillation. Following the peak the potential is increasingly formed by the slow oscillation. It was attempted to separate the EOG-components by mathematical methods in order to study the isolated slow oscillation.

In ischemic retinopathy the slow EOG-oscillations are impaired (Thaler & Heilig, 1977). The fast EOG-oscillations remain unaffected (Thaler et al., 1978). The subtraction of these preserved fast oscillations from the normal electrooculogram should result in the pure slow component.

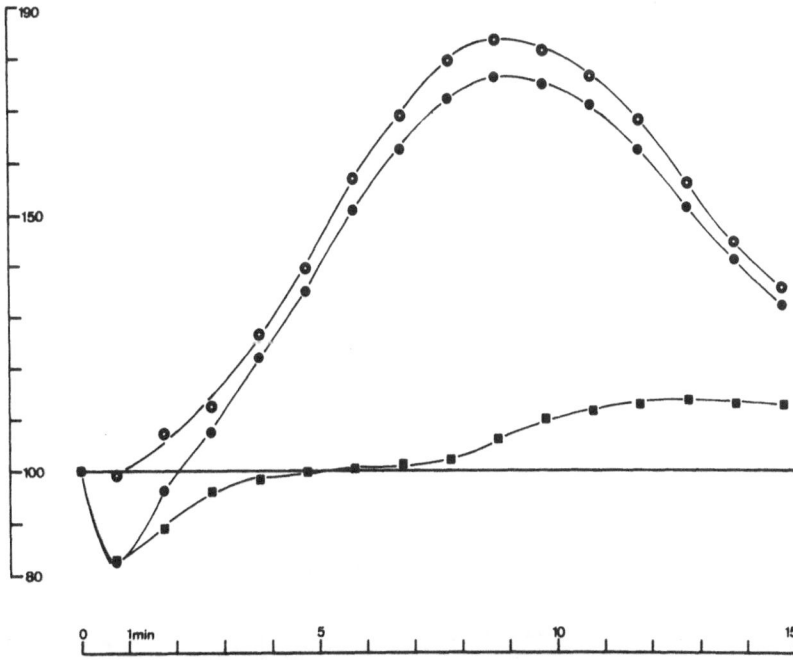

Fig. 1. Mean values of EOG-amplitudes of 30 normal eyes (•), 30 eyes with ischemic retinopathy (■) and 30 calculated pure slow oscillations (○).

*Supported by 'Fonds zur Förderung der wissenschaftlichen Forschung' Grant Nr. 2455 and by 'Jubiläumsfonds der Österreichischen Nationalbank' Grant Nr. 1151.

Table. 1. Mean values (x) and standard deviations (s) of EOG-amplitudes of 30 normal eyes (N), 30 eyes with ischemic retinopathy (P) and 30 calculated pure slow oscillations (N-P).

minutes		1	2	3	4	5	6	7	8	9	10	11	12	13	14	15
N	x	82.9	96.4	107.3	121.9	135.0	150.9	162.3	171.8	175.8	175.0	170.7	162.2	151.2	140.8	131.7
	s	9.0	10.1	9.4	14.5	19.7	24.1	26.4	29.9	30.3	29.2	27.2	27.2	26.9	25.9	23.6
P	x	83.0	88.9	96.2	98.6	99.8	100.4	101.4	102.0	106.4	109.8	111.7	113.1	113.6	113.3	112.6
	s	10.4	8.1	9.6	12.1	12.8	17.0	20.8	24.2	28.1	30.1	29.9	30.9	29.3	29.0	25.1
N–P	x	99.9	107.5	112.7	126.7	139.5	157.1	168.9	179.4	183.5	181.7	176.8	167.9	156.3	144.8	135.4
	s	9.5	8.1	11.2	17.2	21.0	25.5	27.9	31.3	31.5	30.2	28.4	28.3	27.4	24.8	22.6

The recordings were performed in 30 patients with unilateral central retinal artery occlusion. The light induced responses were measured at 45 seconds and at one minute intervals up to the 15th minute. The EOG data of the eyes with ischemic retinopathy were subtracted from those of the normal fellow eyes individually. The subtraction was confined to data smaller than 100%.

The mathematical evaluation revealed that the slow oscillation commences shortly after the peak of the fast oscillation. The slow component does not alter the peak amplitude of the fast oscillation.

REFERENCES

Thaler, A., & P. Heilig. EOG and ERG components in ischemic retinopathy. *Ophthal. Res.* 9: *38–46* (1977).
Thaler, A., P. Heilig & V. Scheiber. Fast oscillation of the corneoretinal potential in ischemic retinopathy. *Ophthal. Res.* 9: *324–328* (1978).

Authors' address:
II Augenklinik der Universität
4 Alserstrasse
Vienna A–1090
Austria

ELECTRO–OCULOGRAPHIC INVESTIGATIONS IN CENTRAL RETINAL VESSEL OCCLUSIONS*

F. PONTE & G. LODATO

(Palermo, Italy)

The behaviour of the electro–oculogram (EOG) in retinal vascular diseases is different if vascular changes are acute or chronic (see François et al., 1974).

In chronic forms the EOG is hardly impaired or not at all. These EOG alterations, however, are always related to the severity of anatomic changes and to the ERG impairment. In acute forms, such as arterial or venous occlusions, the EOG is almost constantly impaired with a slight reduction of absolute amplitude and a pathological Arden's ratio depending on the absence of lightrise.

Although there is almost general agreement on the behaviour of EOG in retinal vascular occlusions, no satisfactory explanation of electro-oculogram impairment in acute pathology of retinal circulation has been proposed.

In the present report we have studied some cases of central retinal vessel occlusions with the purpose of finding an explanation of EOG alteration in these vascular diseases.

MATERIAL AND METHODS

Thirty-nine patients with retinal vessel occlusions were studied: 29 venous obstructions (branch or total occlusions) and 10 arterial obstructions (branch or total occlusions). All the subjects had complete ocular and systemic examinations, including electrophysiological tests (ERG and EOG) and intravenous fluorescein fundus angiography. Patients, of both sex, aged 44–81, presented diffuse arteriosclerosis (general and in fellow eye).

The EOG was recorded for each eye by an EEG apparatus (Neuroaverager Mod. 1172 OTE Biomedica) with a time constant of 0,3 sec. The technique of testing is reported elsewhere (Ponte & Lauricella, 1971).

RESULTS

Twenty-one patients were affected by total retinal vessel occlusions (15 venous and 6 arterial). In these cases Arden's ratio was greatly altered in almost all patients. In 2 cases showing fundoscopic and fluoroangiographic pictures of central venous thrombosis caused by a primitive venous occlu-

* This paper has been supported by Grant No. 72.00851.04 of the Consiglio Nazionale delle Ricerche, Roma, Italy.

sion (venous stasis retinopathy: Hayreh, 1976; pre—occlusive syndrome: Sedney, 1976) the EOG was normal. The base value was almost always lower in the affected eye than in the fellow eye but it did not seem to depend on Arden's ratio changes.

Eighteen patients had branch occlusions (14 venouw and 4 arterial). The Arden's ratio was altered in the affected eye when three venous branches were occluded or when retinal oedema, caused by a branch arterial occlusion, involved half or more of the retina. The base value variations were independent from Arden's ratio changes being indifferently lower, equal or higher in the affected eye with respect to the fellow one.

DISCUSSION

Our results show that in total retinal vessel occlusions (either venous or arterial) the EOG is pathological: while the base value is slightly reduced the Arden's ratio is very pathological in consequence of the absence of light-rise. Only two subjects affected by a primitive venous occlusion showed a normal EOG.

In partial occlusions the EOG impairment corresponds with the number of branches involved: if one or two venous branches are occluded the EOG is normal, while if the occlusion concerns three branches the EOG is subnormal. In partial arterial obstruction the EOG impairment is dependent on the extention of ischemic retinal oedema.

It is difficult to explain the typical alterations of EOG in these retinal vascular diseases since the origin of light—sentitive component of EOG (light-rise) is still uncertain.

Some authors thought that the origin of the light-rise of EOG is in visual cells and pigment epithelium: as evidence of this theory there are EOG alterations in all diseases of the outer retinal layers and of the choroid. Others supposed that the origin of light—rise also depends on the activity of the internal retinal layers (see François et al., 1974). Imaizumi et al. (1968) proposed that the function of the internal retinal layers has some relation to the appearance of light—rise mainly originating in the outer layer of the retina.

If the origin of light—rise is only in the more external retinal layers, the EOG alterations in the central retinal artery occlusion or in the venous one consequent to a primitive arterial impairment could be explained by supposing that there is a concomitant ischemia of choroidal circulation. In this case, however, it should be admitted that ischemia of one of these circulations must be always coupled by ischemia of contiguous circles.

In ischemic papillopathy, on the contrary, caused by a Zinn-Haller's circle obstruction, there is neither ischemia of the retinal circulation because the fundus picture is normal, nor of the choroidal one because the EOG is normal (François et al., 1957; Ponte & Lauricella, 1971). Moreover, in central retinal venous thrombosis consequent to a primitive venous impairment, the possible occlusion of shunts between the choroidal veins and the central retinal one, it should be easily compensated by vortex veins drainage.

If the function of the internal retinal layers as well as of the outer layers, has some relation to the appearance of light-rise, its alteration would be easily explained by a retinal ischemia.

If this is true, it is possible to discriminate with EOG the two clinical forms of central retinal venous thrombosis identifiable at present with respect to the aetio-pathogenetic picture (Ponte et al., 1977):

1) with flat EOG, more frequent, typical of aged patients with arteriosclerotic diseases. Clinical features (haemorrhagic overflowing, retinal oedema) are a consequence of tissue hypoxia and metabolic acidosis caused by a primitive ischemia;

2) with normal EOG (also called venous stasis retinopathy, or pre-occlusive syndrome) typical of young patients. The pathogenesis is primitively venous as a consequence of a thrombotic occlusion: the tissue ischemic damage is subsequent and tardive, the visual acuity is better preserved.

SUMMARY

The EOG was studied in 21 patients with total retinal vessel occlusions (15 venous and 6 arterial) and in 18 patients with branch occlusion (14 venous and 4 arterial). In total occlusions light-rise is mainly affected: in branch occlusion the EOG alterations are related to the number of impaired branches. The authors think that EOG alteration can be a consequence of ischemia in internal retinal layers whose functional integrity is necessary to the appearance of light-rise in outer retinal layers. Therefore, it is possible to distinguish, by EOG recording, two clinical features of retinal vessel occlusions:

– the first, with flat EOG caused by a primitive arterial impairment;

– the second, with normal EOG caused by a primitive venous impairment.

REFERENCES

François, J. A. De Rouck, E. Cambie & A. Zanen. L'electrodiagnostic des affections retiniennes. *Bull. Soc. Belge Ophthal.* 166, (1974).

Hayreh, S. S. So-called 'Central retinal vein occlusion'. *Ophthalmologica* 172: *1–13*, (1976).

Imaizumi, K., F. Takahashi, G. Yoshida & K. Ogawa. The origin of electro-oculogram (EOG). VIth ISCERG Symposium, 1967. In: Advances in Electrophysiology and -pathology of the Visual System. Thieme, Leipzig, (1968).

Ponte, F. & M. Lauricella. L'elettro-oculografia nella pratica clinica. Casistica e considerazioni. Atti 53° Congresso S. O. I., Malta, (1971).

Ponte, F., C. Bruno, G. L. Casano & V. Abbadessa. La terapia medica delle occlusioni del circolo ottico-retinico. Atti 11° Congresso S. O. M., Palermo (1977).

Sedney, S. C. Photocoagulation in retinal vein occlusion. Thesis. *Docum. Ophthal.* 40 (1976).

Authors' address:
Clinica Oculistica dell 'Università
Via L. Giuffre 13
Palermo
Italy

Docum. Ophthal. Proc. Series, Vol. 15

SOME CONSIDERATIONS REGARDING THE EFFECT OF ANTIMALARIAL DRUGS ON THE EOG AND THE 'MACULAR EOG'

H. FRANCK, J.C. MULLER & A. BRONNER
(Strasbourg, France)

Since the early work in electrooculography performed by Arden and François, little real progress has been made, either from a theoretical point of view or in the clinical applications of the test. Amplitude changes give information about the standing potential, but, in fact, we still know very little about the mechanisms involved. The 'Arden ratio' has a clinical value insofar that it allows the detection of pigment alterations. The EOG also allows us to follow the progression of patients being treated with potentially retinotoxic antimalarial drugs. Traditionally, the only parameter measured is 'amplitude', In this paper, we want to draw attention to the 'time' parameter. Only a few authors have taken this time parameter into consideration (Arden & Barrada, 1962; Gliem, 1971; Krogh, 1975).

For present purposes we wish to consider two parameters: first, the real amplitude of the dark trough and light peak, which means the difference of the mean value of the two first minutes of examination, dark or light to the trough or peak; and second, the length of time from the beginning of dark adaptation to the dark trough, and from the beginning of illumination to the light peak. The technique of recording normal EOG has been reported in an earlier paper (Bronner, Franck & Müller, 1977).

For the 'macular EOG', small eye deflections sustending 10 degrees were elicited by following a moving target on a panel illuminated first with light, and, secondly, with red light (625 nm). Before each examination, the patient was dark adapted for 10 minutes. The EOG was recorded using the same technique as mentioned above.

These studies have been performed on patients treated with antimalarial drugs. The results were compared, on the one hand, with those of a control group and, on the other, with those of a group of patients suffering from pigmentary retinal dystrophy. This was done to see whether the parameters of time and amplitude were related to the degree of intoxication of the pigment epithelium in the first case, and, if they also depended on the degree of destruction of the pigmentary epithelium in case of pigmentary retinal dystrophy. The statistical test used was the 't' test.

ANALYZED PARAMETERS

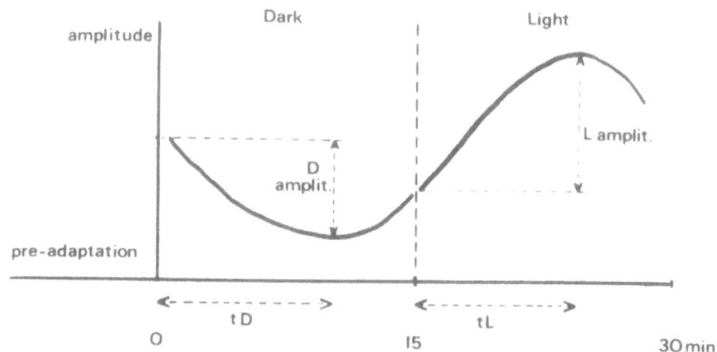

NORMAL EOG

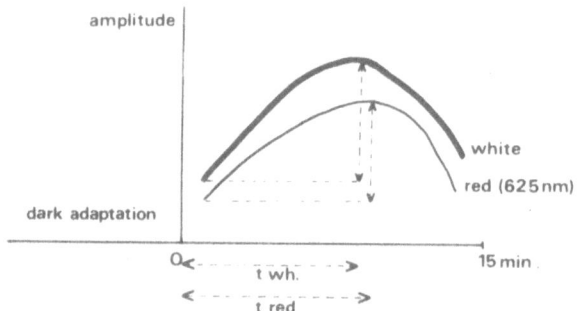

MACULAR EOG

Fig. 1.

RESULTS AND DISCUSSION

The patients treated for varying periods with antimalarial drugs (A.M.D.) were divided in two groups by their Arden ratio: those having a normal ratio, over 180, and those having a pathological ratio below 180; The group of patients with pigmentary retinal dystrophy had a pathological ratio below 120. All people of the control group had a normal Arden ratio greater than 180.

Results of parameter 'amplitude'

There appears no statistically significant difference between the means of the control group and the group of patients (Arden ratio over 180) treated with antimalarial drugs, for dark amplitude and for light amplitude. The group of patients with an abnormal Arden ratio also showed no significant difference in amplitude for dark and light response when compared to the normal EOG. Nevertheless, the difference became significant with 'macular EOG' for white (P = 5%) and red (P = 2%) illumination. Comparing the mean values of amplitude belonging to the group of patients having pigmented retinal dystrophy versus the control group, the parameter amplitude of dark, light, white and red appeared to be statistically highly significant (Fig. 2).

Results of parameter 'time'

Considering the parameter 'time' under the same conditions as parameter 'amplitude', it appears that the group of patients treated with antimalarial drugs and having a normal Arden ratio presents, for the normal EOG technique, a statistically significant diminution of time for the dark trough and for the light peak. It was not possible to notice any difference with the 'macular EOG' technique.

The group of patients having an Arden ratio below 180 presented the same significant results for the normal EOG, but with a higher degree of significance. In the 'macular EOG' technique, only the time of red peak diminished remarkably.

Patients with pigmentary retinal dystrophy presented a significantly high difference versus the control group, for normal EOG as well as for the 'macular EOG' (Fig. 3). Thus, it seems that the diminution of time, especially the time of the light peak, seems to be related to the functional state of the pigment epithelium and the visual cells.

Fig. 2.

PARAMETER 'AMPLITUDE'

		PRD $L/_D$ < 180		Control	AMD $L/_D$ < 180		AMD $L/_D$ > 180	
		P	mean au	mean	P	mean au	P	mean au
normal EOG	Dark	1%	065	241	ns	141	ns	169
	Light	1%	0.77	819	ns	727	ns	774
macular EOG	white	1%	230	580	5%	300	ns	477
	red	1%	036	415	2%	152	ns	481

a.u = arbitrary units

161

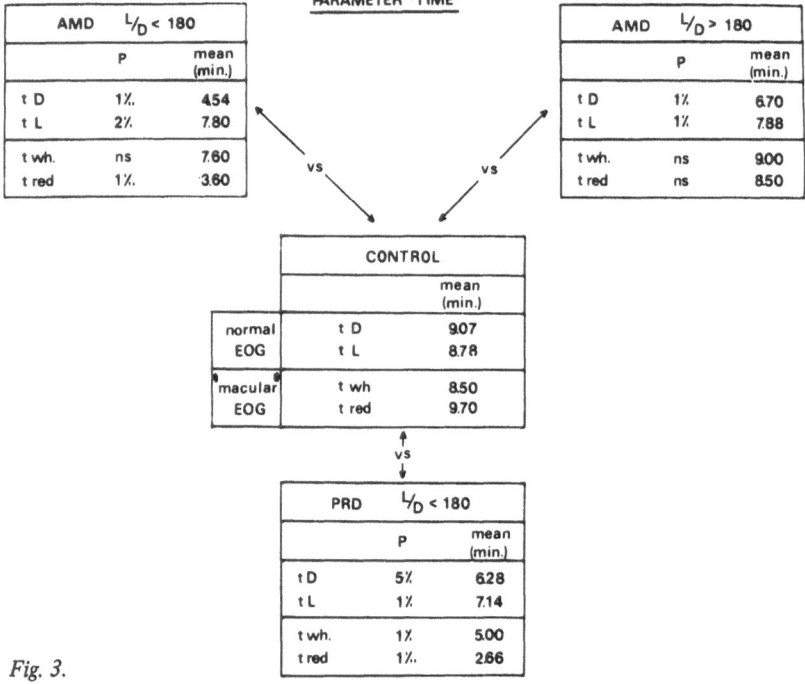

Fig. 3.

The damage induced by chloroquine and derivates occurs at the level of the pigmentary epithelium and the visual cells. As noted in experimentally induced retinopathy (Bernstein, 1967), it is probable that an important factor in the development of toxicity is related to the binding of the drug to the intracellular nuclear proteins. Enzyme systems may be involved. Thus, it seems that the parameter of time may be able to provide additional information relative to EOG dynamics.

CONCLUSIONS

It appears that the parameter 'time' is more sentitive than the parameter 'amplitude', or the Arden ratio. Time is affected, even if the Arden ratio is normal. Secondly, it seems that the shortening of time, especially for the light peak, is related to the amount of pathologic alteration of the retinal pigment epithelium. The shortest time to reach the light peak appears with the group of patients having a pigmentary retinal dystrophy.

SUMMARY

Parameters of 'time' and 'amplitude' have been tested on a group of patients treated with antimalarial drugs and on a group of patients having pigmentary retinal dystrophy. Parameter time appears to be more sensitive to alterations of the pigmentary epithelium than parameter 'amplitude' or Arden ratio.

REFERENCES

Arden, G.B. & A. Barrada. *Br. J. Ophthal.* 46: *468–482* (1962).

Bronner, A., H. Franck & J.C. Müller. *Soc. Ophtal. de l'Est* (in press).

Gliem, H. Abhandlung aus dem Gebiete der Augenheilkunde. Monographien 40. Thieme, Leipzig (1971).

E. Krogh. *Acta Ophthal.* 53: *563–575* (1975).

Authors' address:
Centre Hospitalier Régional
Clinique Ophtalmologique
Service d'exploration fonctionnelle électrophysiologique
1 Place de l'Hôpital
Strasbourg
France

VISUAL EVOKED RESPONSES TO
SQUARE WAVE REVERSING PATTERNS

W.R. BIERSDORF & C.C. WHISTLER
(Columbus, Ohio, USA)

The impetus for this study was in the clinic, to find a good technique for testing visual evoked responses of patients with visual acuity losses. One objective was to use pattern reversal stimulation to avoid contamination from luminance responses. Literature studies on pattern reversal stimulation of visual evoked responses have utilized two types of reversal. One type is sine wave reversal, such as employed by Spekreijse (1966), Behrman et al. (1972) Sokol & Bloom (1973) and others. Another type of stimulation is abrupt or 'square-wave' reversal, utilized by Armington et al. (1971), Johnson et al. (1966), Regan & Richards (1971) and Halliday et al. (1972). We decided to compare these two types of pattern reversal on the same normal subjects, to let us know what we might expect from patients. The evoked responses obtained were analysed by means of narrow band electronic filters and comparisons drawn between the two types of stimulation.

METHOD

The stimuli were checkerboard transparencies of the Vectograph type with adjacent squares linearly polarized at right angles. Two types of analysing shutters were used. The first type was a rotating disc of linearly polarizing material, producing a sinusoidal reversal of contrast when placed in the light beam containing a Vectograph. The second type of shutter was an electronic shutter modified to switch two pieces of linearly polarized material at 90° in the light beam. This produced the abrupt or square wave reversal of checkerboard contrast. The transition time for this reversal was 6 msec. An additional fixed analyser in the beam could be adjusted slightly to ensure luminance equality of the two sets of checks. Noise from a ventilating fan masked auditory shutter clicks for the subject. The projector light source and shutters were outside the shielded recording room. The light beam entering through a wall aperture illuminated Fresnel lens and ground glass diffusors to then illuminate a Vectograph by transmission. The subject viewed the illuminated checkerboard through a circular aperture in the same plane of 7.5° visual angle. The subject was seated at a distance of 1 meter from

*This research was supported in part by Grant EYO0454 from the National Institutes of Health.

the checkerboard in an otherwise dark room. The checkerboards of 20 cd/m² average luminance were viewed monocularly. Contrast defined in the usual manner was held constant at 0.87.

Recording of the evoked potentials was monopolar from O_z (International 10-20 EEG System) to one ear lobe. A ground electrode was attached to the mastoid. Band pass of the amplifiers was from 0.2 to 50 Hz. The evoked responses from sinusoidal stimulation were simultaneously analysed by narrow band electronic filters (Krohnhite) set at minimum bandwidth with amplitude decreases on both sides of peak at 24 db per octave. Simultaneous measures of fundamental and second harmonic response were obtained. Responses (64) were averaged by an average response computer (Hewlett-Packard 5480) and permanent records obtained by an x-y recorder.

Most of the data presented are on two subjects, while essential findings were confirmed on two additional subjects. All subjects had normal acuity (20/20 or better) and no evidence of visual system disease.

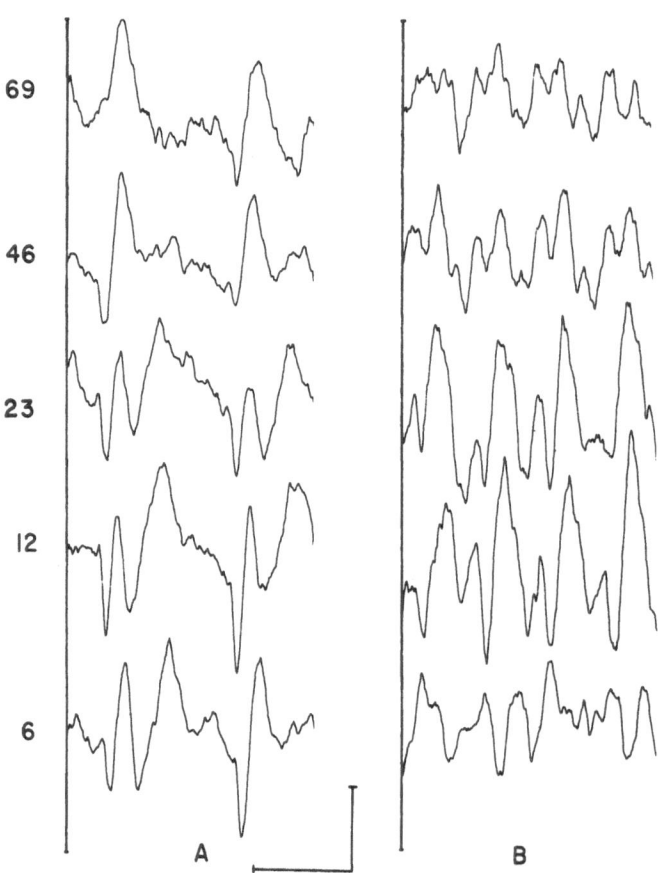

Fig. 1. Evoked responses to square wave reversal (A) and sine wave reversal (B) at four reversals per sec. Check size in minutes of arc at left. Calibrations differ: (A) 10 microvolts and 200 msec; (B) 5 microvolts and 400 msec. Positive upward. Subject C W.

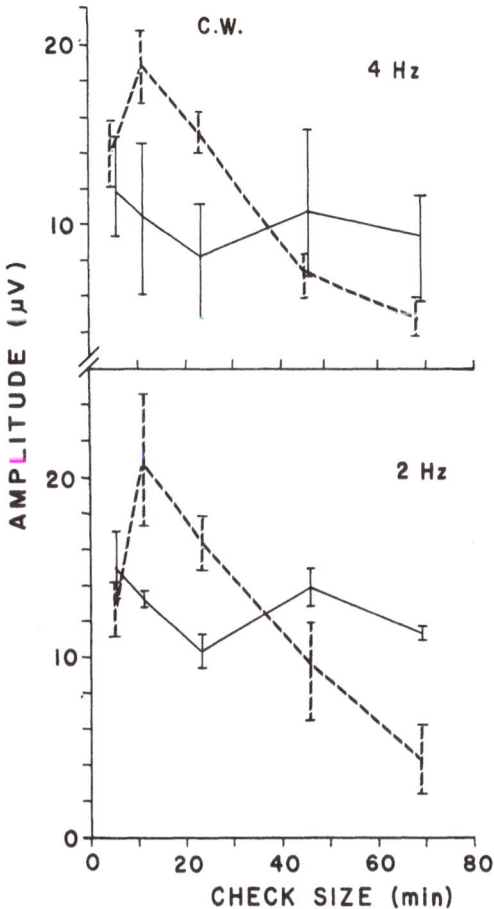

Fig. 2. Amplitudes of square wave reversal for N_1-P_1 (solid line) and N_1-P_2 (dashed line) at two reversal rates. Vertical lines indicate range. Check size (abscissa) in minutes of arc. Subject C W.

RESULTS

Evoked responses to five check sizes are presented in Fig. 1. On the left are responses to square wave reversal, and on the right to sine wave reversal. Both reversal rates are at 4 Hz (4 reversals per sec) but the left column illustrates 2 reversals, while the right shows 4 reversals with a different analysis time. Check size is represented in minutes of visual angle. Inspection of the sine wave column (B) for the middle check sizes shows 4 large peaks ('fundamental') alternating with 4 small peaks originating as the second harmonic of the stimulation frequency. The sine wave responses were measured from these potentials after passage through narrow band filters set at the fundamental and second harmonic of the stimulation rate.

For the middle check sizes, each square wave reversal (A column) produced two prominent positive peaks (P_1, P_2) each preceded by a negative peak (N_1, N_2). Amplitudes of these peaks were measured from the preceding peak, or from the baseline for N_1. Examination of these amplitudes showed two different functions of check size. N_1, and P_2 showed amplitude functions reaching a maximum at an intermediate or small check size. In contrast, P_1, and N_2 showed amplitude functions nearly constant, relatively independent of check size. To show the differences between these two functions, we have plotted the two positive peak amplitude functions measured from a common N_1 in the following figures.

Figure 2 illustrates evoked potential amplitude from square wave reversal from the same subject as the previous figure. Two reversal rates are shown at 2 Hz and 4 Hz. At each rate there is a solid line representing the amplitude of the 100 msec positive peak (P_1) and a dashed line representing the 200 msec potitive peak (P_2). The variance indicated is the range of the average data for each of 3 days runs. P_1 is roughly constant amplitude across check sizes, while Pz reaches a peak at a middle check size (12 min) with decreasing amplitudes for smaller and larger check sizes. Looked at more closely, P_1 is larger than P_2 for the largest checks. P_2 then increases for the middle check sizes to become larger than P_1. For the smallest check size used (6 min), P_1 increases to reach a small peak. Similar results held for the 2 and 4 Hz reversal rates. Stimulation was also performed at an 8 Hz rate, but only one peak could be recorded, as P_2 from the previous reversal interfered with P_1 from each alternation.

Figure 3 illustrates evoked potential amplitudes also from square wave reversal for a second subject. Again, we see a rough constancy of amplitude

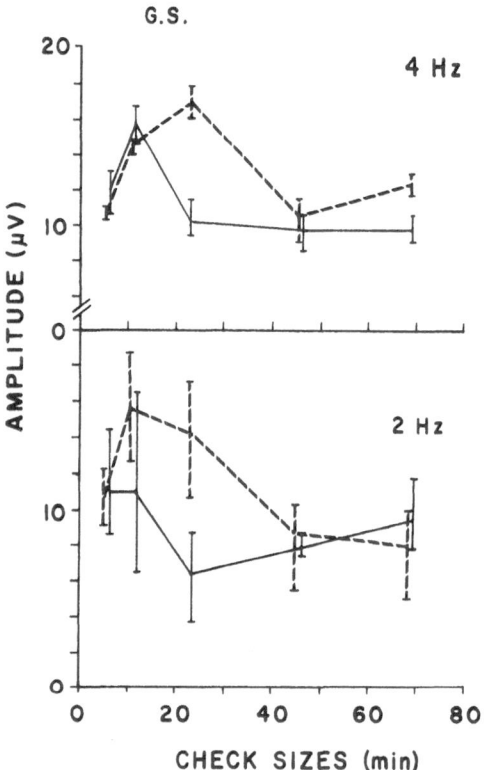

Fig. 3. Amplitudes of square wave reversal for subject G S. Legend as in preceding figure.

Table 1. Peak latencies of P_1 and P_2 components.

Check size	69	46	23	12	6
P_1					
2 Hz	96	92	96	102	111
4 Hz	102	101	98	102	115
8 Hz	103	100	100	104	116
P_2					
2 Hz	202	193	204	205	212
4 Hz	215	219	222	214	226

for P_1 with a peak amplitude for P_2 at a middle check size. A more detailed inspection shows P_1 reaching a peak at a smaller check size than does P_2, as was also the case for the previous subject.

Table 1 shows the peak latencies for the two positive peaks. These are the averages of the two subjects in Fig. 2 and 3. Both P_1 and P_2 latencies tended to be somewhat shorter for the middle check sizes and become somewhat longer for the smallest check sizes.

Figure 4 shows the filtered amplitudes from sine wave reversal stimulation. These are averages of three subject's data for the fundamental and second harmonic components. Four different reversal rates were employed. The shape of these curves are similar to that previously reported from sine wave reversing gratings (Behrman et al., 1972). An 8 Hz rate produced the highest amplitudes for the fundamental with higher and lower rates producing smaller responses. For the second harmonic, 8 Hz also produced the maximum response. For both components, maximum response is obtained for the middle check sizes of 12 or 23 min.

In Figure 5, we have a comparison of the amplitude of the fundamental sine wave response with P_1 from the square wave stimulation. As in the pre-

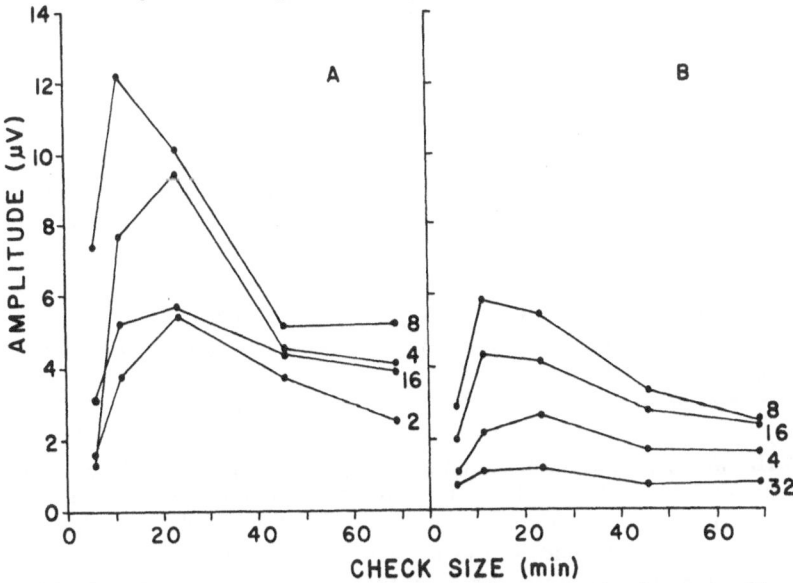

Fig. 4. Sine wave reversal amplitudes (A) fundamental or stimulus frequency, (B) second harmonic. Parameter is reversals per sec. Average CW, GS, CM.

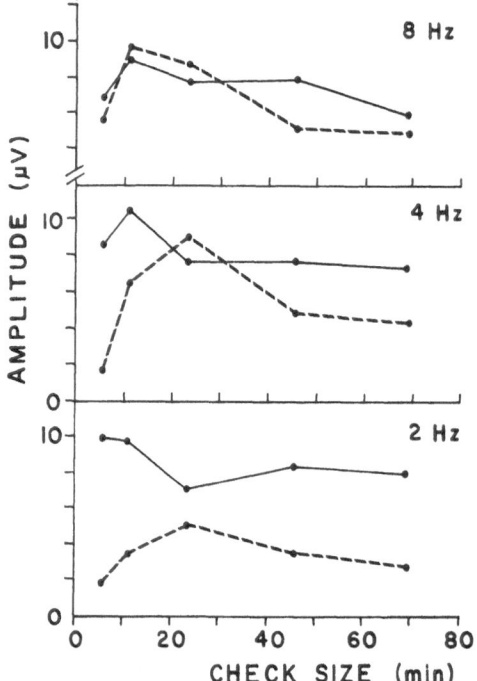

Fig. 5. Comparison of N_1-P_1 amplitudes square wave (solid line) with fundamental amplitudes sine wave reversal (dashed line) at three reversal rates. Average CW & GS.

vious figures, P_1 amplitude (solid line) is approximately constant, regardless of the reversal rate (2, 4 or 8 Hz), or of check size. It reaches a small peak at or near 6 min. In contrast, the sine wave response peaks at a middle check size of 12 or 23 min. In addition, it is considerably larger at the faster reversal rates than at 2 Hz, as was shown in the previous figure.

DISCUSSION

What is the relation between the evoked potentials obtained from these two types of stimulation? Both the late positive peak (P_2) from square wave reversal and the sine wave reversal curves show amplitude curves peaking for the middle check sizes of 12 or 23 min. There is a difference between the two in that P_2 amplitude is larger than the sine wave fundamental response. However, the shapes of the curves are similar. If the time course (duration) of the two responses are considered, they are very similar. We would like to suggest that the sine wave fundamental response and P_2 of the square wave reversal are basically the same response.

In an attempt to test this possibility, we estimated the duration of the N_1-P_2 response as about a quarter of a second and set the electronic filter at 4 Hz. We then analyzed the square wave reversal responses with this filter. At both 2 and 4 Hz stimulation rates, this filter produced sinusoidal responses containing apparently only one frequency. It was peaked as a function of check size in the middle sizes like the sine wave reversal data. For 8 Hz stimulation rate, however, the 4 Hz filter produced a response indicating two interfering frequencies. This was apparently due to the interference of

170

P_2 with P_1 at this fast stimulation rate. In attempting to isolate the P_1 response, we set the filter at 8 Hz and analysed the square wave reversal responses. This time the amplitude function was flat as a function of check size and similar to the P_1 data.

Is there a correlate of the P_1 component in the sine wave reversal data? The answer seems to be negative. P_1 amplitude as a function of check size is relatively constant, remaining large for large check sizes, and reaching a small peak amplitude at a check size smaller than that for P_2. This cannot be equated with the second harmonic of the sine wave response. The second harmonic basically has the same shape of curve vs. check size as the fundamental sine wave response. Electronic filtering of the sine wave reversal responses with the 8 Hz filter produced an amplitude curve peaked for the middle check sizes, rather than flat, as was the case for P_1 of the square wave reversal responses.

The waveform of the responses obtained here with two negative and two positive peaks to square wave reversal is similar to that reported for abruptly appearing sine wave grating patterns by Kulikowski & Leisman (1973). Kulikowski has suggested an interpretation of these two peaks based on recent animal research (1976). Two different types of retinal ganglion cells have been identified in the cat. Human psychophysical research has also provided evidence for separate visual detectors for pattern and for flicker or movement. For large gratings, the sensitivity for movement is higher than that for pattern.

The amplitude of P_1 is higher than P_2 in this region of large checks and, thus, may be identified as the flicker or movement VER. On the other hand, the late positive P_2 was identified as the pattern response (Kulikowski & Leisman, 1973). Recently Kulikowski has proposed subtracting the reversal VER from the on-off VER to obtain the pattern response (1976). In this interpretation, both peaks are present in the pattern response.

As this manuscript was being prepared, we found a recent report on sudden appearance of sine-wave gratings (Parker & Salzen, 1977). These authors also measured two positive peaks in their VER's. The amplitude functions of check size were similar to what we have found for square wave reversing checkerboards. P_1 was of relatively constant amplitude for bar widths down to near the minimum perceptible. P_2, however, reached a peak amplitude for a middle bar size with decreases for both small and large bar widths. Peak latency findings were somewhat different from our results in showing a monotonic increase in latency for decreasing bar width. Higher contrast gratings showed smaller latency increases, however.

Thus, the waveforms obtained here to high contrast wave pattern reversal at low rates appear to be similar to those reported by other investigators for square wave appearance of grating patterns. It is suggested the second positive peak may be the same response obtained at stimulation frequency for sine wave reversal stimulation.

SUMMARY

Visual evoked responses were obtained to high contrast reversing checkerboard patterns from 4 normal subjects. Two types of reversal were employed: sine wave, and abrupt or square wave. Rates of reversal were 2, 4 and 8 Hz for square wave, and 2, 4, 8, and 16 Hz for sine wave. The VER's from square wave reversal showed prominent positive peaks near 100 and 200 msec, each preceded by negative peaks. As a function of check size, the second positive peak (P_2) showed a peak amplitude for check sizes 12 to 23 minutes of arc, with decreasing amplitudes for larger and smaller check sizes. The first positive peak (P_1) amplitude was relatively constant over check size, although reaching a small peak near 6 minutes. P_1 and P_2 amplitudes were independent of reversal rate. The VER's from sine wave reversal showed amplitudes versus check size similar to that of P_2, but were dependent on reversal rate. Maximum amplitudes were obtained at 8 Hz with lower amplitudes at higher and lower rates. Second harmonic responses from sine wave reversal showed functions similar to the fundamental, although smaller. Evoked response waveforms are compared to previous research.

REFERENCES

Armington, J. C., T. R. Corwin & R. Marsetta. Simultaneously recorded retinal and cortical responses to patterned stimuli. *J. Opt. Soc. Am.* 61: *1514–1521* (1971).

Behrman, J., S. Nissim & G. B. Arden. A clinical method for obtaining pattern visual evoked responses. In: The Visual System (ed. G.B. Arden), Plenum, New York. pp. 199–206 (1972).

Halliday, A. M., W. I. McDonald & J. Mushin. Delayed visual evoked response in optic neuritis. *Lancet* 1: *982–985* (1972).

Johnson, E. P., L. A. Riggs & A. M. L. Schick. Photopic retinal potentials evoked by phase alternation of a barred pattern. In: Clinical Electroretinography. Pergamon London pp. 75–91, (1966).

Kulikowski, J. J. Methods for separating pattern and movement-related evoked potentials. *J. Physiol.* 257: *2–3P* (1976).

Kulikowski, J. J. & G. Leisman. The effect of nitrous oxide on the relation between the evoked potential and contrast threshold, *Vision Res.* 13: *2079–2086* (1973).

Parker, D. M. & E. A. Salzen. The spatial selectivity of early and late waves within the human visual evoked response. *Perception* 6: *85–95* (1977).

Regan, D. & W. Richards. Independence of evoked potentials and apparent size. *Vision Res.* 11: 679–684 (1971).

Sokol, S. & B. Bloom. Visually evoked cortical responses of amblyopes to a spatially alternating stimulus. *Invest. Ophthal.* 12: *936–939* (1973).

Spekreijse, H. Analysis of EEG responses in man evoked by sine wave modulated light, Thesis. Univ. Amsterdam (1966).

Authors' address:
Department of Ophthalmology, and
Institute for Research in Vision
Ohio State University
Columbus, Ohio 43212
USA

Docum. Ophthal. Proc. Series, Vol. 15

UNFAMILIAR EFFECTS OF FLICKER ON THE HUMAN EEG*

G. DAGNELIE, T. J. T. P. VAN DEN BERG & D. REITS

(Amsterdam, The Netherlands)

INTRODUCTION

Over the past two decades, many clinicians have adopted the use of averagers to measure visually evoked responses. Apart from light flashes, the principal stimuli for these measurements have been sine wave modulated homogeneous fields, introduced in electrophysiology by Kamp et al. (1960). The value of this easily definable stimulus has been proved over the years, e.g. by Spekreijse (1966), who proposed models for the human luminance system based on studies using this stimulus.

In the case of flash stimulation a variability in amplitude and/or latency of the evoked response has been reported in literature, and various authors have tried to specify the nature of such fluctuations: Trehub (1965) argued that the amplitude of responses to photic stimulation fluctuates, Swadlow & Waxman (1975) found a variability in conduction latencies of optic tract axons following antidromic stimulation. Also, considerable effort has been spent on the description of fluctuations in the EEG subsequent to flash stimulation (e.g. Ciganek, 1969) and in spontaneous EEG. Fluctuations of responses to sine wave modulated light have received very little, if any, attention; however, in our experiments we have occasionally observed the following phenomena, especially at low stimulus intensities:

In an apparently normal subject measurement of an average evoked response is started; initially, an average response seems to develop, but after a certain time it gradually declines and finally may even disappear; alternatively, at a later stage in the procedure, the shape of the average response may differ markedly from the one that seemed to develop initially. Since these results seemed to indicate the presence of fluctuations, we have set up a series of experiments in which fluctuations of the response and changes in background EEG related to sinusoidal stimulation were the main points of interest.

An example of the appearance of both phenomena is given in Fig. 1: by alternating periods of sinusoidal stimulation and of steady illumination, we obtained the two power spectra shown in this figure, permitting a

*Part of this research was supported by the Organization of Health Research (TNO), The Hague, The Netherlands.

reliable comparison of the EEG signals in the two situations. One expects to find peaks at the stimulus frequency and at the second harmonic in the spectrum obtained during modulation; however, there also is an increase of background activity, and around the first harmonic 'sidebands' can be observed. The increase in background activity was found to be strongest in the alpha frequency range, irrespective of the stimulus frequency, and amounted to a factor of 2 in power. In this paper, however, we will devote our attention to the sidebands, since these may have been caused by response fluctuations.

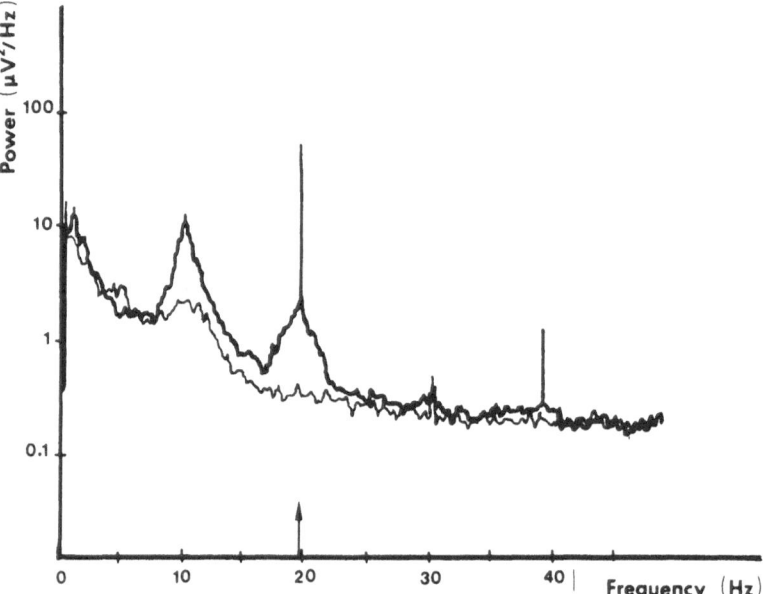

Fig. 1. Power spectra calculated from the EP of a normal female subject (inion-ear derivation) during a 10 min experiment in which alternating 8 s periods of sinusoidal modulation and steady illumination were presented. Average stimulus intensity was 600 lux, stimulus frequency 19.5 Hz (arrow), modulation depth 50%. Power is plotted on a logarithmic scale. The alternation of modulated and steadily illuminated periods eliminates the influence of gradual changes in background EEG on the results. Stimulus generation and signal analysis are controlled by the same computer time base in order to prevent imperfect sampling.

ANALYSIS AND RESULTS

If the amplitude of a sinusoidal signal is modulated in time, the peak in its power spectrum will be flanked by symmetrical sidebands; this fact may be familiar to many readers from AM radio technique. One can obtain similar sidebands by modulation of the delay time of a sinusoidal signal with constant amplitude; in this case some periods of the signal are stretched in time and others are compressed proportionally, a situation resembling the Doppler effect in sound. This point is illustrated in part 1 of Fig. 2, where three signals and their power spectra are compared as a model; the addition of noise symbolizes the presence of background EEG activity in a response signal.

174

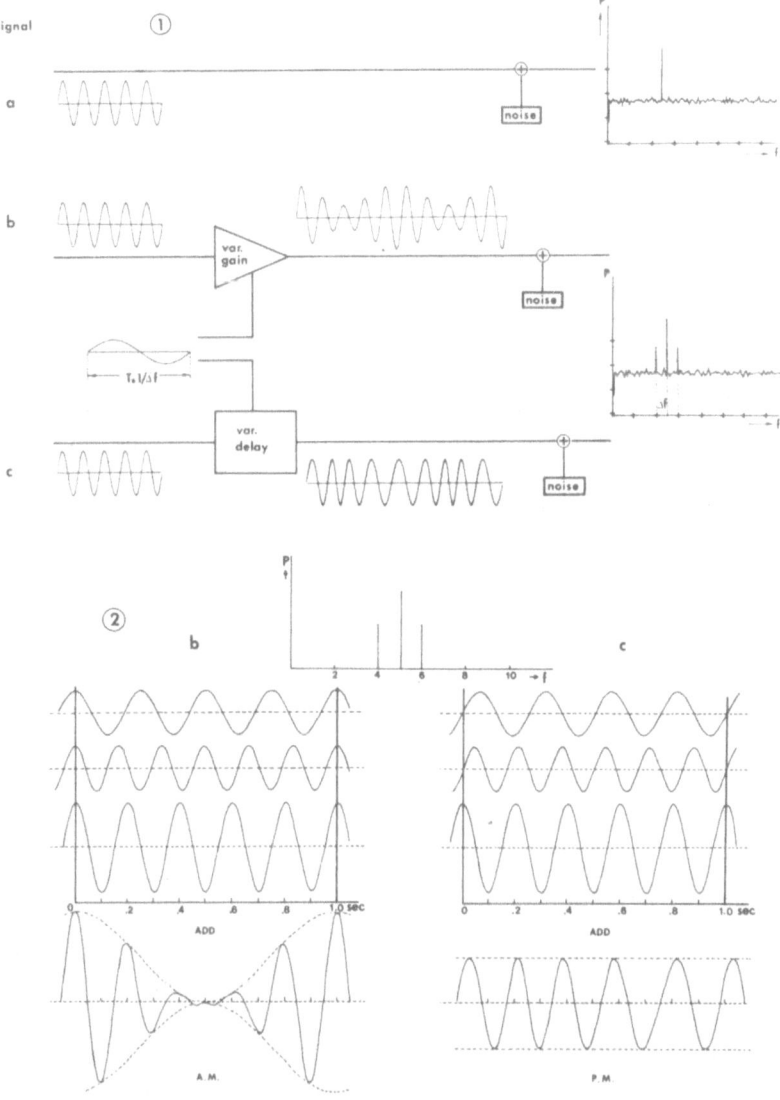

Fig. 2. Part 1: Spectral analysis of: a) sinusoidal signal plus noise; b) amplitude modulated (AM) sinusoid plus noise; c) latency (or phase) modulated (PM) sinusoid plus
noise. Situations b) and c) have indistinguishable power spectra, since they contain the
same symmetrical sidebands. Part 2: Situations b) and c) from part 1 can be
distinguished if the relative phases of the principal component and the symmetrical
sideband components are considered. Only the noise-free situation is shown.
Note: the power spectrum of situation c) is only valid to a first approximation. Higher
order terms, leading to smaller peaks at larger distances from the principal component,
are needed for exact calculation, but these do not affect the validity of the analysis
demonstrated here.

175

Situation a) represents an undistorted response, resulting in a power spectrum with a single peak superimposed on the noise spectrum.

In situation b) the signal enters an amplifier modulating its amplitude sinusoidally around the incoming value, with a frequency Δf. As a result of this modulation the power spectrum of the output signal shows two symmetrical sideband peaks. The power of these peaks is determined by the strength of the fluctuations, their distance to the principal peak is just Δf; therefore, the slower the fluctuations, the closer the side components lie to the principal component.

In c) the signal enters a delay that varies sinusoidally, with the same frequency Δf as in b) ; the amplitudes of input and output signal are equal. The latency modulation, visible in the signal as wavelength distortion, results in sideband peaks similar to those in b) (to a first approximation). The width of the sidebands is again determined by the modulation frequency Δf, their size depends on the difference between shortest and longest delay times.

Although the power spectra in b) and c) are identical, a distinction between the two can be made on the basis of the phase relationship between the three components (Dagnelie, 1977). This is illustrated qualitatively in part 2 of Fig. 2, where noise has been left out for simplicity, and decomposition of a power spectrum like that in b) and c) of part 1 is shown. Both situation b) and c) show a decomposition into a 5 Hz sine wave, corresponding to the principal component, and smaller 4 and 6 Hz sine waves, corresponding to the side components, but the relative positions (phases) of the components differ between the two situations. If, as is the case in b), the *maxima* of the side components coincide at T = 0 with the maximum of the principal component, then the maxima of the side components will, after a certain period (in this case after 1 s), coincide again with another maximum of the principal component. A comparable rule can be found for c), where *zero crossings* of the side components coincide at T = 0 and T = 1s with a maximum of the principal component. However, a change from b) into c) will never occur, as one will readily accept when realizing that the sum of the three components on the left is indeed signal b (amplitude modulation), whereas the sum of the signals on the right is equal to signal c (latency modulation).

Discrimination between amplitude and latency fluctuations is, therefore, possible on the basis of the relative phases of symmetrical side components and the principal component. In practice, two additional facts should be considered: first, fluctuations will never be sinusoidal, but may be expected to have a random character and to contain a band of frequencies, giving rise to sidebands like those found in Fig. 1. There one expects slow fluctuations to be predominant as the sidebands are strongest next to the principal peak, and one can analyze such sidebands by pairs of components. Secondly, the presence of noise complicates the analysis; therefore significant results with EEG signals require impractically long experiments if signal to noise ratios (SNR) are poor. This is the main reason why most of our results have been obtained in the medium frequency range, where relatively good SNR values can be found.

Two examples of the results of our analysis are shown in Fig. 3. In one case the analysis indicates strong fluctuations in amplitude, in the other case latency fluctuations seem to have been present in the evoked response.

DISCUSSION

From the left half of Fig. 3 it can be concluded that the amplitude of one or more harmonic components of a visually evoked response may vary considerably. If one considers the largest response to be a significant measure for the VEP amplitude, one may end up with an averaged response amplitude that is much lower than the desired value; also the shape of the averaged response will be distorted if not all harmonic components fluctuate to the same extent.

From the right half of Fig. 3 it may be concluded that latency fluctuations are relatively unimportant at medium frequencies, compared to the response period (in our case 55 ms). One should, however, be careful, since in our analysis Δf is at least 0.25 Hz. In that case fluctuations whose periods exceed 8 s will contribute very little to the sidebands; their activity is mainly stored in the principal component. Comparison of averaged responses from many short intervals may reveal these slow fluctuations; we have been able to show that such fluctuations do occur and that they can be latency fluctuations. In some cases they reduced the average of medium frequency responses as measured after a long time to less than half the actual size. It is clear that severe distortion of response shapes is probable in those cases, since the reduction is strongly frequency dependent.

The main purpose of this paper is to issue a warning: one should not consider an averaged evoked response the result of a static phenomenon; there

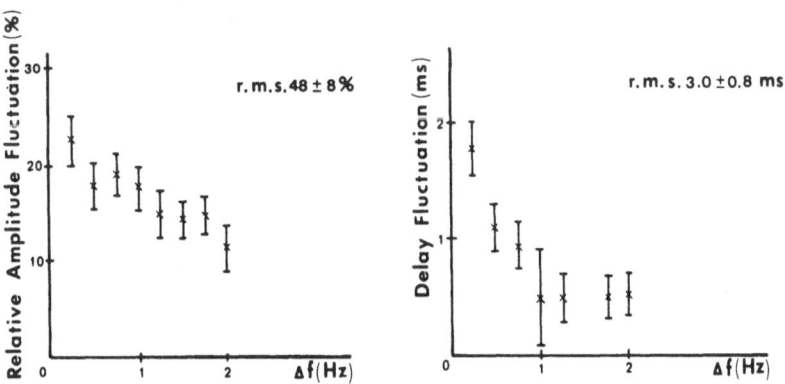

Fig. 3. Two examples obtained as a result of sideband analysis. Δf represents the frequency difference between the principal component and each of a pair of side components, and is equal to the frequency of the fluctuations.
Left: Analysis of the signal whose power spectrum is shown in fig. 1 indicates the presence of strong amplitude fluctuations.
Right: Analysis of an experiment using 18 Hz stimulation (closed eyes) indicates the presence of latency fluctuations.

is always a possibility that its shape has been influenced by the averaging procedure itself. In order to obtain an indication of the degree to which responses fluctuate, it is advisable to calculate power spectra of the EEG signals, even if one does not have the means to analyse sidebands. Preferably, power spectra should be obtained using alternating periods of stimulation and of steady illumination.

REFERENCES

Ciganek, L. Variability of the human visual evoked potential: normative data. *E. E. G. Journal* 27: *35–42* (1969).

Dagnelie, G. Non-stationary aspects of the visually evoked response to sinusoidally modulated light. Master's thesis, Amsterdam (1977).

Kamp, A., C. W. Sem-Jacobsen, W. Storm van Leeuwen & L. H. van der Tweel. Cortical responses to modulated light in the human subject. *Acta physiol. scand.* 48: 1–12 (1960).

Spekreijse, H. Analysis of E. E. G. responses in man evoked by sine wave modulated light. Thesis, Amsterdam (1966).

Swadlow, H. A. & S. G. Waxman. Observations on impulse conduction along central axons. *Proc. Nat. Acad. Sci.* 72: *5156–5159* (1975).

Trehub, A. Spontaneous slow modulation of flicker-evoked response in human brain. *E. E. G. Journal* 19: *182–184* (1965).

Authors' address:
The Netherlands Ophthalmic Research Institute
104, Eerste Helmerstraat
Amsterdam
The Netherlands

ELECTRO–PERIMETRY BY MEANS OF THE SCOTOPIC VECP*

E. ADACHI–USAMI, M. MISAGO & N. KANAYAMA
(Hamamatsu, Japan)

It is well-established in the human scotopic vision that psychophysical studies on the different parts of the retina show close correspondence to the anatomical data, i.e. distribution of rods in the retina (Østerberg, 1935).

Recently it has been shown that measurements of latency of a scotopic VECP recorded from the scalp above the occipital cortex in man confirmed such psychophysical data of spectral sensitivity function, sensitivity in the course of dark adaptation, temporal and spatial summation (Vaughan et al., 1966; Adams et al., 1969; Wooten, 1972; Huber & Adachi–Usami, 1972; Adachi–Usami & Kellermann, 1973).

In 1973 we reported that spatial summation measured with the scotopic VECP latency was similar to that measured by sensory thresholds for a field up to 9° around the fixation point. For technical reasons larger fields have not been tested. Therefore, in the present study the peripheral scotopic VECP and possibility of sensitivity mapping or perimetry were investigated using the two following approaches: (A) mapping from the center of the retina to its periphery using small circular stimuli, and (B) concentric sensitivity contouring by displacing concentric ring stimuli centered around the fixation point radially at the retina.

METHODS

The optical system is shown in a previous paper (Adachi, 1977). Light from a xenon arc was brought to focus at the shutter to produce a test stimulus with a duration of 100 msec, then, it was led to the remodelled Goldmann perimeter with a glass fiber guide of 10 mm in inner diameter. Stimuli were manually triggered at random with an average rate of about 0.5 Hz. The terminal of a glass fiber guide was inserted into the cylindrical cabinet at the upper part of the sphere where the original source should be. The original light source was, then, replaced to the lower part of the sphere and used as adapting light. The visual angle of the target was set at $1°30'$ and $5°30'$. A red light emitting diode of $15'$ visual angle was placed at the center of the sphere as a fixation light.

A circular stimulus of a $14°11'$ radius and ring stimuli of 5°, 10°, 15°, 20°,

* Supported by grant No. 187013 from the Ministry of Education, Japan.

25°, 30° inner radi: respectively having equal areas to the area of a circular stimulus of a $14°11'$ rdius were formed with the diaphragm put at the position where the beam passed through lens$_4$ of the previous paper, and projected onto the screen situated 25 cm from the eye. In order to exclude stray light, the screen, excepting a projected circular or ring area, was covered with black paper. A light emitting diode was placed in the center of the presented stimuli as a fixation light. The other device was the same as the one described above.

The VECP was recorded with an electrode placed 3 cm above the inion, the indifferent electrode was on the earlobe. Potentials were amplified with a bandpass of $1.5-300$ Hz and fed into an averager. Two hundred responses were averaged.

The subject, whose right eye was dilated, lay in a completely dark room. the eye was exposed to a constant white light of 2.0 log ft−L for 5 minutes which was followed by 20 min dark adaptation. Measurements began with the determination of the sensory threshold. A test light illumination was then increased in 0.15 log steps. Following each step, a VECP was recorded. All experiments were done with central fixation. Seven normal observers served as subjects. For each subject at least three runs were performed.

All measurements reported here referred to the latency from the onset of the stimulus to the second negative trough N_2 of the scotopic VECP. Criterion latency for determination of the retinal illumination was 250 msec. Positivity of the scalp electrode is shown as an upward deflection.

RESULTS

Mapping experiments on the temporal retina with small circular stimuli

Scotopic VECPs to the test fields of $1°30'$ and $5°30'$ in diameters were measured for different retinal eccentricities, $5°$, $8°$, $9°$ . . . temporal from the fovea on the horizontal meridian.

Scotopic VECPs to a circular stimulus of $1°30'$ in diameter

Figure 1 shows scotopic VECPs in response to stimuli falling on the different parts of the temporal retina and Figure 2 demonstrates N_2 latency vs the log of test light illumination obtained from Figure 1. This subject, Y.M., was found to have VECP sensitivity up to the farthest peripheral retina, $10°$ from the fovea among seven subjects.

From these records, (1) all records had N_2 latency of around 250 msec, (2) amplitudes decreased as the stimulus was moved from the center to the periphery, and (3) VECP sensitivity increased with moving the stimulus from the center to its periphery, were observed. The increase of the sensitivity at the peripheral retina was also found by sensory measurements. The VECP threshold (test light illumination necessary for obtaining N_2 latency of 250 msce) was, however, 1.6 log units higher than the sensory threshold. Three subjects out of seven showed the detectable VECP being restricted to the retina within $10°$ peripheral retina from the fovea, and the other four only up to $5°-8°$.

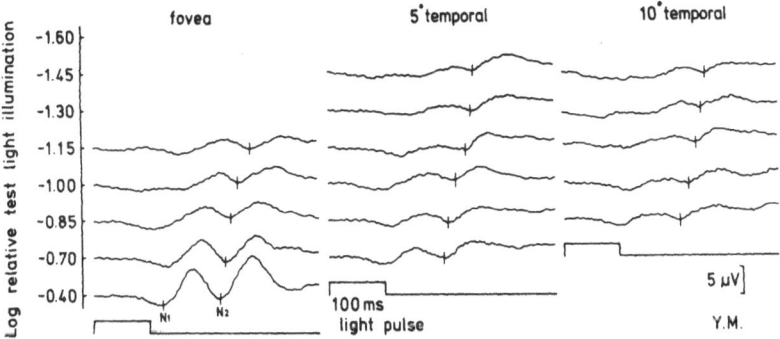

Fig. 1. Scotopic VECPs to a green (λ = 522 nm) test light of a 1°30′ diameter for three different retinal positions stimulated. Stimulus duration (100 msec) is indicated below records. Short lines on the records are points measured as N_2 latency (period between the onset of the stimulus and N_2). No VECP is obtainable with stimulation on the retina over 10° apart from the fovea. Sensory threshold values are indicated with arrows in Figure 2.

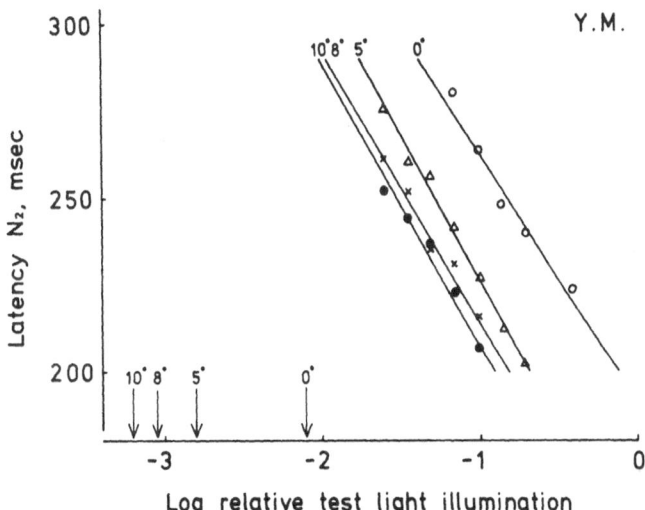

Fig. 2. Measurements of the scotopic VECP N_2 latency vs the log of relative test light illumination for a test field of a 1°30′ diameter falling on the central retina (open circles), horizontally 5° temporal from the fovea (triangles), 8° (crosses) and 10° (filled circles). Arrows indicate data of sensory measurements. Subject, Y.M.

The VECP amplitude disappeared with stimulation of over those critical perimetric angles.

Circular stimulus of 5°30′ in diameter

Instead of a test field of 1°30′, a stimulus of 5°30′ was tried in the subject, Y.M.. It was seen in the result that no VECP could be obtained with stimulation of temporal eccentricities of over 10° and in the range where the VECP was detectable (0°–10°), N_2 latency vs the log test light illumination

181

curves were displaced leftward by 0.5 log units compared to the curves for 1°30' stimulus.

The ratio of a test field area of 1°30' stimulus to that of 5°30' was 1.13 log units, a spatial summation index of 0.44 was obtained. This meant that Piper's law was proved by means of the scotopic VECP in this retinal position.

Next place, using higher test light illumination which was 2.5 log units above the absolute threshold, the VECP at a peripheral region was studied in the subject, M.T., whose VECP sensitivity was restricted to the retina at 5° from the fovea. Though VECPs were clearly observed even for stimulation at 50° periphery, no difference in amplitudes and latencies was seen in each record. Besides, the fact that the subject reported flashing of the whole sphere suggested that the responses recorded were caused by stray light falling on the whole retina.

In order to exclude stray light, a constant adapting light of −1.05 log ft-L was given during VECP recordings. In this way, no VECP could be obtained with over 5° peripheral stimulation.

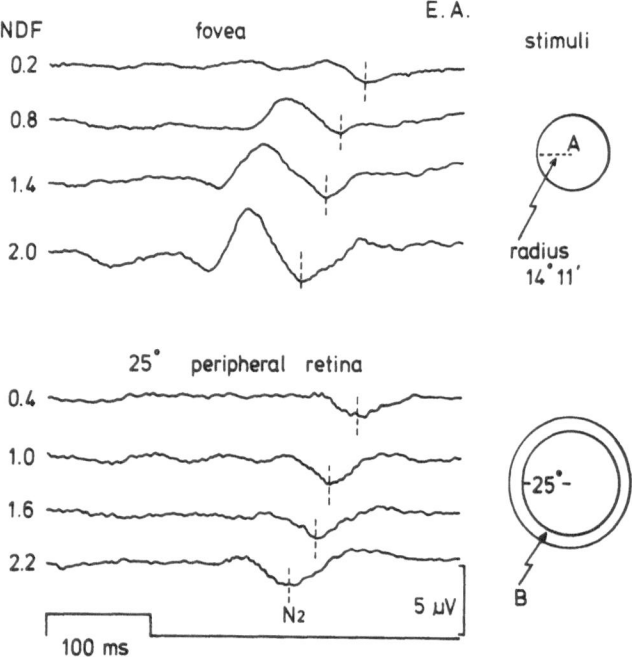

Fig. 3. Scotopic VECPs to a circular stimulus of a 14°11' radius and those to a ring stimulus having 25° inner radius and 28°44' outer radius whose exposed area (B) is equal to the circular area of a 14°11' radius (A). Both records were measured under central fixation. Numbers besides records denote the log of stimulus illumination, zero being equal to the sensory threshold for the ring stimuli. Dashed lines are the N_2 latency measured. A green ($\lambda = 522$ nm) stimulus of 100 msec duration is given at random. Subject E.A.

Prior to study of the sensitivity contouring, fundamental scotopic properties such as spectral sensitivity, sensitivity in the course of dark adaptation were confirmed for the VECP at a peripheral retina using concentric ring stimuli. The results are not given here.

Concentric sensitivity contouring using the equal areal ring stimuli

With a circular stimulus of $14°11'$ radius and ring stimuli of $5°$, $10°$, $15°$, $20°$, $25°$ inner radii and $15°02'$, $17°21'$, $20°38'$, $24°31'$, $28°44'$ outer radii, respectively, whose areas were equal to the circular one, sensitivities at different retinal regions were studied. Some of them involved a part of the disc region.

Figure 3 and 4 show the result of the subject, E.A.. This data was reproducible in the same subject, but the data of the other subjects, N.K. and M.M., showed quite different tendencies. The data of subject E.A. showed that the VECP sensitivity increased as the stimulated retinal area moved from the center to the periphery as the sensory data showed. On the other hand, the data of subject N.K. demonstrated that the VECP sensitivity remained equal with changing stimulating retinal position and in subject

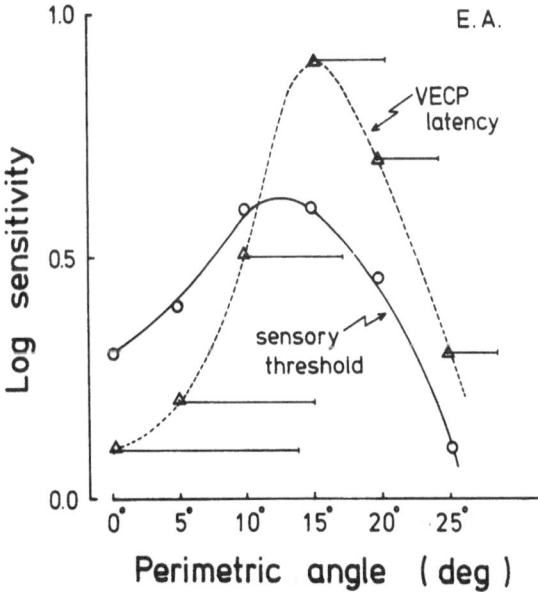

Fig. 4. Log relative sensitivity (relative stimulus illumination required for sensory thresholds and for the criterion VECP latency of 250 msec) plotted against the perimetric angle of the retina stimulated. Stimuli ($\lambda = 522$ nm) have $5°$, $10°$, $15°$, $20°$ and $25°$ inner radius and $15°02'$, $17°21'$, $20°38'$, $24°31'$ and $28°44'$ outer radius respectively whose areas are equal to the circular stimulus of a $14°11'$ radius. Horizontal lines drawn on the VECP data denote the perimetric widths of ring stimuli. The data of the sensory threshold are displaced downward by 2.0 log units in order to facilitate comparison. Subject E.A.

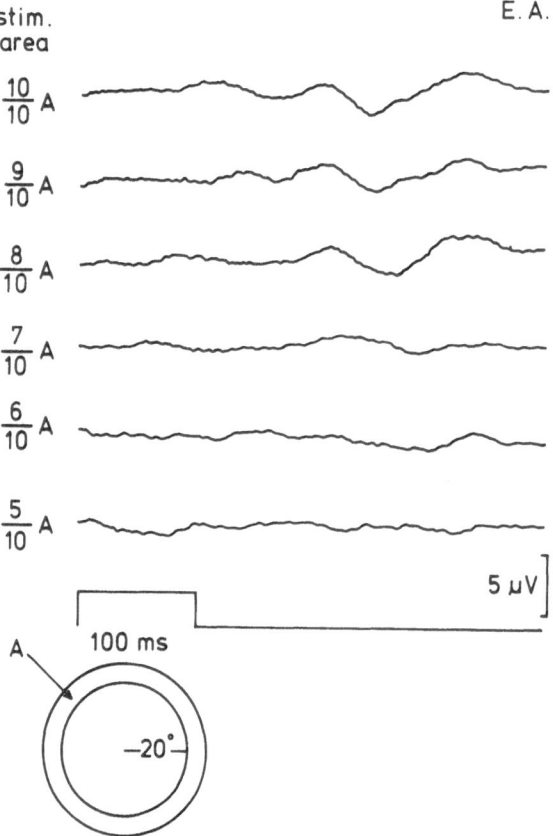

stim.
area

E. A.

$\frac{10}{10}$ A

$\frac{9}{10}$ A

$\frac{8}{10}$ A

$\frac{7}{10}$ A

$\frac{6}{10}$ A

$\frac{5}{10}$ A

5 µV

100 ms

A

−20°

Fig. 5. Effects of stimulus area at the peripheral retina on the scotopic VECP. A green (λ = 522 nm) ring stimulus having a 20° inner and 24°31' outer radius (Area A) is divided into ten arcs and 10/10, 9/10, 8/10 ... 1/10 of area A are presented on the retina respectively, central fixation. Area A is equal to the circular area of a 14°11' radius. Stimulus illumination, 1.8 log units above each sensory threshold. Subject E.A.

M.M. the VECP amplitude was not recognizable when stimuli fell at 10° temporal retina.

Spatial summation effect on the scotopic VECP

A ring stimulus of 20° inner and 24°31' outer radii where the disc region was excluded (indicated as A in the Figures 5 and 6) was divided into ten arcs with equal areas and the scotopic VECPs for 10/10 x A, 9/10 x A, 8/10 x A ... 1/10 x A were studied, respectively.

In subject E.A. the amplitude disappeared when the stimulus area became half the full ring. A similar result was obtained when the turn of cutting 1/10 fraction was altered.

Thresholds for both sensory excitation and N_2 latency of 250 msec were plotted against the log area of the stimuli for the temporal retina between 20° and 24°31' radially (Fig. 6). VECP data could show only three points due to the great reduction of the amplitude with decreasing the area.

184

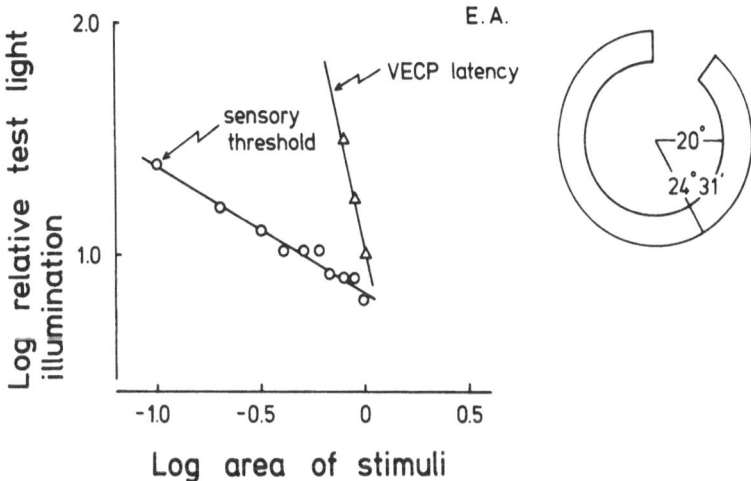

Fig. 6. Log relative stimulus illumination vs the log area of stimuli at the temporally peripheral retina between 20° and 24°31' from the fovea. Log area of stimulus, 0 is a full ring having a 20° inner radius and 24°31' outer radius. The others are the arcs of 9/10, 8/10, 7/10, 6/10 . . . 1/10 of the full ring. VECP data are obtained from illumination necessary for a criterion latency of 250 msec (triangles) and sensory data are indicated by circles. The data of the sensory threshold are displaced upward by 1.6 log units in order to facilitate comparison. Subject E.A.

DISCUSSION

It has been shown psychophysically by Hecht et al. (1937), Pirenne (1948), and Hallett et al. (1962) that sensitivity at different parts of the retina is closely related to the rod distribution.

Our data from mapping of the scotopic VECP showed good agreement with them within the retinal range of 10° in radius as far as the VECP was detected. However, we had to conclude from observation on obtained VECPs that the VECP could not penetrate to the electrode with stimulation of over 10° from the fovea. It could be understood that such results were due to the anatomical projection of the retina onto the cortex. This fact was also supported by results that the peripheral response was not detectable even with increased test light illumination.

Further, with regard to the electrode position, recording the VECP at various positions on the scalp was tried, at positions around a semicircle of 6 cm in radius centered at the inion. However, no improved result was found.

Thus, it must be concluded that VECP experiments with smaller circular stimuli could not go further in the retinal range of over 10° from the fovea.

Sectioning of ring stimuli was used to find the inhomogeneity of the sensitivity, excluding the spatial summation effect. Regrettably we measured only six points owing to a too long experiment period. Results obtained were also collectively miserable, since two out of three subjects showed ambiguous results. But we believe that the result from subject E.A.

was reliable due to the following reasoning. Maximum sensitivity position of the subject, E.A., was around $20°$ from the fovea, when the outer part of the ring contributed mainly to its visual threshold (Adachi-Usami & Kellermann, 1973). This was quite understandable by referring the psychophysical data and the rod distribution.

Since the subject showed the detectable response to a ring stimulus of a $25°$ inner radius and $28°44'$ outer radius and no response was obtained with a circular stimulus of a $5°30'$ diameter for a retinal region of over $10°$ eccentricity from the fovea, Figure 5 is of interest to connect the two phenomena above. It can be clearly seen in the figure that the amplitude decreases and latency prolongs with a decrease of the stimulus area. To be more precise, sensory thresholds decreased by 0.3 log units when the area was reduced to a half, while the VECP to a test light of 1.8 log units higher illumination than the sensory threshold diminished in its amplitude and N_2 latency prolonged appr. 70 msec. The prolonged value of 70 msec suggested the great value of the summation index.

This tendency can also be seen in the curve for the VECP of Figure 6, which consists of only three data points obtained from the same subject with a good reproducibility. Nevertheless, these data were not enough to evaluate spatial summation effects quantitatively.

A possible explanation of why the scotopic VECP for peripheral stimulation of over $10°$ was obtained with ring stimuli and not with circular ones is that, in the former, the VECP output amplitude may become great enough to compensate the attenuation of the potential from the cortex to the electrode position. The greater output in the former case is proved by the fact that ring stimuli have a greater area, i.e. 2.55 log units greater than the circular stimulus of $1°$ $30'$ diameter, and 1.6 log units greater than $5°$ $30'$ and this suggests extraordinary great spatial summation effects.

Reasons for establishing these hypotheses are based on the fact that spectral sensitivity determined by N_2 latency suggested the scotopic characteristics of the VECP in the present study and the result showed the considerably great summation effect.

CONCLUSION

Judging from the present study, the feasibility of perimetry by means of the scotopic VECP which must provide the effective resolution of retinal sensitivity for clinical use may be pessimistic. However, sensitivity contouring methods of the peripheral retina might offer some information in the view of clinical perimetry. Because our data could not conclude it impossible.

REFERENCES

Adachi-Usami, E. & F.-J. Kellermann. Spatial summation of retinal excitation as obtained by the scotopic VECP and the sensory threshold. *Ophthal. Res.* 5: *308–316* (1973).
Adachi, E. Perimetry by the human scotopic visually evoked cortical potential – Critical eccentricity of the stimulating retinal area. *Acta Soc. Ophthal. Jap.* 81: *340– 346* (1977).

Adams, W.L., G.B. Arden & J. Behrman. Responses of human visual cortex following excitation of peripheral retinal rods. Some applications in the clinical diagnosis of functional and organic visual defects. *Br. J. Ophthal.* 53: *439–452* (1969).

Hallett, P.E., F.H. Marriott & F.C. Rodger. The relationship of visual threshold to retinal position and area. *J. Physiol.* 160: *364–373* (1962).

Hecht, S., C. Haig & G. Wald. The dark adaptation of retinal fields of different size and location. *J. gen. Physiol.* 19: *321–337* (1936).

Huber, C. & E. Adachi-Usami. Scotopic visibility curve in man obtained by the VER. In: The visual system: neurophysiology, biophysics and their clinical applications. Proc. XIth IUPS-ISCERG Symp. Birghton 1971. Plenum, New York, pp. 189–198 (1972).

Østerberg, F. Topography of the layer of rods and cones in the human retina. *Acta ophthal.* Suppl. 6 (1935)

Pirenne, M.H. Vision and the Eye. Chapman and Hall, London (1948).

Vaughan, H.G., Jr., L.D. Costa & L. Gilden. The functional relation of visual evoked response and reaction time to stimulus intensity. *Vision Res.* 6: *645–656* (1966).

Wooten, B.R. Photopic and scotopic contributions to the human visually evoked cortical potential. *Vision Res.* 12: *1647–1660* (1972).

Authors' address:
First Dept. of Physiology
Hamamatsu University
School of Medicine
Hamamatsu
Japan

Docum. Ophthal. Proc. Series, Vol. 15

THE OPTIC NERVE IN ENDOCRINE ORBITOPATHY

H. W. SKALKA
(Birmingham, Ala., USA)

Distension of the meninges of the orbital optic nerve occurs routinely with increased intracranial pressure, whether papilledema be present or, as when optic atrophy supervenes, not demonstrable. This meningeal distension is due to the presence of a perineural cuff of cerebrospinal fluid under pressure. Using A-scan ultrasonography, we have found the dural-surface to nerve-surface distance about the retrobulbar optic nerve to be enlarged in a variety of local ocular or orbital conditions. Included among these are processes causing physical changes within the nerve itself, such as drusen of the disc or optic atrophy; perineural affections, such as orbital cellulitis or perineural tumors; and local alterations of fluid dynamics as would be induced, for example, by ocular hypotony. The widened intervaginal space in these latter conditions is presumably secondary to local alterations, and is independent of the systemic cerebrospinal fluid pressure. The technique of measurement has been described elsewhere (Skalka, 1977), but, briefly, is as follows: the A-scan probe is placed at the lateral canthus and angled back until the sound beam strikes the optic nerve perpendicularly, returning a strong double echo from each surface of the nerve. The inner echoes represent the nerve surface, and the outer echoes the dural sheath. Differences greater than 1.50 mm. between nerve and dural diameters may be considered abnormal.

We have also found a consistently widened nerve-surface to dural-surface distance about the orbital optic nerve in the immediate retrobulbar area in patients with endocrine orbitopathy, whether they be hyper-, hypo-, or euthyroid by general physical examination and conventional laboratory tests at the time of examination. This has been an invariable finding in the involved orbits of some three dozen such patients. Those with monocular involvement (as determined by absence of clinical symptoms and signs and absence of extra-ocular muscle thickening on A-scan biometry) have had only monocular enlargement of this subdural perineural space.

The distance from nerve-surface to dural-surface in patients with endocrine orbitopathy tends to increase as the degree of extraocular muscle involvement (as determined by A-scan biometry of rectus muscle thickness) increases. It is not known for certain whether this is due to thickening of the meninges about the orbital optic nerve or to fluid accumulation in the intervaginal spaces. Histopathologic study of one case by Dr. Lorenz Zimmerman of the Armed Forces Institute of Pathology suggested a slightly enlarged subdural space which was felt to have been filled by a watery fluid in vivo (pers. comm.)

Clinically, most of the endocrine orbitopathy patients we have examined had normal visual acuity, unremarkable-appearing optic discs, normal fields and color vision. Recently, we have begun to evaluate the VER in these patients with the poorly understood auto-toxicity of Graves' disease-patients whose visual function appears clinically normal, but who have enlarged perineural spaces about their orbital optic nerves.

We have obtained clinical VER determinations in approximately a dozen patients with endocrine orbitopathy and enlarged perineural optic nerve measurements. Testing was performed using either the DISA 1411 apparatus with Grass photostimulator, at two flashes per second, averaging 128 responses consisting of 500 data points on a 200 msec sweep; or the Nicolet CA 1000 apparatus with pattern-reversal black and white check or flash stimulation at 3.75 reversals or flashes per second, averaging 256 responses consisting of 1024 data points on a 200 msec sweep. Some patients were examined with both instruments. Our electrode was placed 1 cm. above the inion in the midline and referenced to the mastoid bone. Findings were compared with results obtained in a normal population.

As recorded amplitudes were found to be quite variable from day to day, even for the same individual, and as no systematic effect on amplitude caused by endocrine orbitopathy (in the absence of frank visual compromise) was seen, evaluations were based on implicit times measured to the first positive peak of the VER recording.

Implicit times with the pattern-reversal black and white checks using the Nicolet CA-1000 system with television stimulator were all in the nineties of milliseconds in our normal population, and averaged 98.59 msec OD, 98.40 msec OS, and 93.68 msec OU. Implicit times using television screen flash stimuli yielded values in the hundred and tens of msecs, with our OU average at 118.07 msec. DISA 1411 recordings of Grass photostimulator flash stimuli showed somewhat more variability among our normals, implicit time values OD ranging from 91.4 to 116 msec, with an average of 102.6 msec; OS from 92.8 to 120 msec, with an average of 108.7 msec; and OU from 108.0 to 120.0 msec, with an average time of 115.0 msec.

All our endocrine orbitopathy patients with normal visual acuities, fields, and color vision had VER implicit times in the normal range. Amplitudes varied, but were of similar voltages and variability as that seen in the normal population. Patients with monocular involvement of endocrine orbitopathy showed no difference, on average, between eyes in their latencies or voltages on VER testing. Our endocrine orbitopathy patients with acuity and visual field compromise due to media changes (mainly cataract) showed normal implicit times, although recorded voltages were, as expected, somewhat low. One patient with severely depressed acuity (20/70 OD, CF OS), markedly constricted fields, glaucoma, disc cupping, and arteriolar sheathing OU, showed both very low voltage and significantly prolonged latency in the 136-142 msec range with flash stimuli using both our DISA and Nicolet protocols).

190

What might be termed the orbital 'auto-toxicity' of Graves' disease does involve the intervaginal space about the retrobulbar optic nerve, in mild cases as well as in cases of 'malignant exophthalmos'. Ultrasonographic biometry consistently and reproducibly demonstrates this. Although we have not yet had the opportunity of performing VER testing on a patient in the acute, florid stage of malignant exophthalmos, there is no reason to doubt that the severe optic nerve compromise often accompanying this condition would lead to correspondingly severe VER abnormalities. However, the ultrasonographically demonstrable perineural alterations in the usual clinical presentation of endocrine orbitopathy, with or without extraocular muscle restrictions, but without significant acuity or field alterations, does not produce detectable alterations in the latencies (or voltages) of the clinically recorded VER.

REFERENCES

Skalka, H. W. Quantitative ultrasonographic determination of perineural optic nerve Cerebrospinal fluid in ultrasound in medicine. Vol. 3–a, Clinical Aspects. 1029-1042. Plenum New York (1977).

Docum. Ophthal. Proc. Series, Vol. 15

THE VISUAL EVOKED POTENTIAL IN PATIENTS
WITH CATARACTS

C. R. S. THOMPSON & G. F. A. HARDING
(Birmingham, England)

Of recent years there has been a marked emphasis on the use of pattern reversal as the appropriate stimulus for studies of the Visual Evoked Potential (VEP), particularly in normal subjects or co-operative adult patients. Early studies of the clinical value of the VEP usually used flash as the stimulus, but the inherent crudity of an undifferentiated flash of light discouraged many workers from continuing with this stimulus or from using flashed patterns as an alternative stimulus. However, as we indicated in previous studies (Harding et al., 1970), the flash evoked potential is most useful in identifying gross field defects in patients who cannot or will not fixate a pattern. Thus, the technique is of use in very young children, grossly handicapped patients, and in conditions of opacity of the eye. Dense opacities of the optic media prevent full clinical assessment of the retina, and there is, therefore, a problem of whether cataract surgery will result in improved vision.

Fricker (1971), using fast intermittent photic stimulation of patients with unilateral cataracts, demonstrated the utility of the cortical response in predicting the visual outcome of cataract surgery. We have previously reported early trials of the flash evoked potential as a predictor of postoperative visual efficiency in patients with dense cataracts (Harding, 1974).

This paper reports our studies of the predictive value of the flash visual evoked potential in 21 patients with dense unilateral cataracts. All patients had previously undergone a general ophthalmological examination and were considered suitable for surgery. They were referred for investigation of their VEPs, the results of which did not influence the decision for surgery. One patient subsequently refused surgery. The remaining 20 patients had a wide age range from 10 to 94 years, with a majority of patients over 60 years of age. The normal or non-cataract eye of each of the patients had usually a best corrected vision of 6/9 to 6/6 except for three patients whose acuity was 6/24.

METHODS

A Grass PS.22 photostiumulator, which had been modified by the addition of an opal diffuser, produced a transient light flash from a Xenon flash tube at a range of stepped intensities from 68 to 483 nit seconds. The photostimulator was placed 30 cm from the patients eyes, which were stimulated monocularly in a random sequence. The size of the pupil and precise state of refraction were not controlled.

Silver-silver chloride electrodes were arranged acoording to the International 10-20 system (Jasper, 1958), and a special VEP montage (Fig. 1) which allows differentiation of the occipital sources was used (Harding, 1974). The EEG was recorded using an SLE 8 or 12 channel machine and the output signal was averaged using a TMC Computer of Average Transients (CAT). A

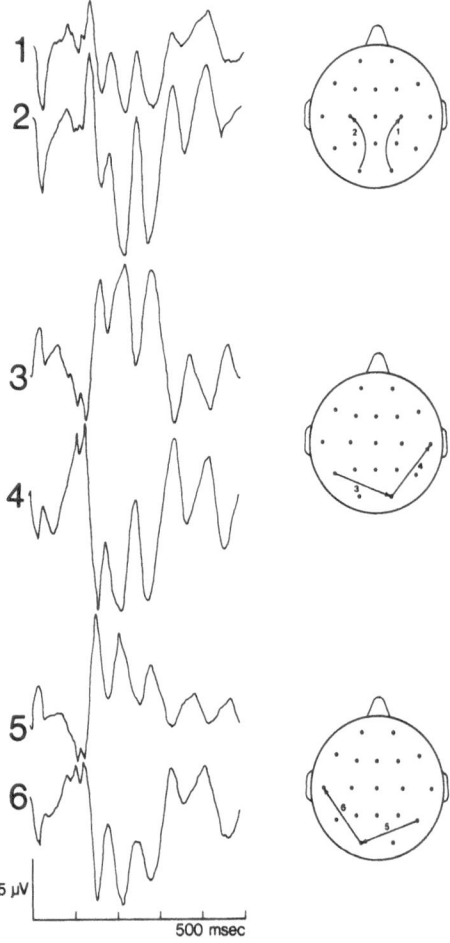

Fig. 1. Localisation and visual evoked potential. This figure shows the VEP from a 20 year old normal subject. Channels 1 and 2 shows the response from the right and left occiput, respectively, when compared to relatively indifferent central electrodes. Channels 3 and 4 show phase reversal of the VEP from the right occipital electrode, which is common between the two channels. The left occiput is mid-way between the two electrodes of channel 3, and therefore, the signal arising from the left occiput does not significantly contribute to the write-out in channel 3. Channels 5 and 6 show the phase reversal of the left occipital evoked potential in a similar way. (From Harding, 1974).

5 μV calibration pulse was induced onto the electrode leads (Lindley & Harding, 1974). The output of the CAT was plotted on an XY plotter from which measurements of latency and amplitude were derived.

RESULTS

The visual evoked potential results were independently rated by two observers, one observer had no knowledge of the clinical history, age or post-operative acuity of the patients. Intra-individual comparisons of the VEP from the cataract and non-cataract eyes were made, according to our normal criteria of amplitude difference between the two eyes of not more than 33% (2 s.d.), and a latency difference of not more than 12 msecs and localisation at the two occiputs. On the basis of these objective criteria the VEP was rated into 3 Grades.

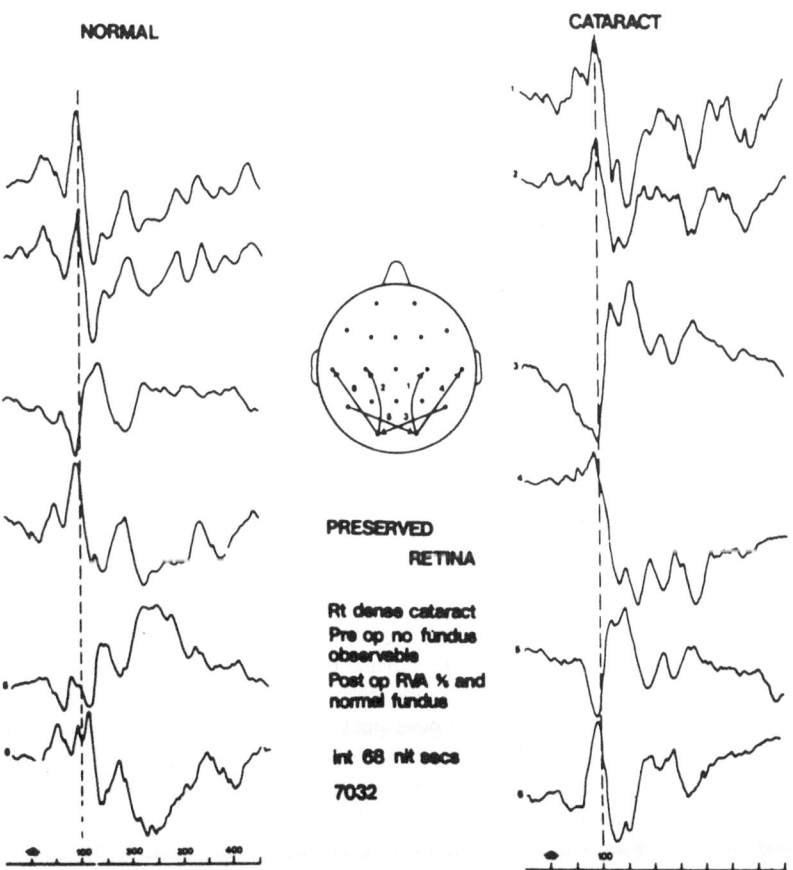

Fig. 2. Shows the response from the normal and cataract eye of a patient who obtained good post-operative visual acuity. The VECP was recorded post-operatively, and showed similar responses from both eyes with little reduction in amplitude and clear phase reversal to both occiputs. At that time the patient had a dense cataract making clear observation of the retina impossible.

195

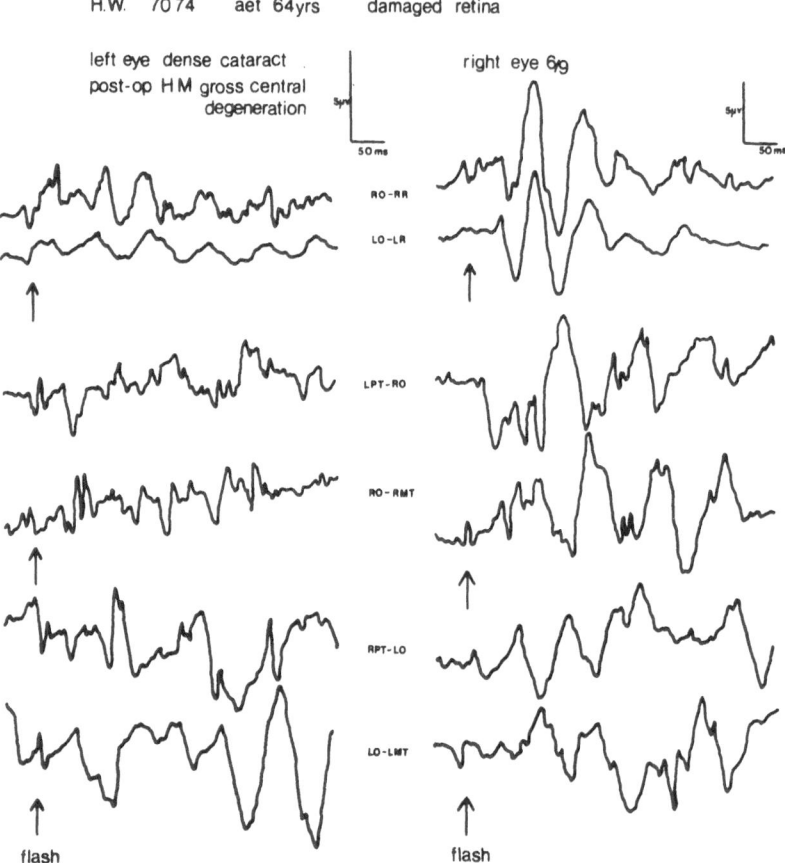

H.W. 70 74   aet 64yrs   damaged retina

left eye dense cataract
post-op H M gross central
degeneration

right eye 6⁄9

RO-RR

LO-LR

LPT-RO

RO-RMT

RPT-LO

LO-LMT

flash

flash

Fig. 3. Shows the response from a patient who had poor post-operative vision. Preoperatively the VEP from the left eye was markedly reduced without clear or consistent components, and without clear phase reversal to either occiput.

A Grade 1 VEP was used to predict good visual acuity. The response from
the cataract eye was similar to the normal eye with a small, or no reduction
in amplitude. All the main components phase reversed to both occiputs,
(Fig. 2). Grade 3 VEP predicted poor post-operative vision. There was a no-
tice-able reduction in amplitude compared with the good eye with no clear
localisation of the major components at the right or left occiput (Fig. 3). A
Grade 2 rating was used to represent a category of VEP where judgment was
difficult and quenstionable. Generally, there was a significant reduction in
amplitude and phase reversal was only inconsistently obtained. In some of
these cases stimulation of the good eye produced visual potentials of unusual configuration, thus providing an inadequate comparator.

Baseline to peak measures were taken of P1, N2, P2 and N3 components.
The early and late components were extremely variable, and did not appear

196

to show any consistent trend with either VEP grading or post-operative vision. This was particularly true in the older patienst who show the reported trend (Dustman & Beck, 1969), of high amplitude early components, which do not relate to visual acuity. The P2 component showed least variability, and was most predictive of post-operative results. The mean percentage reduction or percentage increase in the amplitude of the P2 component from the cataract eye compared to the normal eye is shown in Fig. 4.

Twelve patients had Grade 1 VEPs. Five of these patients had a larger P2 component from the cataract eye than the normal eye. This was possibly due to the diffusing effect of the cataract, and the greater amount of alpha rhythm in the background EEG record. At 68 nit/seconds intensity, nine patients had a reduced P2 from the cataract eye and in four this reduction was around 50%, beyond our normal criteria. However, increasing the flash intensity to 96 nit/seconds improved all the results of the Grade 1 patients, and there was less difference between the two eyes. At this intensity the

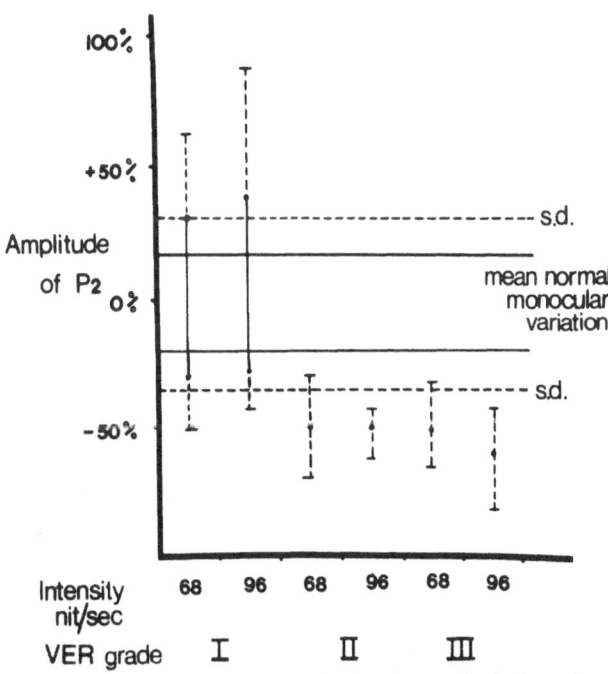

Fig. 4. Shows the percentage reduction or increase in amplitude from the cataract eye when compared to the normal eye for visual evoked response Grades 1, 2 and 3, at two intensities of the Grass Photostimulator. The mean amplitudes and the ranges are shown compared to the normal mean monocular variation ± two standard deviations (s.d.). The Grade 1 responses are shown to approximate closely to the normal limits, and also to increase in amplitude with intensity. In Grades 2, and 3 there is no increase in amplitude with increase in intensity, and the mean latencies fall outside the normal range.

greatest reduction seen in only two eyes was 42%. A further increase in flash intensity was not effective.

Three patients had a Grade 2 VEP. At 68 nit/seconds one patient who did in fact have a final visual acuity of 6/6 had a large 70% reduction in P2 amplitude. In the other two, the difference was around the normal limits. Increasing the intensity did not increase the amplitude of the response from the cataract eye.

In Grade 3 VEPs, amplitude provided useful criteria with four of the five patients showing a significant reduction of more than 45%. Increasing the intensity increased the difference in response amplitude from the two eyes. In the one patient with only 33% reduction at 68 nit/seconds and 42% at 96 nit/seconds, the amplitude of the cortical response evoked from the good eye was only 3–4 μV, and this may contribute to the apparently small reduction in amplitude.

The use of amplitude alone as a predictor of post-operative visual acuity was not effective in seven of the twenty patients. The normal criteria of greater than 12 msec latency difference of the P2 component evoked by monocular stimulation was exceeded by a significant number of patients in all VEP Grades, and did not in general relate to post-operative visual acuity. When the amplitude criteria was borderline, and the latency was not excessively delayed, phase reversal of P2 to the right and left occiput was

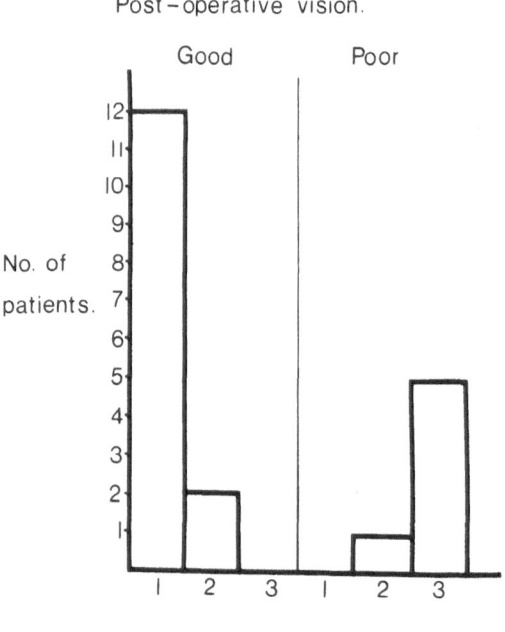

Fig. 5. Shows the relation of the VEP Grades to the post-operative finding of good vision (6/12 or better), and poor vision (6/24 or worse). The VEP proves to be an accurate predictor of visual outcome (P = 0.007).

useful in resolving the prognosis. In all patients with good post-operative visual acuity, P2 was located in both hemispheres, either at 68 or 96 nit/ seconds intensity. This included two patients with significantly reduced and delayed responses who were therefore placed in the Grade 2 category. None of the Grade 3 patients, all of whom had post-operative poor vision, showed any consistent localisation of the P2 component.

The post-operative vision of the twenty patients who underwent surgery was arbitrally divided into good vision -6/12 or better, and poor vision -6/ 24 or worse. The visual evoked potential prognostic grade was then compared to the actual vision after surgery (Fig. 5).

Fourteen patients had good vision, their ages range from 22 to 94 with a mean of 66 years, and the history of the cataract varied, but was most frequently an old trauma. Twelve of these patients had Grade 1 VEPs, and the two patients with Grade 2 VEPs were both elderly, aged 78 and 87, and we have little experience of normal controls of this age. One of these patients also had early lens opacities and senile macular degeneration in the so-called good eye and a visual acuity of 6/24.

Six patients had poor post-operative vision. The age range was 10 to 64, mean 38 years, and again the most common etiology was old injuries to the eye.

Of the five patients with VEP Grade 3, two only had perception of light, and a third showed gross central myopic degeneration. The youngest aged 10, had a congenital cataract and her vision was 6/36. It was unexpected to record such abnormal flash visual evoked potentials with this clinical history. The one patient with a Grade 2 VEP had an early traumatic cataract at age 4, and the eye was also slightly divergent. Post-operative the fundus was good, and there was no technical reason why the vision was only counting fingers. The surgeon concluded that the eye was amblyopic.

DISCUSSION

The correlation between the visual evoked potential grade and the post-operative vision was significant at the 0.007 level, but 14% of our prognostic results were false negative, and 16% false positive, although all fell in the 'doubtful' Grade 2 category. The effect of the cataract alone on the amplitude and latency of the VEP appears to be minimal, and corrected by an increase in intensity of 50%, that is, from 68 to 96 nit/seconds intensity (Fig. 6) The greatest problem is the difference in the background EEG when the cataract eye is being stimulated. The VEP may be obscured by the alpha rhythm, or alternatively, synchronous alpha waves may be identified as a cortical evoked potential. This difficulty is not resolved by simulating the diffusing effect of the cataract.

Due to the inherent variability of the flash VEP, the main difficulty is in identifying the normal or degenerated eye at the extreme of the overlapping ranges, either in terms of amplitude or latency.

Post-hoc, it seems that the greater number of criteria used in assessing the VEP grade, the more reliable the prognosis. Thus, an amplitude reduction of 45% or more, a latency delay of more than 20 msecs, a failure to phase re-

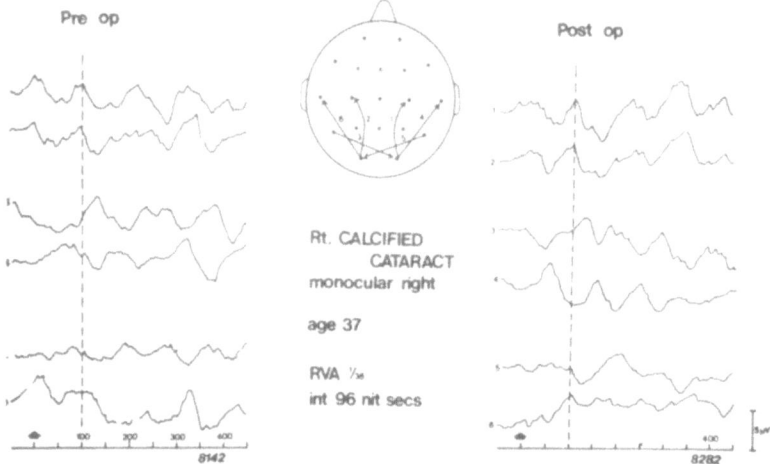

Fig. 6. This figure compares the visual evoked potential obtained pre and post-operatively in a patient with a calcified cataract of the right eye. It can be seen that a vague negative component is obtained around 100 msecs. and a later positive component is obtained around 150 msecs. The findings are similar in the pre and post-operative condition, although the same intensity of stimulation was used on each occasion.

verse to either occiput of the P2 component is indicative of poor post-operative vision.

From this and previous studies it appears that the flash VEP is not useful in predicting post operative acuity, if the patient history is suggestive of amblyopia, especially in the presence of strabismus. With this reservation, it appears that the flash evoked potential can provide a useful prognosis for vision in dense cataracts.

ACKNOWLEDGEMENTS

We are grateful to Mr. John Pearce, Ophthalmic Surgeon, Bromsgrove Hospital, for referring the patients and providing the post-operative assessments of vision as well as for his continued encouragement. This work was partly supported by the Paul S. Cadburry Trust to whom we are also most grateful.

REFERENCES

Dustman, R. E. & E. C. Beck. The effects of maturation and ageing on the waveform of visually evoked potentials. *Electroenceph. Clin. Neurophysiol.* 26: *2–1* (1969).

Fricker, S. J. Analysis of the visual evoked response by Synchronous Detector techniques. *Invest. Ophthal.* 10: *5* (1971).

Harding, G. F. A. The Visusal Evoked Response. *Adv. Ophthal.* 28: *2–28* (1974).

Harding, G. F. A. C. R. S. Thompson & C. P. Panayiotopoulos. Evoked response diagnosis in visual field defects. *Proc. Electrophysiol. Technol. Ass.* 16: *159–163* (1970).

Jasper, H. H. Report of the committee on methods of clinical examinations in electroencephalography. *Electroenceph. Clin. Neurophysiol.* 10: *370–375* (1958).

Lindley, J. & G. F. A. Harding. A simple on-line calibrator for use in averaging evoked potentials. From: Proceedings and Journal of the Electro-Physiological Technologists' Association. Vol. 21, No. 1. (1974).

Authors' address:
The University of Aston
Gosta Green
Birmingham B 47 ET
England

Docum. Ophthal. Proc. Series. Vol. 15

THE ERG AND VEP IN PATIENTS WITH SEVERE EYE INJURY

S.J. CREWS, C.R.S. THOMPSON & G.F.A. HARDING

(Birmingham, England)

Severe ocular trauma presents a number of problems in diagnosis and management. The visual potential of the eye has to be predicted and weighed against the risk of sympathetic ophthalmia and the chances of a blind painful eye, and on this balance an early decision must be made whether to enucleate. In addition, there is an increasing interest in the possibility of major reconstructive surgery in the early post-operative stage after primary repair.

Clinical assessment is frequently restricted by the opacities of the media. Subjective responses are limited not only by these optical problems, but also by the psychological effect of the trauma, the unreliability of communication in young children and cerebral damage in patients with multiple injuries. Objective tests are also of value in patients who do not speak a known language and in medico-legal problems.

Consensual pupil responses in the unaffected eye may detect an afferent defect. Ultrasonography is of obvious use in the study of structural changes, especially when planning further surgery. Earlier work (Crews et al., 1975) had suggested that the ERG and VEP might be of value in predicting visual outcome. We therefore conducted a prospective study of severe perforating and blunt injuries in 64 eyes of 60 patients present at the Birmingham & Midland Eye Hospital, where opaque media prevented examination of the posterior segment.

METHODS

All electrodiagnostic assessment was performed within 1 month, usually within 2 weeks of the trauma, that is, after primary repair of any perforating injury.

Skin, rather than corneal ERGs were performed to avoid damage by a corneal electrode, using a Devices or Grass photostimulator and either a Medelec or Datalab digital averager. The skin electrodes were placed on the mid position of the lower lid and were referred to a reference electrode on the outer canthus.

Flash evoked cortical potentials were recorded from scalp electrodes placed over each occiput and referred to the right and left central electrodes. For the visual evoked potential the intensity of flash stimulation was varied from Grass Mark 2 (68 nit secs) to Grass 16 (483 nit secs).

RESULTS

The electrodiagnostic findings were compared to the best visual outcome. We have used the term best vision since in some cases it was not practicable to give a final visual outcome, follow-up varied from 4 years to 6 months, the vast majority being more than 18 months. However, in most of the cases a final visual outcome has been achieved. Four of the eyes showed subsequent deterioration of vision − 3 of them related to complications of subsequent surgery.

The best visual outcome was graded between 1−4:

Grade 1a − 6/6 − 6/12
Grade 1b − 6/18 − 6/60
Grade 2   − less than 6/60 with accurate projection
Grade 3   − inaccurate projection
Grade 4   − no perception of light.

Included in this latter category are the enucleated eyes both with retina detached and with retina in situ.

ERG

The scotopic ERG was graded from 1−4 according to the b wave amplitude as compared to the other eye when uninjured or to a mean normal value when both eyes were injured.

Grade 1   − 75 to 100 $\Big\}$ b-wave amplitude as per cent of
Grade 2   − 50 to 74   fellow eye or of mean normal value
Grade 3   − 25 to 49

Seventy-three per cent of patients in ERG Grades 1 and 2 achieved Grade 1 vision and of these 43% gained good (6/6−6/12) vision (Fig. 1). Of the 2 eyes with a good ERG who had no perception of light, both were found to have lesions of the visual pathway. The other 3 eyes were enucleated, but found to have the retina in situ. In ERG Grades 3 and 4 only one achieved useful vision and the vast majority went blind or were enucleated.

VEP

The VEP was independently rated by two observers, one of whom had no knowledge of the clinical history of the patient. From past experience we had found that the amplitude and latency of the P2 or P100 component was the most reliable indicator, being relatively unaffected by other factors such as age (Harding, 1974).

The VEPs were also divided into 4 Grades:

Grade 1 − normal latency and amplitude when compared to the uninjured eye or normal age matched criteria.
Grade 2 − less than 50% reduction in amplitude and no marked delay.
Grade 3 − reduction in amplitude of more than 50% or VEPs with a marked delay well outside the normal range (greater than 30 m.secs.).
Grade 4 − absence of the VEP or a vastly reduced (less than 1.5 μV) and delayed evoked potential only obtained at highest intensity of stimulation.

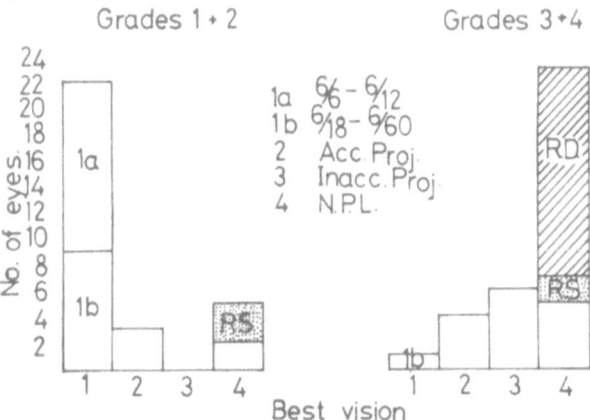

Fig. 1. ERG Grades in relation to visual outcome. Seventy-three per cent of eyes with ERG Grade 1 and 2 achieved a visual acuity of between 6/6 and 6/60. Of the eyes with ERG Grade 3 and 4, only one patient achieved a vision better than 6/60.

The visual grading is shown in the centre table, and corresponds to the numbers on the abscissa.

NPL = No perception of light; RS = Enucleated retina in situ; RD = Enucleated retina detached.

Figure 2 shows the relation between the VEP Grades and best vision. Sixty-seven per cent of those in VEP Grades 1 and 2 achieved useful vision (Grade 1); the only patients in these VEP grades who had their eyes enucle-

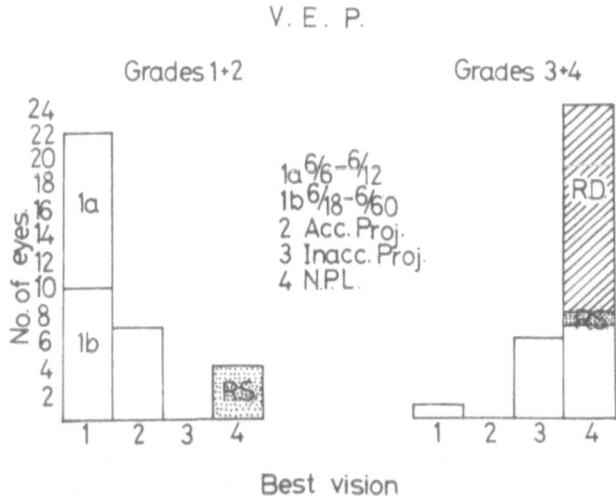

Fig. 2. Shows the relation of the visual evoked potential grade to the visual outcome. Sixty-seven per cent of eyes with VEP Grade 1 and 2 achieved Grade 1 vision, and all eyes in the Grade 1 and 2 VEP category had visual potential, since all enucleated eyes had retina in situ.

ated were found to have the retinu in situ, and therefore had visual potential. One patient, who had a blunt injury, had a good visual outcome 12
months later. As with the ERG the vast majority (94%) with VEP grades 3
and 4 went blind or were enucleated.

The latencies of the P2 component of the VEP from the severely injured
eyes were compared to those of a normal control group and a group of
patients convalescing from traumatic hyphaema. (Fig. 3). The latency of the
P2 component does not clearly differentiate between visual outcome 1a and
1b and is not significantly different in visual outcome Grade 2. However, a
poor visual outcome (Grades 3 and 4) is clearly predicted by the latency,
patients in these groups showing shorter latencies, also having markedly reduced amplitude evoked potentials.

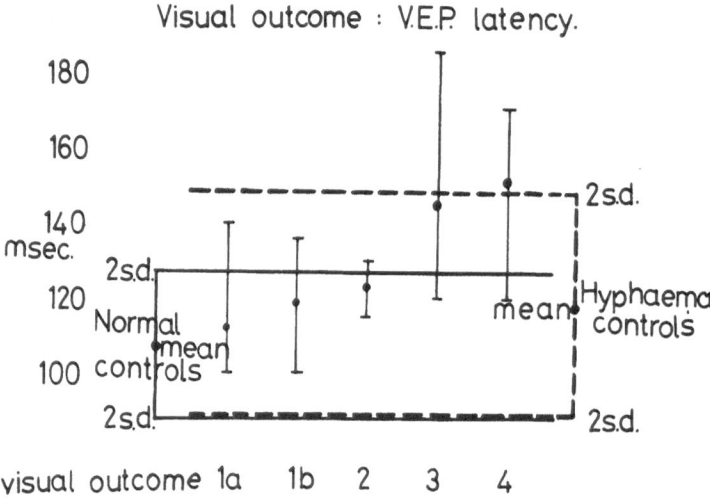

Fig. 3. This figure shows the relation between the visual outcome and the latency of
the major positive (P2 component of the VEP). The visual outcome grading 1a–4 is the
same as in other figures. The mean latency and the range is shown for each visual outcome group. This is compared to the mean latency ± 2 standard deviations of normal
controls and a control group with hyphaema. Only eyes with a visual outcome of inaccurate projection (Grade 3) and no perception of light (Grade 4) show marked
delayed latencies of the major positive component.

Combined ERG-VEP

If the results of the electrodiagnostic investigations are simply combined by
addition the predictive value of the scores is increased. Patients who were
previously missed by the ERG due to optic nerve damage or cerebral blindness are correctly identified (Fig. 4) and the 2 patients who had a good
visual outcome with poor ERG or VEP are now correctly identified (Fig. 5).
Ninety per cent of the eyes with visual potential fall within the combined
score 2–4 whereas 91% of eyes with no visual potential are within range
5–8.

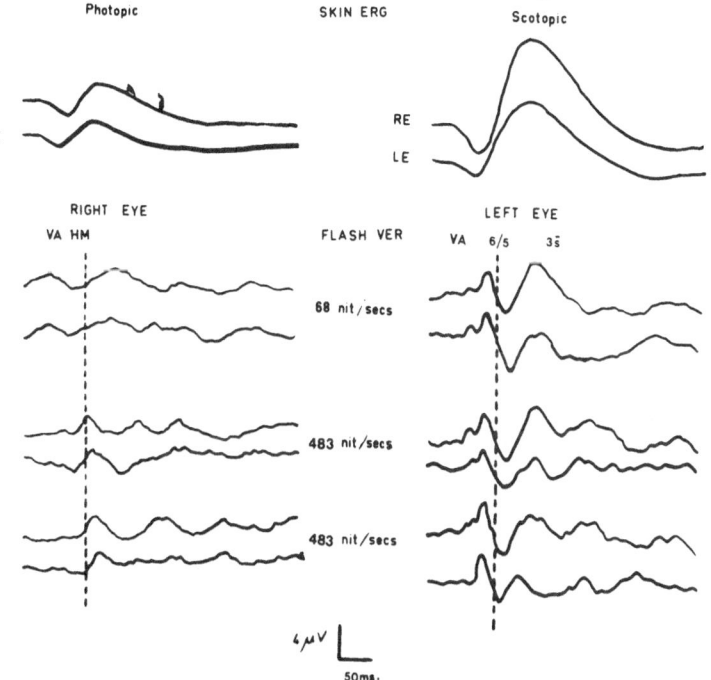

MAJOR TRAUMA SERIES

J.M. aet 26

Right IOFB with traumatic cataract.
Scar near macula, embedded in optic nerve.

Photopic   SKIN ERG   Scotopic

RE

LE

RE

LE

RIGHT EYE   LEFT EYE

VA HM   FLASH VER   VA 6/5   3s̄

68 nit/secs

483 nit/secs

483 nit/secs

4μV

50ms.

Fig 4. Shows the photopic and scotopic skin ERG and VEP at various intensities obtained on a patient who had suffered a penetrating wound to the right eye, with residual intraocular foreign body. The patient subsequently developed a traumatic cataract, and was found postoperatively to have a scar near the macula with foreign body embedded in the optic nerve. The VEP from the right eye is almost absent, with a vague negative component (150 msecs). Both the photopic and scotopic skin ERGs are within normal limits.

E.R.G. V.E.P. Combined score.

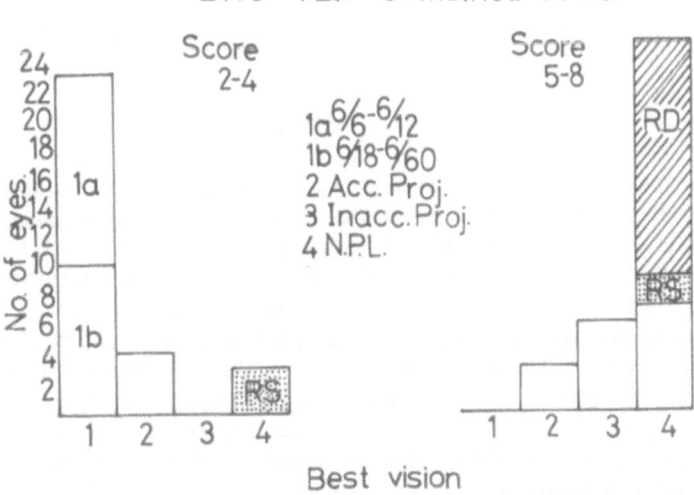

Score 2-4

Score 5-8

1a 6/6-6/12
1b 6/18-6/60
2 Acc. Proj.
3 Inacc. Proj.
4 N.P.L.

No. of eyes

Best vision

Fig 5. Shows the combined ERG and VEP score in relation to visual outcome. The combined score correctly identifies all patients with visual potential and ninety-one per cent of the patients with poor visual outcome.

The 21 enucleated eyes were examined histologically and 16 were found to have the retina detached; all of these had Grade 4 ERGs. Fourteen of the 16 had Grade 4 and two of the 16 Grade 3 VEPs.

Five of the enucleated eyes were found to have retina in situ with well preserved retina and an attempt was made to correlate electrophysiological data with the histology.

Enucleation retina in situ

Patient	ERG	VEP	Histology
M.W.	2	1	Reaction to sutures
			Normal retina
J.C.	1	3	Commotio retinae posterior pole
			Normal peripheral retina
G.P.	2	2	Exit perforating wound
			Early panophthalmitis
N.K.	4	2	Uveitis Pigment Epithelial changes in retina
W.S.	4–2*	2	Intra-retinal separation

* Repeat investigation.

All the five eyes had inaccurate projection of light. In the first patient with good VEP and reasonably good ERG the retina throughout appeared normal, but in the second patient (a contusion injury) with a poor VEP and good ERG there was a traumatic maculopathy, but normal peripheral retina.

In the third patient an undiagnosed exit wound was associated with commencing panophthalmitis. In the fourth patient an improving ERG may have been associated with a curious traumatic intraretinal separation of the outer segments of the receptors. The fifth patient showed an extensive pigment epitheliopathy which might explain the very poor ERG, but reasonable VEP.

Thus all 5 eyes would seem to have some visual potential, though it is difficult to be sure if the eyes could have been saved.

SUMMARY

In conclusion, the combination of the ERG and the VEP offers a diagnostic enhancement of the initial visual clinical assessment in predicting visual potential following major eye injury. It appears to us that the more parameters studied the better the predictive value of the electrodiagnostic assessment. Electrodiagnostic tests performed in the early post-traumatic period and combining both skin ERG and VEP gave accurate prognosis of visual outcome. A skin ERG showing reduction of b-wave amplitude of less than 50%, a VEP with amplitude reduction also less than 50% and without latency delay, invariably predicted a good visual prognosis. In five cases with enucleated eyes with retina in stiu, the electrophysiological findings correlated well with histology.

ACKNOWLEDGEMENTS

We are grateful to the consultant surgeons of the Birmingham & Midland Eye Hospital for allowing us to study their patients, and to Peter Good and Richard Carter for Technical Assistance.

REFERENCES

Crews, S.J., S. Hillman-Jeffrey & C.R.S. Thompson. Electrodiagnosis and ultrasonography in the assessment of recent major trauma. From: Transactions of the Ophthalmological Societies of the United Kingdom. Vol. XCV, Part 11 (1974).
Harding, G.F.A. The visual evoked response. *Adv. Ophthal.* 28: *2–28* (1974).

Authors' address:
Birmingham & Midland Eye Hospital, and
University of Aston
Gosta Green
Birmingham B47 ET
England

Docum. Ophthal. Proc. Series, Vol. 15

PREOPERATIVE EVALUATION OF TRAUMATIC EYE LESIONS WITH VISUAL EVOKED CORTICAL POTENTIALS IN RESPONSE TO SINE WAVE MODULATED LIGHT

CH. HUBER & M. KNUS

(Zürich, Switzerland)

Perforating injuries to the eye may produce a wide assortement of ocular lesions. Generally, the pathology of the eyes' optics is accessible to surgical repair. The pathology of the retina and optic nerve, however, is often not accessible to surgery insofar as the function of the macular area and visual acuity are concerned. As the necessary operations are often numerous and costly in terms of patient discomfort and hospital time, a preoperative forecast of macular function is of interest.

Visual evoked cortical potentials (VECP) have been measured in response to light flashes before cataract operation with only a gross prognostic value (Bider, 1970). Fricker (1970) has shown that latency and amplitude measurement in VECP to flickering lights may have more information value about visual acuity.

We have measured the amplitude of VECP in response to sine wave modulated light as a function of stimulus frequency in patients with severe ocular trauma who were planned for surgical therapy. The reason for the choice of stimulus frequency as a variable parameter is that optical defects have an unknown effect on the intensity of the light reaching the retina. The frequency of the light however is not affected. The use of patterned stimuli is impossible through the destroyed optics. Luminance responses, as we shall show are little affected by the optical opacities encountered in most traumatic cases.

It has been shown that affections of the optic nerve or large macular lesions do reduce the VECP to flickering lights (Milner, Regan & Heron, 1974; Abe, Kojima, Namba & Iwata, 1974; Huber, 1977), particularly in the higher frequency range. A reduction of visual acuity due to amblyopia alone is compatible with a normal VECP to flickering light.

Our aim was not to predict preoperatively the visual acuity but to separate hopeless cases from those where a reasonable increase in visual function could be expected to result from surgery. The preoperative evaluation of patients with unknown retinal function after trauma includes in our clinic A and B Scan Echography, Electroretinography and VECP. We shall refer here only on the VECP results.

MATERIAL AND METHODS

VECPs are recorded from an occipital electrode on the midline 5 cm above the inion, refered to the earlobe. The EEG is averaged over 128 sweeps. The duration of the single EEG period is always longer than a single period of the light stimulus to allow a better discrimination of VECP from artifact at high frequencies.

The light stimulus is a homogeneous field of 40° angular subtense whose-intensity is sine wave modulated in time around a mean luminance level of 50 cd/m². The modulation depth of the light stimulus is 97%, the stimulus frequency is continuously variable from 4 to 55 Hz (see Huber, 1977). The large stimulus size is necessary in patients with very low vision and uncertain fixation to insure a stimulation of the central retina.

VECPs are recorded at increasing stimulus frequencies until the response amplitude is no more measurable or the maximal stimulus frequency of our apparatus (55 Hz) is reached. The amplitude of the monocular VECPs are plotted as a function of the frequency on a half logarithmic plot. As we do not use any narrow band filtering, the responses often include a second harmonic component.

RESULTS

Normals

In Fig. 1 and 2 are plotted the individual measurements of VECP amplitude as a function of frequency in 80 subjects with clear ocular media and normal visual acuity in 8 age groups. Surprisingly, there is little difference in the amplitude values from childhood to old age. The spread of interindividual amplitude is maximal in the low frequency range from 5 to 10 Hz. Unfortunately this is also the frequency range where the responses are of maximal amplitude and, therefore, easiest to measure. A single amplitude measurement in this frequency range cannot show whether the response is reduced or of normal amplitude. At higher stimulus frequencies the amplitude variability is less. In each group two single amplitude-frequency plots have been outlined to show that the slope of the curve is also very variable. From these data and from results on patients with optic nerve atrophy we have drawn on the diagrams a criterion line, defined by two points at 5 10 Hz and 0 microvolt, 25 Hz. Those subjects whose VECP curves are all to the right of the criterion line are considered as normal, if the VECP curve is partly or totally to the left of the criterion line it is considered as pathological. This criterion line is empirical and certainly dependent on the stimulus conditions but it allows preoperatively to separate unfavorable from favorable cases.

Regan (1968) and Gavrisky (1974) have shown that the high frequency responses are more dependent on the absolute luminance values than the low frequency responses. Fig. 3 shows the amount of light intensity reduction needed to reduce the VECP curve to criterion line values in a normal

212

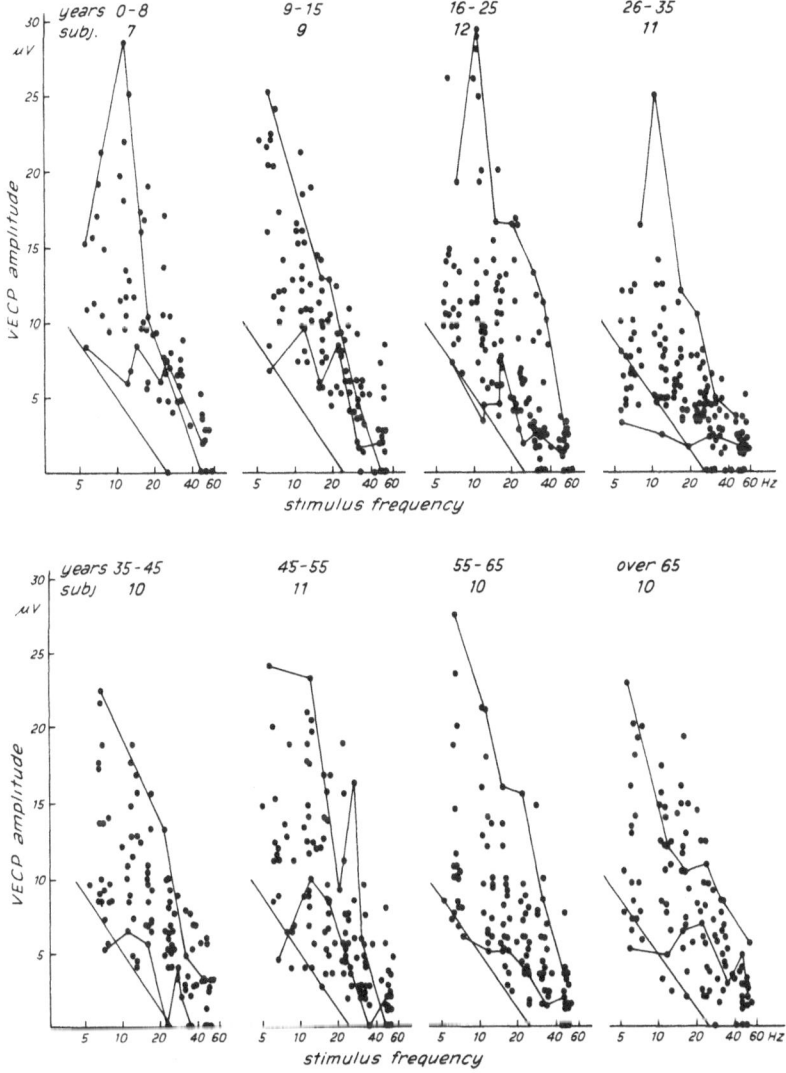

Fig. 1, 2. Amplitude of monocular VECP in healthy subjects as a funtion of stimulus frequency. The points are the single amplitude measurements. Two individual VECP curves have been drawn in each group to illustrate the range of variation in normal subjects. The straight line is the empirical criterion line used to separate preoperatively favorable from unfavorable cases.

subject. Cataract patients and most of the traumatic cases suffer from a severe degradation of optical imagery, but the unpigmented scars and opacities encountered are rarely of high optical density. We admitted, therefore, that a moderate amount of intensity reduction between 2 and 3 logarithmic units would not greatly affect the VECP curve and we expected a possible attenuation of VECP amplitude to be due to retinal or neural pathology which would be little accessible to surgical therapy.

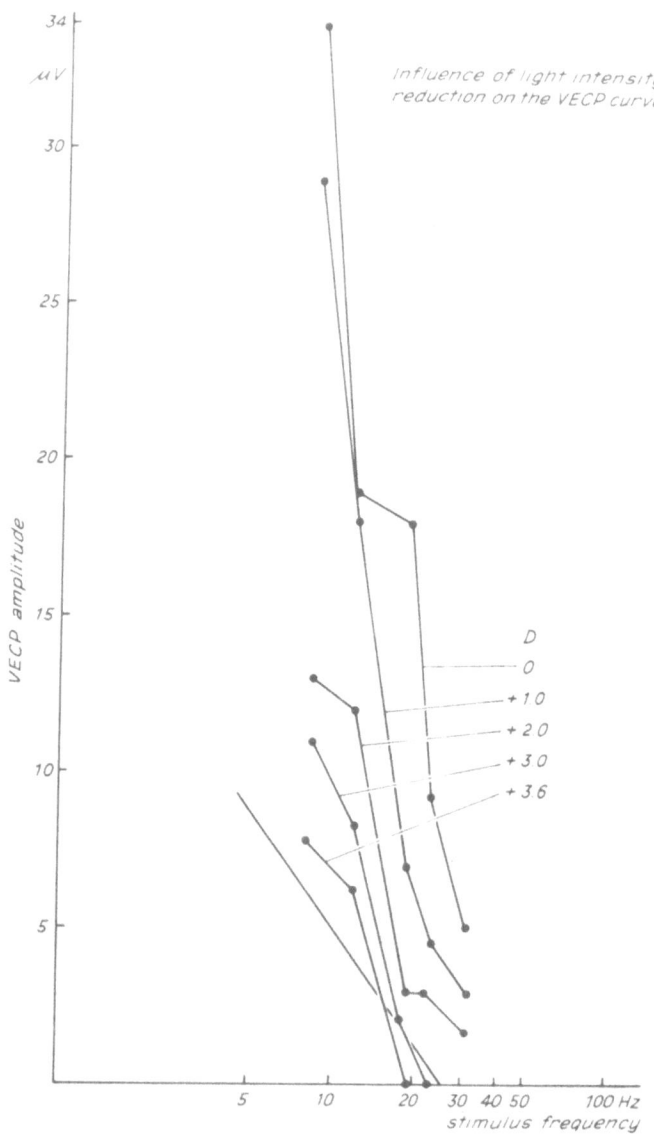

Fig. 3. Influence of the attenuation of stimulus intensity on the VECP curve. The stimulus reduction was performed through the insertion of neutral density filters in the projector. The density of the filter used (logarithmic units) is indicated beside the corresponding curve (D).

214

One group of patients that can have high density opaque media are diabetics with fresh vitreous haemorrhages; they are not included in this report.

Preoperative evaluation of traumatic lesions

This paper includes data on 20 patients with severe ocular injuries. The common point in all cases is that preoperatively the retina was difficult or impossible to see and a visual evaluation of the macula impossible. All but one case had visual acuities reduced to a level of finger counting or less in the affected eye. Only subjects who underwent surgical therapy are included and the visual function after improvement of the optics correlated to the preoperative VECP.

In 13 cases the lesions were due to perforating injuries with intraocular foreign bodies, in 4 cases to perforation without intraocular foreign body and in 3 cases to a blunt contusion. In most cases the intraocular foreign body had been extracted before the time of reconstructieve surgery. The patients have been separated in two groups according to the position of the VECP curve in relation to the earlier defined criterion line.

Patients with unfavorable VECP prognosis (Fig. 4)

The VECP curves in these 10 eyes are entirely or mainly to the left of the criterion line. The insert on the figure shows the type of operation, the postoperative visual acuity and the type of retinal pathology encountered at the time of operation. The best postoperative acuity is low. Case 2 is

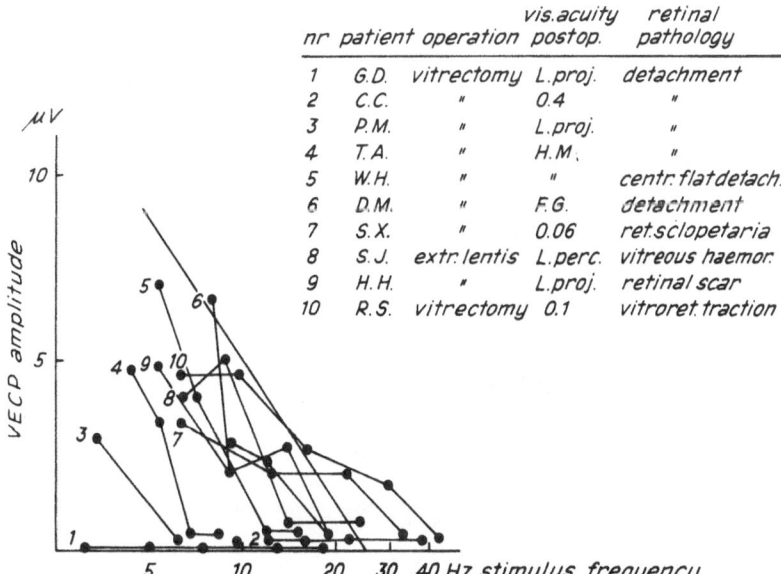

nr	patient	operation	vis.acuity postop.	retinal pathology
1	G.D.	vitrectomy	L.proj.	detachment
2	C.C.	"	0.4	"
3	P.M.	"	L.proj.	"
4	T.A.	"	H.M.	"
5	W.H.	"	"	centr. flat detach.
6	D.M.	"	F.G.	detachment
7	S.X.	"	0.06	ret. sclopetaria
8	S.J.	extr. lentis	L.perc.	vitreous haemor.
9	H.H.	"	L.proj.	retinal scar
10	R.S.	vitrectomy	0.1	vitroret. traction

Fig. 4. Preoperative VECP curves in 10 eyes with trauma and unfavourable VECP prognosis. The postoperative best visual acuities are indicated and the kind of retinal pathology discovered at the time of surgery.

obviously a wrong VECP prognosis and is one of the not to frequent cases whose visual acuity increased markedly after reattachment of a central detachment. Case 10, whose acuity is 0.1 has the best VECP curve of the group and is a borderline case for our VECP classification. The macular pathologies described were seen only at the time of surgery. In no cases did the operative procedure reveal an intact central retina. Case No. 8 was not reoperated and its macular morphology is still unknown.

Patients with favorable VECP prognosis (Fig. 5)

The VECP curves in these 10 eyes are all to the right of the criterion line. The insert in the figure includes the type of operation and the preoperative and postoperative visual acuities. The range of visual acuities is much better than in the first group but there is still one case with a vision of only light perception due to a central proliferative vascular retinopathy with detachment (No. 5), and one case with an acuity of only 0.1, due to a small macula scar (No. 7).

Comparison of injured and sound eyes

One way to get around the large interindividual variability is the possibility to compare the sound eye with the injured eye in those cases with only unilateral pathology. In Fig. 6—7 the monocular VECP curves are plotted in both eyes in three patients with favorable and 3 patients with unfavorable

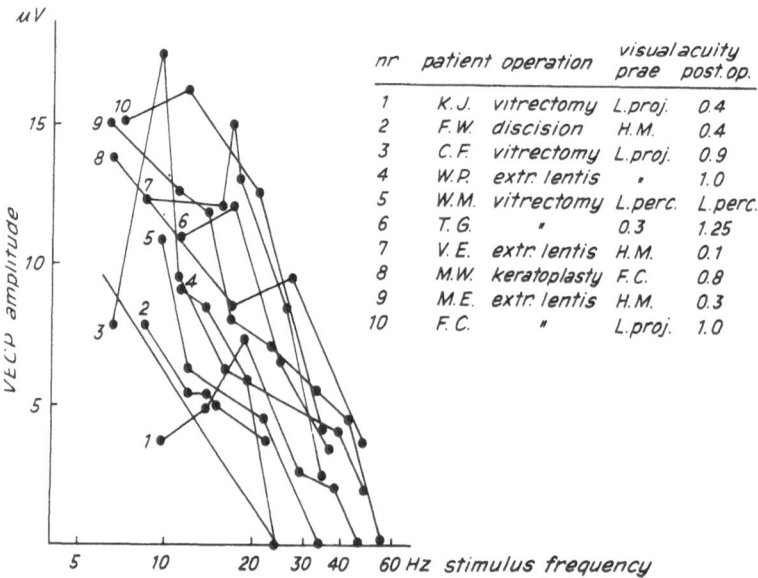

Fig. 5. VECP curves in 10 eyes with trauma and favorable VECP prognosis. The kind of operation and the postopeative increase in visual acuity is indicated.

216

prognosis taken from the two previously described groups. The large distance on the frequency scale between the sound and the injured eye in the unfavorable cases is obvious compared to the similar amplitude attenuation curves in spite of the extreme differences in visual acuities at the time of the VECP measurement in the favorable group (in all three cases with favorable prognosis 1.0 visual acuity in one eye and less than 0.1 in the other eye).

CONCLUSION

The prognostic value of this type of VECP evaluation is not the prediction of any visual acuity in the usual sense, but it seems possible to separate those cases where the best results after surgery will be an increase of visual field only, from those more fortunate cases where the visual function may be above 0.1 and allow the patient to go about by himself. This is possible even in the absence of a sound eye for comparison. In borderline cases where the VECP curve lies very near or astride the criterion line the sound eye can be used as a reference. The VECP curves are very similar in both

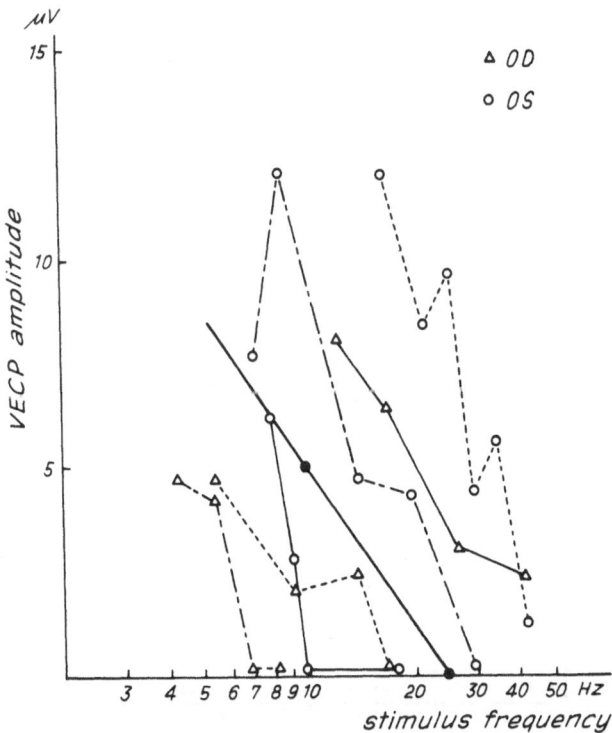

Fig. 6. VECP curves in both eyes from three subjects of Fig. 4 the two curves with similar line drawing belong to the same subject. Notice the large asymmetry between sound and injured eye. The curves of the injured eyes are to the left of the criterion line.

eyes of normal subjects and a large difference in amplitude value speaks for retinal or neural pathology.

In relation to the electroretinogram and echography the VECP information can be used either to substantiate the results of the other methods or to add information not obtainable with ERG or echography alone. A flat retinal detachment in an eye with thick vitreous membranes may be difficult to detect by echography. An extinct electroretinogram as in retinitis pigmentosa is compatible with a normal VECP curve if the optic nerve is intact. The echogram helps the surgeon to decide what he will do. The ERG and VECP may tell him whether it is worthwhile to do it or not.

SUMMARY

Retinal function in patients with traumatic opacities of the ocular media can be judged roughly with a subjective evaluation of light perception and projection or objectively with the electroretinogram. Both methods give little information about macular function. The different kinds of visual evo-

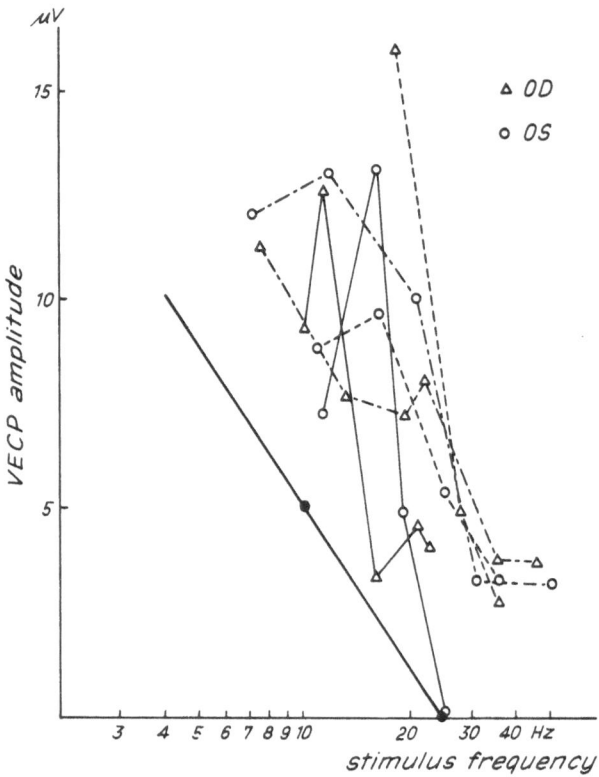

Fig. 7. VECP curves in both eyes from three subjects of Fig. 5. In the patients with favorable prognosis the attenuation curves are similar in the sound and injured eye in spite of large differences in visual acuity.

ked cortical potentials (VECP) share the advantage that the potentials are elicited by the macular area. Flash VECP may be affected by opacities of the ocular media alone. Pattern stimulation is not possible through the disturbed optics. The frequency of a flickering light is not affected by the opacities. It is possible to separate favorable from unfavorable cases before surgical intervention by the position of the frequency dependent attenuation curve of VECP amplitude along the frequency scale. Large macular lesions, detachment and lesions of the optic nerve strongly reduce the high frequency part of the VECP curve whereas opacities of the ocular media alone do not. Amblyopia, macular oedema or even a small macular scar cannot be detected behind opaque ocular media.

ACKNOWLEDGEMENT

This work was supported by a grant from the Schweizerischer Nationalfonds zur Förderung der wissenschaftlichen Forschung Nr. 3.020.73.

REFERENCES

Abe, H , M. Kojima, K. Namba & K. Iwata. Flicker and VER. Studies on the flicker VER in patients with lesions of the visual pathways. *Acta Soc. Jap.* 79: *117–129* (1974).

Bider, E. Visual evoked responses in optic cortex in the presence of macular degeneration. *Ophthalmologica* 161: *187-195* (1970)

Fricker, S. Analysis of VER with synchronous detector techniques. *Invest. Ophthal.* (1971).

Gavrisky, V. Investigation about high rate flicker visual evoked cortical potentials by humans. *Agressologie* 15: *455–460* (1974).

Huber, C. Amplitude versus frequency characteristics of visual evoked cortical potentials to sine wave modulated light in diseases of the optic nerve. Proc. Docum. Ophthal. Proc. Series. Vol. 13. pp. 69–78 (1977). 14th ISCERG Symposium, Louisville Junk, The Hague (1977).

Milner, B., D. Regan & J. R. Heron. Differential diagnosis of multiple sclerosis by visual evoked potential recording. *Brain* 97: *755–772* (1974).

Regan, D. A high frequency mechnism which underlies visual evoked potentials. EEG at clin. *Neurophysiol.* 25: *231–237* (1968).

Authors' address:
University Eye Clinic
Zürich
Switzerland

Docum. Ophthal. Proc. Series, Vol. 15

OPTIC NEUROPATHY DUE TO ALCOHOL ABUSE AND EVOKED CORTICAL POTENTIALS

G. VAN LITH & S. VIJFVINKEL-BRUINENGA
(Rotterdam, The Netherlands)

During the past two years we have seen 22 patients with visual complaints, probably caused by alcohol abuse, at the electrophysiological department of the Rotterdam Eye Hospital. All 22 patients were accustomed to a daily intake of at least one pint of whisky, cognac or genever. It might be better to speak of tobacco-alcohol abuse, since 16 patients were also heavy smokers, 3 patients were moderate smokers, while the smoking habits of the others were not known. Interestingly in this respect is that during the last 10 years a patient with a misuse of tobacco only was never referred to us.

Tobacco-alcohol optic neuropathy is, apart from a social problem, a scientific problem as well. Scientific, because its existence is questionable and its cause problematic. Excellent surveys were presented by Potts in the Friedenwald Memorial Lecture in 1962 and by Dunphy in the De Schweinitz Lecture in 1969. The latter author provides us with anecdotes and theories from older literature, starting with Aristotle and Pliny the Elder; Potts discusses more the etiological problems. Both authors refer to the excellent work of Carroll (1935, 1937), which seemed to prove without doubt that tobacco-alcohol neuropathy is indirectly caused by a vitamin B deficiency. The social behaviour of the patients of Carroll and of ours points also in this direction. Reading Carroll's papers, it is as if we hear the stories of our own patients: unemployment, problems at home, much drinking and smoking, poor nutrition.

Is it surprising that this disease crops up again now that there is so much unemployment? After being found so often in the first part of this century, its existence very probably dropped during World War II. Potts had to write in his lecture: 'to the best of my memory I have never seen an 'authentic' case of the disease.' He attributes this: 'to the fact that as a wartime measure all cereals in this country, i.e. in the U.S.A., were fortified with vitamins and that even a person with severe chronic alcoholism ate large amounts of bread.' Most probably none of the patients we saw ate very healthily, so a deficiency was very likely to exist. However, apart from this indirect effect, direct effects on the visual system may also exist.

Ikeda (1963) found as a direct effect that the retina behaved more scotopically: the scotopic b-wave became higher, the FFF lower, the a-wave being less influenced. The Scandinavian group of Nilsson et al. (1977), Knave et al. (1974) and Skoog (1974) investigated the standing potential in correlation with the c-wave; both phenomena increased when alcohol was used. As to the visually evoked cortical potentials, only light flash evoked potentials were investigated: Müller & Haase (1967) described longer latencies, Lewis et al. (1964) and Rhodes et al. (1969) a decrease in amplitude of the later components of the VECPs.

In our group of patients the ERG, as well as flash and pattern evoked cortical potentials were investigated. These patients were referred to the electrophysiological department because of visual complaints, often of unknown cause. Remarkably, only some of them had a clearly lowered visual acuity, as well as the typical centrocaecal scotoma, but all were habitual and heavy drinkers. In Figures 1 and 2 retinal and cortical potentials of 2 patients (B and C) are presented together with those of a normal subject (A). The first patient, 48 years old, was a welder, having absolutely no visual problems. In November 1976 he became unemployed as the factory he worked for went bankrupt. Since then he started to drink more and more, from the time of getting out of bed, i.e. at lunchtime, till he went to bed again, while eating almost nothing.

Now he has a visual acuity of 0.5 in both eyes, with a centrocaecal scotoma of 10 degrees and a central sensitivity loss in the visual field of half a log unit. Compared to these data, the cortical potentials are much more disturbed (Figure 2, B) All VECPs, whether made by pattern stimulation or by light flash stimulation, can hardly be recognized. The 2 Hz pattern reversal was carried out according to Halliday's method, in order to see if latency shifts could be found (Halliday et al., 1972). The very low amplitudes, however, make a reliable measurement of the latencies impossible.

Apart from these gross abnormalities in the VECPs, the ERGs are also abnormal (Figure 1B). The Ops are lowered as well as the photopic b-wave, the scotopic b-wave not being clearly pathological. These ERG-results are in

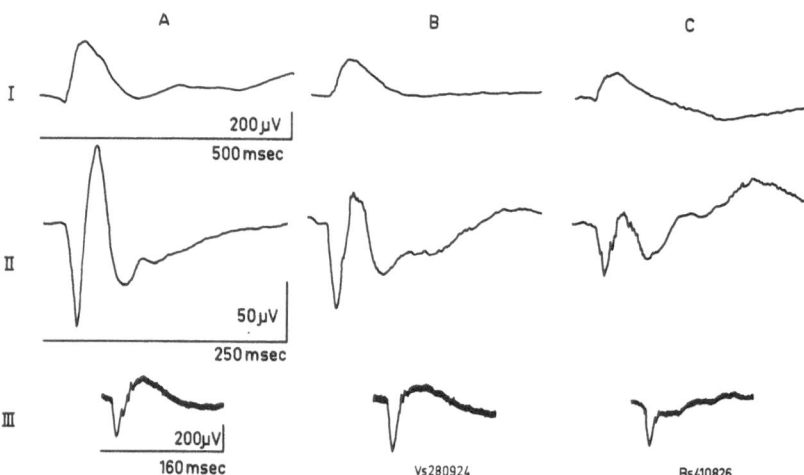

Fig. 1. Scotopic (I) and photopic (II) ERGs, together with a registration of the oscillatory potentials (III) in a normal subject (A) and two patients with alcohol abuse (B,C).

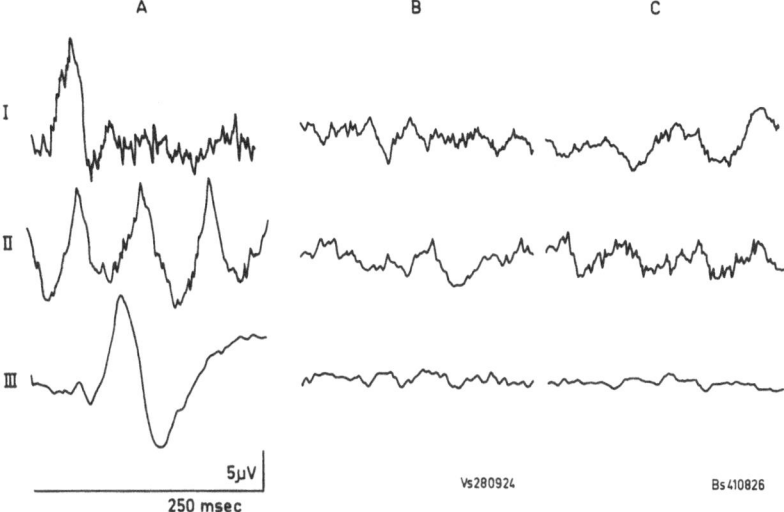

Fig. 2. Cortical potentials, elicited with light flashes in a frequency of 2 Hz (I) and with a pattern reversal stimulus of 4 Hz (II) and 2 Hz (III) in the same three subjects as in Figure 1.

accordance with Ikeda's findings and even more clearly present in the second case.

This patient is 35 years old and has drunk at least a pint of whisky every day for 10 years. At the time of examination visual acuity was 0.8 and 0.4 for the right and left eye respectively. The OPs are absent, the photopic b-wave is very much lowered in any case much more than the scotopic b-wave and the a-wave (Figure 1C). There are still some cortical potentials of a very low amplitude.

A lowered ERG is not a consistent finding. We found it in 7 patients, but if present the abnormalities were as described: abnormal OPs, the b-wave more disturbed than the a-wave and the photopic system more than the scotopic system. The data of the cortical potentials elicited with a 4 Hz pattern reversal stimulus of the whole group of patients are collected in Figure 3. In one patient these responses were not determined. The amplitudes are plotted against visual acuity: the mean value of our normal subjects is 10 μV; as a lower limit of the normal range we consider 7 μV. According to this limit, 7 patients had normal values, 11 patients definitely had too low responses, while 3 patients were borderline cases. Furthermore, there is some relation between visual acuity and the height of the responses.

From this group of patients it seems that subjective visual complaints are the first symptoms, since all patients had complaints, but neither visual acuity nor electrophysiological results were always disturbed. It might be that latency times, determined according to Halliday's method, are more sensitive in this aspect. In this group of patients this method was applied only in four cases: in two of them amplitudes were too low to measure latencies; the two other latency times were increased. In an experimental situation, like Ikeda and the Scandinavian group did for the retina and

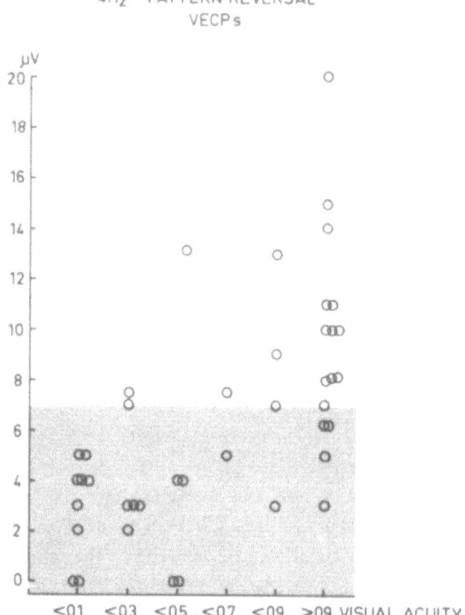

Fig. 3. Amplitude of cortical potentials, elicited with a 4 Hz pattern reversal stimulus, plotted versus visual acuity.

Müller & Haase for flash evoked cortical potentials, we registered pattern evoked potentials after a fast intake of 35% alcohol (genever) in three subjects. A 1 Hz pattern reversal was applied (Figure 4). Apparently, the amplitude of the maximum decreases, its latency becomes longer (from 116 msec

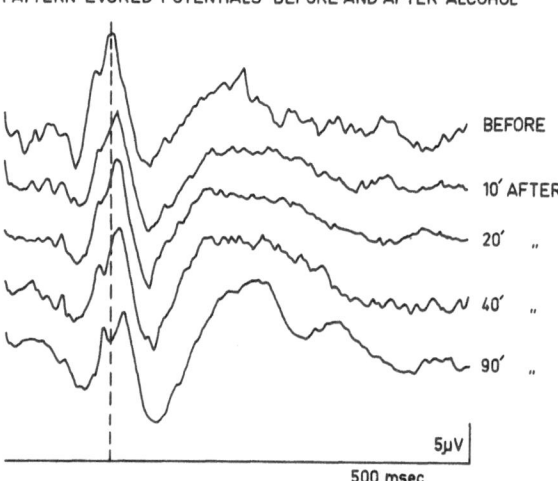

Fig. 4. Cortical potentials to a 1 Hz pattern reversal stimulus before and after intake of 200 cc genever (35% alcohol).

to 127 msec) and the negativity increases. These data from acute experiments make it very likely that alcohol also affects the retina and conductive system directly. This implies that Carroll's conclusion, based on his experiments with chronic alcoholics, is probably too definite. He only describes a recovery of the visual acuity after vitamin B administration; other, more refined, tests on the visual system had not been done at that time.

SUMMARY

In a group of 22 patients with visual complaints, probably caused by alcohol-tobacco abuse, not only the VECPs, but also the ERGs were often abnormal. From acute experiments it seemed very likely that, apart from an indirect toxic effect, a direct toxic effect of alcohol on the visual system may exist.

REFERENCES

Carroll, F.D. Analysis of fifty-five cases of tobacco-alcohol amblyopia. *Arch. Ophthal.* 14: *421–434* (1935).

Carroll, F.D. Importance of diet in the etiology and treatment of tobacco-alcohol amblyopia. *Arch. Ophthal.* 18: *948–962* (1937).

Dunphy, E.B. Alcohol and tobacco amblyopia: a historical survey. *Amer. J. Ophthal.* 68: *569–578* (1969).

Halliday, A.M., W.I. McDonald & J. Mushin. Delayed visual evoked response in optic neuritis. *Lancet* II: *982–985* (1972).

Ikeda, H. Effects of ethyl alcohol on the evoked potential of the human eye. *Vision Res.* 3: *155–169* (1963).

Knave, B., H.E. Persson & S.E.G. Nilsson. A comparative study on the effects of barbiturate and ethyl alcohol on retinal functions with special reference to the c-wave of the electroretinogram and the standing potential of the sheep eye. *Acta Ophthal.* 52: *254–259* (1974).

Lewis, E.G., R.E. Dustman & E.C. Beck. The effects of alcohol on visual and somatosensory evoked responses. *Electroenceph. clin. Neurophysiol.* 28: *202–205* (1970).

Müller, W. & E. Haase. Das Verhalten der corticalen Antwort unter Alkoholeinwirkung. *Graefes Arch. Ophthal.* 173: *108–113* (1967).

Nilsson, S.E.G. & K.-O. Skoog. Variations of the directly recorded standing potential of the human eye in response to changes in illumination and to ethanol. In: ERG, VER and psychophysics; Proc. 14th ISCERG Symposium, Louisville, 1976; ed. by Th. Lawwill. Docum. Ophthal. Proc. Ser. 13: 99–109 (1977).

Potts, A.M. Retinotoxic and choroidotoxic substances. *Invest. Ophthal.* 1: *290–303* (1962).

Rhodes, L.E., F.W. Obitz & D. Creel. Effect of alcohol and task on hemispheric asymmetry of visually evoked potentials in man. *Electroenceph. clin. Neurophysiol.* 38: *561–568* (1975).

Skoog, K.-O. The c-wave of the human D.C. registered ERG. III. Effects of ethyl alcohol on the c-wave. *Acta Ophthal.* 52: *913–923* (1974).

Authors' address
Eye Hospital
Erasmus University
180 Schiedamsevest
Rotterdam
The Netherlands

VISUAL EVOKED RESPONSE ANOMALIES IN A PATIENT WITH FRIEDREICH's ATAXIA

KARL J. FRITZ, JOHN L. TRIMBLE, RAMESH C. TRIPATHI & CAROL S. FRITZ

(Chicago, Ill., USA)

ABSTRACT

Steady state visual evoked responses were studied in a patient with the clinical diagnosis of Friedreich's ataxia. Ophthalmologic examination revealed no anomalies including visual acuity of 6/6 in both eyes, full visual field in both eyes, normal screening color vision, absence of optic atrophy and absence of nystagmus. Steady state VER revealed a monocular moderately attenuated signal in the left eye at 12 and 16 Hz and a markedly attenuated signal at 20 and 25 Hz. This contrasted with a normal VER in the right eye. The patient died of cardiac failure secondary to cardiomyopathy associated with Friedreich's ataxia. Autopsy examination of the brain revealed a number of structural changes. The spinal cord had the usual severe demyelination and axonal changes associated with Friedreich's ataxia. Histologic examination of the optic nerves showed no abnormality in the right nerve but focal axonal swelling, and some evidence of demyelination in the left optic nerve.

CASE REPORT

The patient's illness began in August 1975, when she was nine years old. There were severe right sided headaches associated with vomiting and a lame feeling in the right hand. These effects would persist for approximately three hours and then vanish. Recurrence of these symptoms occurred two weeks later with a right temporal headache and photophobia. This recurred periodically and a neurological diagnosis of encephalitis was made. A few months later the patient was again examined and epilepsy was diagnosed. At this time there were increased headaches and some incoordination. A brain scan was normal. Electroencephalography showed no changes, however, a second electroencephalogram done shortly thereafter showed abnormalities in the left occipital cortex. Computerized tomography was normal. In March, 1976, progressive bilateral hearing loss was diagnosed. A cerebral angiogram, electroencephalogram, lumbar puncture and computerized tomography were all normal. In September, 1976, the patient developed bilateral otitis media and was treated with antibiotics. She was admitted to the hospital in November, 1976, with congestive heart failure associated with nausea and vomiting, and was treated with diuretics and digoxin. The deep tendon reflexes were uniformly depressed and vibration sense in the lower limbs was decreased. The patient was ataxic and showed an intention tremor. Chest X-ray showed cardiomegaly and increased venous congestion. An electrocardiogram demonstrated a first degree AV block and other changes

consistent with myocardial infarction or cardiomyopathy. An echocardio-
gram showed poor contractibility. On the basis of these findings, Friedreich's ataxia with cardiomyopathy was diagnosed. Following this, progressive bilateral nerve deafness, multifocal encephalopathy and transient visual
disturbances were noted. An ophthalmic examination was performed revealing normal visual acuity (6/6) in both eyes, full Goldmann visual fields,
normal color vision and normal fundus features including normal optic nerves. The VER was abnormal with asymmetry between the right and left eye.
By December, 1976, the patient was once again in congestive heart failure
and complained of paresthesias of the face and neck, severe headaches and
nausea. The electroencephalogram showed diffuse dysrhythmia and marked
multifocal encephalopathy. There was decreased conduction velocity in the
ulnar, median, and peroneal nerves. On February 20, 1977, the patient was
again admitted to the hospital with complaints of headache and increasing
hearing loss. An electroencephalogram performed on February 28, 1977,
was considered normal. Patient was again discharged for outpatient follow-
up. Final admission occured on April 6. 1977. The patient had had increased
shortness of breath for the past four days and by the time of admission was
in severe respiratory distress. There was pitting edema off the legs, increased
pulmonary vasculature, and chemical imbalances. On April 7, the patient
suffered a precipitous drop in blood pressure and underwent irreversible car-
diopulmonary arrest.

PATHOLOGY

The disease found at autopsy was marked by focal demyelination of nerves
throughout the body, in particular nerves of the upper limbs, the seventh
cranial nerve, and the sciatic nerve. There was marked axonal degeneration
and demyelination of the dorsal and central spinocerebellar tracts. There
was focal axonal swelling and demyelination of the dorsal lumbar roots, but
with normal ventral lumbar roots. Specific cerebral pathologic changes, demonstrated microscopically, were found in the right frontal cortex where
giant bizarre vesicular nuclei with prominent nucleoli were seen and an occasional group of smaller but similar cells were also seen. These were thought
to be astrocytes. The occipital cortex on both sides showed focal mild spongiform changes in the deep cortex with focal congestion of penetrating arteries. The parietal cortex on the right and on the left showed slight focal
axonal thickening, but the right cerebellum showed subpial basophilic deposits. The dentate nucleus on both left and right sides were normal. The left
and right basal ganglia showed spongiform changes. The midbrain had spongiform changes in the substantia nigra and superior coliculus with a rare giant
neuron in the substantia nigra and superior colliculus with a rare giant neuron
in the periaqueductal gray matter. The upper pons showed mild spongiform
changes in the tegmentum with the medial lemniscus, medial longitudinal
fasciculus and brachium conjunctivum all appearing normal. The midbrain
had mild spongiform changes in the lower pons. The seventh nerve showed
severe changes with focal axonal tufts in the roots near the root entry zone.
There appeared to be some demyelination process occuring in the lower

pons. The medulla oblongata showed demyelination and axonal atrophy of the eleventh nerve. The lower medulla showed no discernable changes. The posterior root ganglia showed focal loss of dorsal root ganglion cells. There was patchy demyelination of the dorsal roots and the dorsal and central spinocerebellar tracts. The most severe demyelination was found in the lumbar spinal cord with superior posterior column and dorsal roots effected.

The eyes were normal under gross and macroscopic examination. The optic tracts showed no significant anomalies in the regions where sections were available. Light microscopic examination of the sections of the optic nerve from both eyes showed an essentially normal structure of the right optic nerve but focal axonal swelling, arborizations of axonal bundles and possible demyelinating changes were apparent in the left optic nerve, (Fig. 1).

ELECTTROPHYSIOLOGY

The VER was recorded using a bipolar configuration with the active elec-

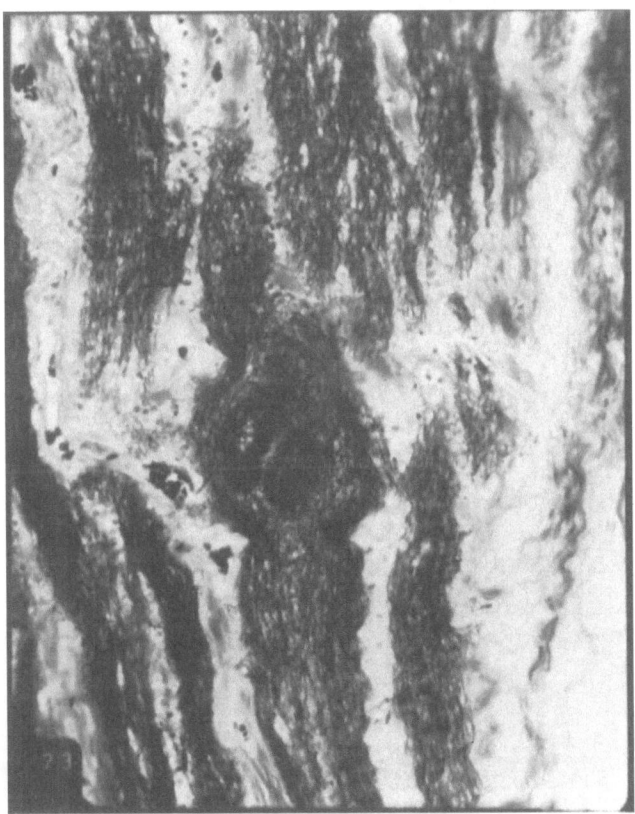

Fig. 1. Focal axonal swelling, arborization of axonal bundles and possible demyelinating changes of left optic nerve.

trode placed just above the inion on the midline, and the indifferent electrode placed on the midline 3 cm anteriorly. The earlobe was used a reference ground. The electroencephalogram was amplified by one hundred thousand, using a Grass P511 AC-coupled preamplifier using a bandwidth of 0.3 Hz to 100 Hz (-3dB points). The stimulus was produced by a Grass P522 photostimulator placed 0.5 meter in front of the patient. The stimulus intensity was set at 16. Frequency of stimulation was controlled by an external pulse generator. Stimulus frequencies of 12, 16, 20, and 25 Hz were used. Stimuli were delivered monocularly with the fellow eye occluded.

The steady state responses obtained showed marked asymmetry between the right and left eyes. The amplitude and waveform regularity were decreased for left eye stimulation at all frequencies up to 25 Hz, (fig. 2).

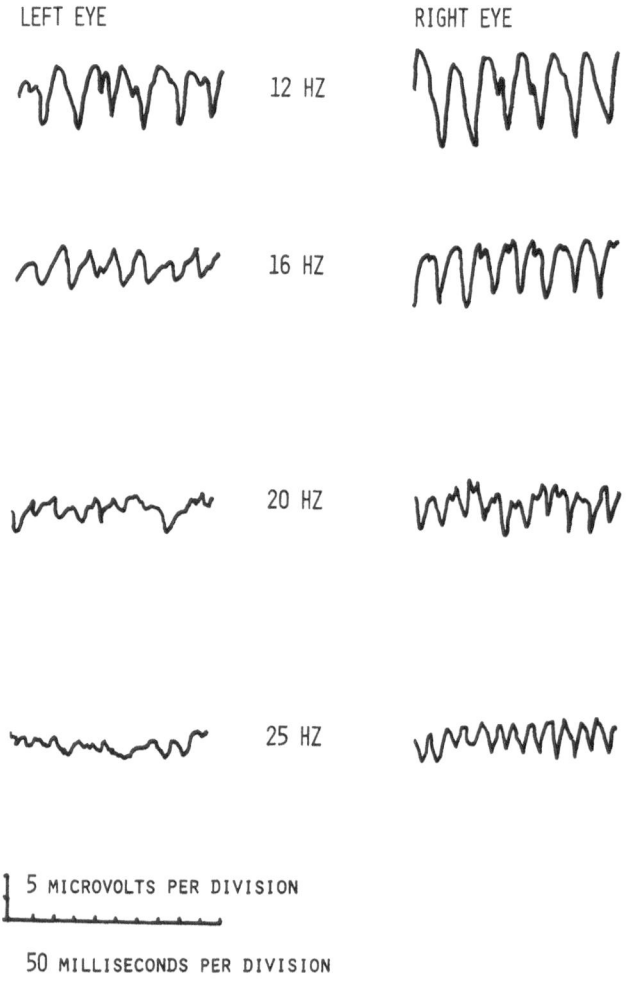

Fig. 2. Asymmetry of steady state VER for left and right eye at 12, 16, 20, and 25 Hz.

230

DISCUSSION

Friedreich's ataxia is a heterofamilial degenerative disease of childhood which is characterized by progressive degeneration of the spinocerebellar tracts, the posterior columns, and the posterior spinal cord roots (Bray, 1969; Ford, 1966; Walsh & Hoyt, 1969). Although this disease is rare, it is the principal type of hereditary ataxia seen in children. Males seem more often affected than females. The exact genetic mode of transmission is obscure.

The usual pathologic changes found at autopsy include a small spinal cord, a cerebellum which seems smaller than usual but does not show degeneration of the pyramidal and dorsal spinocerebellar tracts. It is generally thought that degenerative changes are absent in the cerebrum. However, some authors (Ford, 1966; Walsh & Hoyt, 1969) suggest on clinical grounds that there must be cerebral changes because mental deterioration occurs in late stages of the disease.

Clinically, there are a variety of malformations which may be associated with Friedreich's ataxia. Approximately half of the patients have associated myocardial involvement and there are a variety of chemical abnormalities which may occur. The usual clinical course begins with clumsiness in walking with an onset between six to fifteen years. There is a loss of tendon jerk reflexes in the legs. As the disease progresses, the ataxia becomes worse, the patients become bedridden and there is atrophy of muscle and other deformities. The ocular anomalies found with Friedreich's ataxia may include nystagmus, optic atrophy, optic neuritis, blepharoptosis, Argyll Robertson pupils, ophthalmoplegia, and pigmentary degeneration of the retina.

The patient presented in this paper had none of the usual ocular findings. The only unusual finding associated with vision was the asymmetric steady state visual evoked response. Cerebral disease was symmetric and included spongiosus of the occipital cortex and slight focal axonal thickening in the parietal cortex. The optic tracts were examined in several regions for demyelination but none was found. The optic nerve showed histological asymmetry with myelin stain. The right optic nerve was normal, whereas the left optic nerve demonstrated focal regions of axonal thickening and regions of decoloration similar to those present in dorsal root ganglia.

The source of asymmetric VER may lie in the asymmetry found on histological changes are suggestive of demyelination, further confirmatory studies with electron microscopy are underway to verify derangement of myelin in the left optic nerve.

ACKNOWLEDGEMENT

The authors would like to thank Tina Rainieri, Tati Montesinos, and Mark Golden for preparation of special histologic sections.

REFERENCES

Bray, P.F. Neurology in Pediatrics. Year Book Medical Publishers, Chicago (1969).
Ford, Frank, R. Diseases of the Nervouw System in Infancy and Childhood (Fifth Edition), Charles C. Thomas, Sprinfield (1966).

Walsh, Frank B. & William F. Hoyt. Clinical Neuro-ophthalmology, Williams and Wilkins, Bultimore (1969).

Authors' address:
Dept. of Ophthalmology
University of Chicago
950 E. 59th Street
Chicago, Ill., 60637
USA

INVARIANCES OF THE CONE-DOMINATED ERG
(TREE SHREW AND MAN)

J. M. THIJSSEN & H. J. TER LAAK

(Nijmegen, The Netherlands)

The electroretinogram of a tree shrew (*Tupaia chinensis*) has been investigated (Ter Laak, 1975; Thijssen et al., 1978) and, in some respects, compared to the human photopic ERG (Thijssen & Ter Laak, 1976). The retina of tree shrews contains only cones, hence cone specific aspects of the primate ERG can be clearly demonstrated. The present analysis revealed two invariances. First: the ratio of x-wave to a-wave amplitudes is invariant while changing stimulation and adaptation light intensities or both. The proportionality constant for the tree shrew was found to be 4.3. This is very close to the figure of 4.4 found by Bonaventure et al. (1976) for the chicken ERG. The human photopic ERG appears to reveal the invariance only if the rod system is completely inactive, which can be favoured by using red light stimulation. The proportionality constant for the human ERG appeared to be 2.0.

A second invariance was found when at various adaptation levels the so-called critical time duration, CD (integration time), for flash evoked ERG responses was compared to the critical flicker frequency, CFF, after correction of the latter for the changes in incremental sensitivity. Then, the product of CD times CFF corr. is independent of the adaptation level and it equals on the average 0.6. This figure found for the tree shrew's ERG is very similar to the value of 0.5 obtained from psycho-physical measurements of human foveal vision.

REFERENCES

Bonaventure, N., N. Wioland & P. Karli. Brightness coding of white and chromatic stimuli in the chicken, suslik, and rat electroretinogram: relation to light adaptation. *Ophthal. Res.* 8: *81−92* (1976).

Ter Laak, H. J. Electrophysiological investigations into luminance coding in the retina of a tree shrew (Tupaia chinensis). Thesis, Nijmegen University (1975).

Thijssen, J M., H. J. ter Laak & P. M. A. van Well. Masking, de Lange curves and integration time as revealed by the electroretinogram of a tree shrew (Tupaia chinensis) *Europ. J. Physiol.* 377: *199−204* (1978).

Thijssen, J. M. & H. J. ter Laak. Invariances of the cone-dominated ERG (tree shrew and man). pp. 331−340, in: Docum. Ophthal. Proc. Series Vol. 7 (ed. by A. F. Deutman), Junk, The Hague (1976).

Authors' address:
Biophysics Laboratory of the Institute of Ophthalmology
University of Nijmegen
Nijmegen
The Netherlands.

Docum. Ophthal. Proc. Series, Vol. 15

ERG COMPONENTS OF THE CHICKEN RETINA

N. WIOLAND & N. BONAVENTURE

(Strasbourg, France)

Since the early works of Einthoven & Jolly (1908) and of Granit (1933), the gross ERG has been known to be the sum of several potentials of different signs and amplitudes. A good number of models of component analysis have been published on various species (Granit, 1933; Brown, 1968; Ogden & Wylie, 1971; Rodieck, 1972; Knave et al., 1972).

Our previous results on the chicken retina have shown striking differences in the ERG patterns depending on stimulus wavelength. This was clearly evidenced in the characteristics of the 'a-b function' drawn for white and monochromatic stimuli (Bonaventure et al., 1976). The purpose of the present work is to analyse the characteristics of the ERG subcomponents of the chicken, the retina of which is predominantly photopic.

METHODS

The experiments were performed on 3 to 7 weeks old chickens which were curarized and artificially ventilated. Body temperature was held constant and the electrocardiogram was checked at regular intervals. The pupils were dilated with drops of homatropin and Flaxedil. The retinal potentials were derived in a conventional manner, between two silver-chlorided electrodes and fed into a d.c. amplifier with low drift. Photic stimulation was provided by a xenon source, equipped either with narrow-band interference filters or with a monochromator.

The electroretinogram was recorded for stimuli of various intensities, durations and spectral characteristics.

RESULTS

a and b-waves

Fig. 1a shows the intensity-voltage (I-V) function of a and b-waves elicited by brief (10 msec) and long (3 sec) stimuli of white light. The a-wave is measured from the base-line and b-wave from the trough of the a-wave. The a-wave amplitude increases regularly with log intensity and is completely independent of flash duration. The intensity-voltage functions for the b-wave are more complicated, showing a saturation level, or even a voltage decrease in the middle of their operating range.

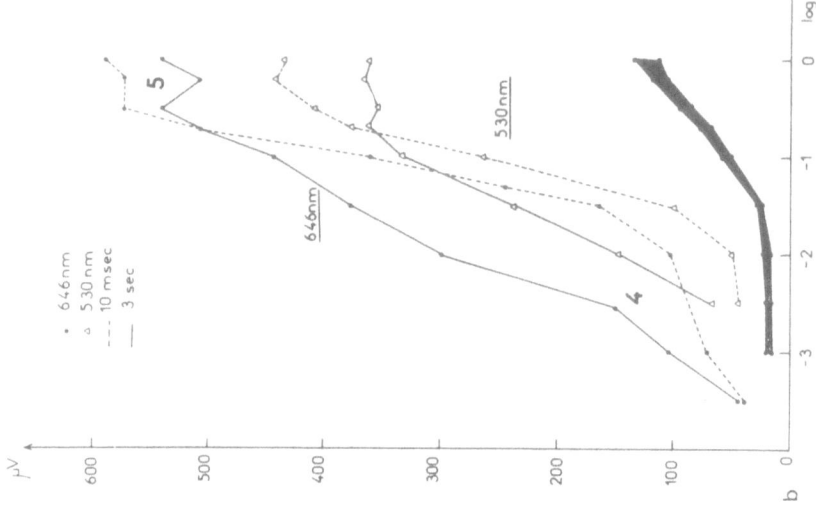

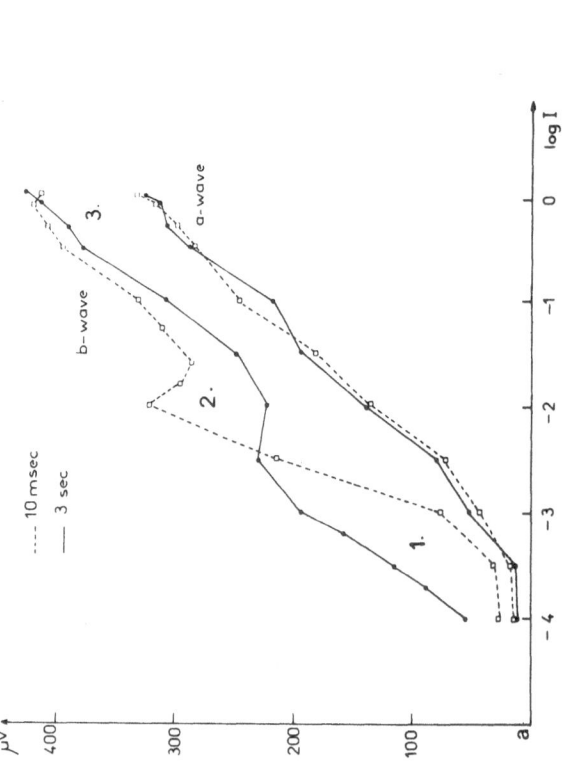

Fig. 1. Intensity-voltage functions for a and b-waves of ERGs recorded in response to flashes of 10 msec and 3 sec duration. The numbers (1 to 5) on the curves refer to Fig. 2. *Fig. 1a.* White light (maximal intensity = 20,000 lux).
Fig. 1b: Monochromatic light. Comparison of two wavelengths, 530 and 646 nm, to which the retina is equally sensitive as proved by equal a-wave amplitudes (all values of a-wave amplitude for both wavelengths and both durations fall in the grey zone).

If the responses to brief and long stimuli are compared, one can distinguish between a low intensity range where the highest amplitudes are obtained by stimulations of long duration, and a high intensity range where the highest amplitudes are obtained by brief flashes. The two curves always cross at an intensity that elicits and a-wave of 70 μV.

The same I-V functions are drawn for 15 different wavelengths (ranging between 420 and 700 nm). Fig. 1b shows an example of two wavelengths, 530 and 646 nm, which are chosen for their equal brightness to the retina, as proved by equal a-wave amplitudes. If one considers the curves drawn for a and b-waves at both wavelengths and both durations, the following observations may be made:

1. The I-V functions for the a-wave are all of the same type: they are independent of flash duration and they are only shifted along the X-axis depending on the wavelength.

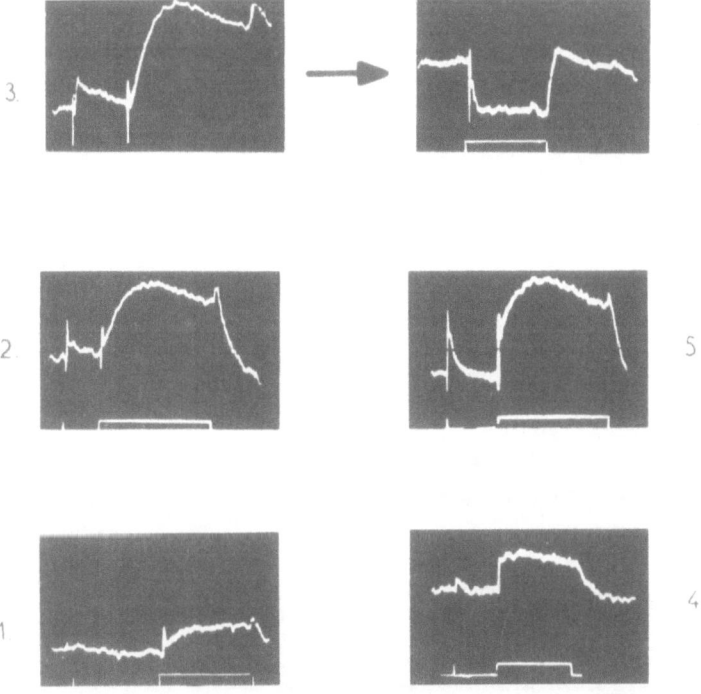

Fig. 2. Each photo shows the ERG patterns in response to a brief flash followed by a long flash. The numbers refer to Figures 1a and 1b. 1. white light, low intensity range; 2. white light, higher intensity, to which the b-wave becomes higher with brief flashes; 3. white light, high intensity range; 4. monochromatic light 646 nm, low intensity range; 5. monochromatic light 646 nm, high intensity range.

In photos 2 and 5, on the one hand, and photos 1 and 4, on the other, the a-waves are of approximately the same amplitude. This permits comparison of ERG patterns for white and monochromatic lights of equal brightness.

Upper right: white light, high intensity and long duration after moderate anoxia, which suppresses the c-wave.

Calibration: 200 μV and 1 sec.

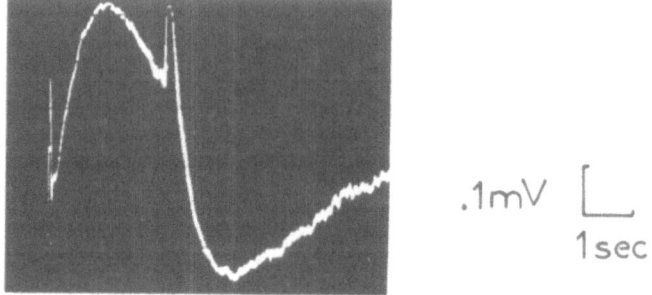

.1mV ⌐
1sec

Fig. 3. C-wave.
Fig. 3a. ERG in response to a flash of white light, high intensity and long duration, showing positive and negative c-waves.

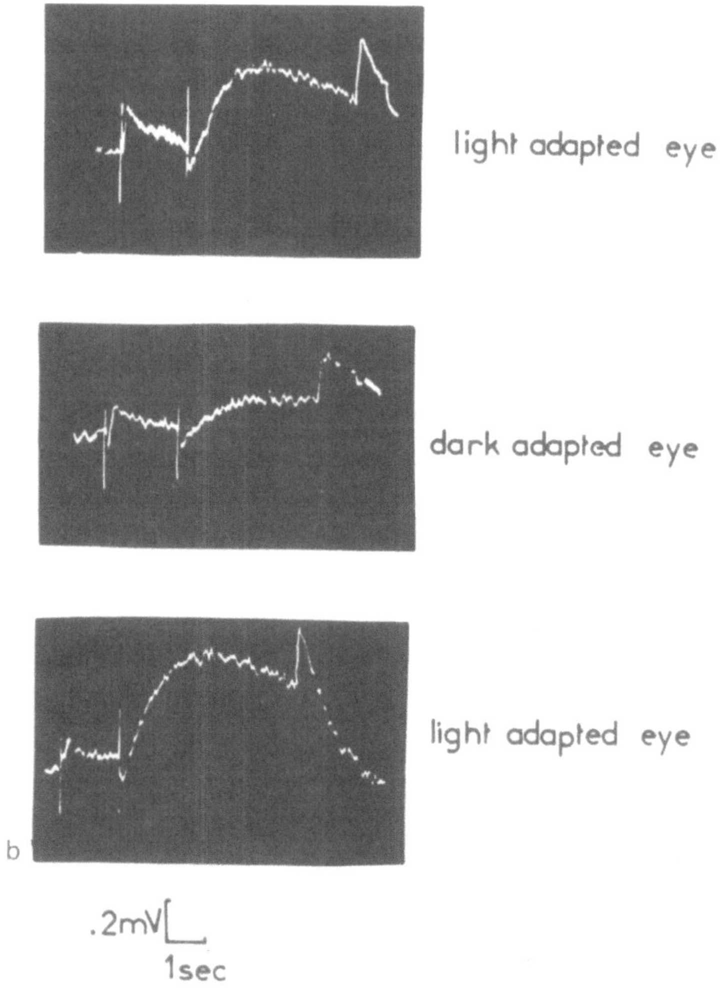

light adapted eye

dark adapted eye

light adapted eye

.2mV⌐
1sec

Fig. 3b. same conditions of recording; upper trace: after light adaptation; middle trace: following 10 min dark adaptation; lower trace: following light adaptation (a series of 10 flashes of high intensity and 5 sec duration each).

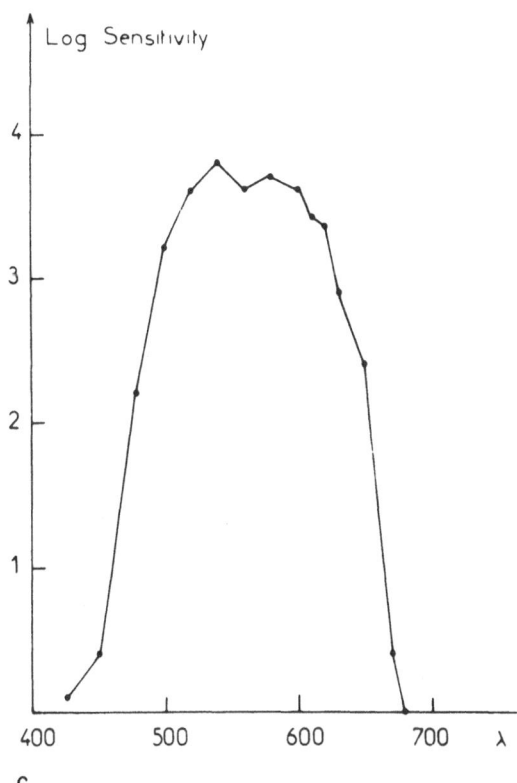

Log Sensitivity

Fig. 3c. spectral sensitivity for the c-wave.

2. The I-V functions for the b-wave show marked differences according to both duration and wavelength. The discrepancy between long and brief stimuli shown for white light, recurs with each monochromatic light. Whatever the wavelength, the crossing point between the two curves is found again at approximately the same level on the x-axis, i.e. at an intensity that elicits an a-wave of about 70 μV.

3. The a-b amplification appears to be wavelength-dependent: for an equal a-wave amplitude elicited by various wavelengths, the b-wave amplitudes are different. The comparison between the two wavelengths of Fig. 1b shows that the b-wave amplitude, which corresponds to a given a-wave amplitude, is always higher for 646 nm than for 530 nm. For the various wavelengths tested, this a-b amplification is higher than for the white light.

c-wave

At high intensities, the c-wave constitutes by far the most prominent element of the response (reaching 800 μV or more, Fig. 3a). A flash duration of at least 10 sec is necessary for complete development of the c-wave. When the light is turned off, a positive 'off-effect' occurs, which is immediately followed by a negative c-wave. The latter is a mirror image of the positive c-wave and behaves in the same manner. The c-wave is increased by light adaptation and decreased by dark adaptation (Fig. 3b). The spectral sens-itivity of this component is shown in Fig. 3c. It culminates around 550 nm.

DISCUSSION

The observation of the patterns of individual ERG's (Fig. 2), as well as the analysis of the I-V functions obtained for various durations and spectral characteristics of the stimulus (Fig. 1a and 1b), indicate that, in chickens like in many other species, the b-wave, measured in the gross ERG, is a com-bination of several components reflecting the activity of various populations of cells.

a-wave

The a-wave is constituted by the leading edge of 'distal P_{III} potential', which is supposed to reflect receptor activity and shows far less temporal integration than the slow P_{III} (Witkovsky et al., 1975). The observation that flashes of 10 msec and 3 sec elicit the same a-wave amplitude confirms that point.

b-wave

The results reported here lead us to propose a model of ERG components in which the b-wave is the sum of 3 processes (in addition to the c-wave, which gives additional interference): the transient b-wave itself and 2 processes of longer temporal integration: a positive d.c.-component and a negative-d.c. component; the relative importance of these subcomponents is dependent on the intensity range, as well as on the duration and spectral characteristics of the stimulus.

Both positive and negative d.c. components are favoured by long duration of the stimulus.

1) *The positive d.c. component* is further favoured by low intensities and by stimulations of long wavelengths (Fig. 2.4). It may be brought in relation to the d.c. component isolated at low intensities in the cat (Brown, 1968), in the sheep (Knave et al., 1972) and in the human eye (Knave et al., 1973; Taümer et al., 1976).

The relative importance in the b-wave of this component could be the origin of:
1) the greater b-wave amplitude elicited by flashes of long duration in the low intensity range;
2) the discrepancy between the various wavelengths (Fig. 1a and 1b).
With white stimulations the positive d.c. component is either very small or masked by a more prominent negative d.c. component (Fig. 2.1.). This may be the reason why Ogden & Wylie (1971) did not isolate a positive d.c. com-ponent in the avian ERG.

2) *The negative d.c. potential*, according to the proposed model, is favoured

240

by high intensities and long durations of the stimulus and is most prominent in the response to white light. A moderate anoxia (Fig. 2, upper right) which suppresses the c-wave, permits clear isolation of this component. The relative importance of the negative d.c. component in the b-wave could explain several features of the I-V functions:

1) The b-wave saturation level results from the decreasing importance of the positive d.c. component, and the increasing importance of the negative d.c. component when higher intensities are reached.

2) Long durations of the stimulus favour the negative d.c. component. This could explain that this saturation level occurs at lower intensities with long flashes than with brief ones.

3) In the high intensity range, the b-wave amplitude is lower with flashes of long duration. This could be a consequence of the increasing predominance of the negative d.c. component.

Furthermore, at these high intensities, the responses to brief flashes may be increased by addition of 'off-effects' and c-waves.

The negative d.c. component described here, shows more resistance to anoxia and to drugs than the other components. Thus, it may be brought in relation with the negative d.c. component described in sheep by Knave et al. (1972) and with 'Proximal P $_{III}$' potential isolated by Murakami & Kaneko (1966) in frog and turtle retinas.

c-wave

In our experimental conditions (curarized animals) the c-wave appears to be a prominent feature of the chicken ERG. Ogden & Wylie (1971) did not record a c-wave in the avian ERG. This fact may be due to the use of general anesthetics. Some recordings performed after administration of thiopenthal (2.5 mg/100 g) induced a transient disappearance of the c-wave, as already shown in the sheep by Knave et al. (1974).

The c-wave which originates in the pigment epithelium, has been classically related to the scotopic system (Brown, 1968; Steinberg et al., 1970). It is absent in pure cone retinas, one exception being the tree shrew (Tigges et al., 1967). It disappears after light adaptation in mixed retinas. The c-wave recorded in the chicken ERG is clearly related to the photopic system: it is increased by light adaptation, it can be recorded for long wavelengths (Fig. 2.5) to which the scotopic system no longer responds, and its spectral sensitivity curve culminates in the photopic range.

REFERENCES

Bonaventure, N., N. Wioland & P. Karli. Brightness coding of white and monochromatic stimuli in the chicken, souslik and rat electroretinogram: relation to light adaptation. *Ophthal. Res.* 8: *81–92* (1976).

Brown, K.T. The electroretinogram: its components and their origin. *Vision Res.* 8: *633–677* (1968).

Einthoven, W. & W.A. Jolly. The form and magnitude of the electrical response of the eye to stimulation by light at various intensities. *Q.J. exp. Physiol.* 1: *373–416* (1908).

Granit, R. The components of the retinal action potential in mammals and their relation to the discharges in the optic nerve. *J. Physiol. Lond.* 77: *207–239* (1933).

Knave, B., A. Møller & H.E. Persson. A component analysis of the electroretinogram. *Vision Res.* 12: *1669–1684* (1972).

Knave, B., S.E. Nilsson & T. Lunt. The human electroretinogram: DC recordings at low and conventional stimulus intensities. *Acta Ophthal.* 51: *716–726* (1973).

Knave, B. & H.E. Persson. The effect of barbiturate on retinal functions. I. Effects on the conventional electroretinogram of the sheep eye. *Acta Physiol. Scand.* 91: *53–60* (1974).

Knave, B., H.E. Persson & S.E.G. Nilsson. The effect of barbiturate on retinal functions. II. Effects on the c-wave of the electroretinogram and the standing potential of the sheep eye. *Acta Physiol. Scand.* 91: *180–186* (1974).

Murakami, M. & A. Kaneko. Differentiation of P_{III} subcomponents in coldblooded vertebrate retinas. *Vision Res.* 6: *627–636* (1966).

Ogden, T.E. & R.M. Wylie. Avian retina. I. Microelectrode depth and marking studies of the local ERG. *J. Neurophysiol.* 34: *357–366* (1971).

Rodieck, R.W. Components of the electroretinogram; a reappraisal. *Vision Res.* 12: *773–780* (1972).

Steinberg, R.H., R. Schmidt & K.T. Brown. Intracellular responses to light from cat pigment epithelium: origin of the electroretinogram c-wave. *Nature* 227: *728–730* (1970).

Taumer, R., N. Rhode, W. Wichmann & J. Röver. Experiments concerning the human c-wave. *A. v. Grafes Arch. klin. exp. Ophthal.* 198: *139–164* (1976).

Tigges, J., B.A. Brooks & M.R. Klee. ERG recordings of a primate pure cone retina (Tupaia glis). *Vision Res.* 7: *553–562* (1967).

Witkovsky, P., F.E. Dudek & H. Ripps. Slow P_{III} component of the carp electroretinogram. *J. gen. Physiol.* 65: *119–134* (1975).

Authors' address:
Laboratoire de Neurophysiologie
Centre de Neurochimie du C.N.R.S.
11 rue Humann
67000 Strasbourg
France

CHANGES IN ERG WAVE FORM OF THE ISOLATED BOVINE EYE DURING LONG TERM PERFUSION

Y. TAZAWA, H. IMAIZUMI, H. MERA, T. OTSUKA,
Y. TAKAHASHI & K. IMAIZUMI

(Morioka, Japan)

INTRODUCTION

The use of isolated retinal preparations in a bathing solution is one of the conventional methods for electroretinographic investigation of the retina. The conditions of the experimental procedure deviate to a considerable extent from the physiological conditions of in vivo studies. We have reported a series of studies of the retinal function and metabolism using a perfusion technique of isolated bovine eyes, the "Living Extracorporeal Bovine Eye" (Imaizumi, 1974; Imaizumi et al., 1972, 1973, 1974; Mera, 1972; Otsuko, 1973; Takahashi, 1974, Tazawa & Seaman, 1972), which is able to maintain the eyes at a nearly physiological state, developed by one of the present authors (Tazawa) in collaboration with Seaman (Tazawa) Seaman, 1972).

We have found no report in the literature of experimental studies concerned with observation of ERG changes of the enucleated whole eye of warm-blooded animals under prolonged perfusion via the ocular blood vessels. The only exception is a study by Hoff & Gouras (1972) on changes in ERG or optic nerve response to anoxia in isolated feline eyeballs maintained under continuous perfusion with tissue culture media. The present study was undertaken to investigate changes in the amplitude and peak time of a- and b-waves and oscillatory potentials in the ERG with time, using isolated bovine eyes maintained by continuous perfusion over an extended period.

MATERIALS AND METHODS

The perfusion technique for the "Living Extracorporeal Bovine Eye" has been described elswhere (Imaizumi et al., 1972, 1974; Tazawa & Seaman, 1972), and only a brief outline is given here.

Bovine eyeballs enucleated immediately after sacrifice were used. A sterile polyethylene tube was passed into the ciliary artery, through which the isolated eye was perfused with heparinized fresh bovine blood saturated with 100% oxygen and filtered through a 10 μ-mesh blood filter. The perfusion was carried out at a pressure of 800 mm H_2O and flow rate of 2 to 2.5 ml per minute.

Electroretinograms were recorded using a pair of non-polarized Zn-ZnSO$_4$ electrodes, one placed on the cornea and the other on the sclera near the optic nerve. A xenon stroboscope for ERG (Nihon Koden Kogyo Co.; Model MSP-2R) which flashed a stroboscopic light into the eye through a 60 cm glassfiber (American Opitics Co., In.; Model LG-5-24), 10 mm diameter, was used. The glassfiber tip was fixed about 1 cm above the corneal surface. The ERG potentials evoked by stroboscopic lights, 1, 730 candela, were amplified (Nihon Koden Kogyo amplifier, Model AVB-2, RC coupling) and observed by means of a cathode ray oscilloscope (Nihon Koden Kogyo Co.; Model VC-7). The amplifier time constants were 0.3 sec for recording a- and b waves and 0.003 sec for tracing oscillatory potentials, respectively.

Both the isolated perfused eye, kept under dark adaptation throughout the experiment, and the blood perfusate were maintained at 32°C. Usually, it took approximately one hour to start ERG tracings after enucleation at the slaughter house and subsequent transportation to the laboratory. The ERG pattern obtained after setting up the eye on the recording devices and adapting to dark for 15 minutes was taken as the control, followed by tracings made at 10 minute intervals.

RESULTS AND DISCUSSION

Influence of prolonged perfusion on a- and b-waves in ERG

As shown in Figs. 1 and 2, the amplitude of a-waves increased progressively, reaching a maximum (approx. 140%) about 60 minutes following initiation of the ERG tracing, and continued at this peak level over the ensuing 60 minutes. This was followed by a gradual decline to the control level about 3 hours after beginning. The ERG showed a further decrease with further time lapse and, at 10 hours after the enucleation, there was only a slight negative component.

The amplitude of b-wave sharply increased during the initial period of about 2.5 hours and reached a maximum level (approx. 190%) about 30 minutes later than the a-waves and remained there for nearly 60 minutes like the a-waves (Figs. 1 and 3). Subsequently, the b-wave amplitude diminished gradually, returning to the control level at about 5.5 hours, followed by a further conspicuous decrease. Positive deflections were no longer demonstrable 10 hours after starting the experiment.

Peak times of a- and b-waves were shortened by almost 10% compared to the control during approximately 90 minutes after starting the experiment as can be seen from Fig. 4. Thereafter, the peak time became prolonged progressively with time. The prolongation of peak time was more pronounced with b-waves than a-waves.

The overshoot phenomenon characterized by transient, marked increases of a- and b-waves observed in the ERG of the isolated bovine eye might be interpreted as an expression of recovery from mild hypoxia incurred during transportation of the eye from slaughter house to laboratory, which required about one hour. During transportation, it was inevitable for the perfusion pressure to decrease to 550-600 mmH$_2$O. Our previous study (Imaizumi et

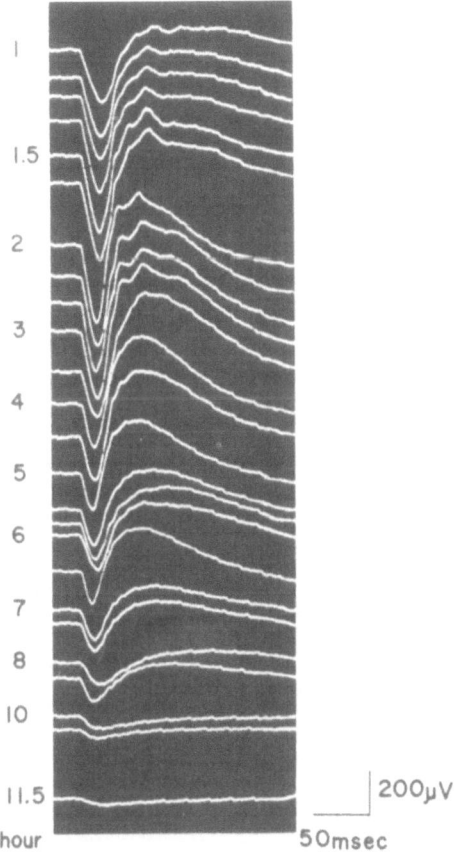

Fig. 1. Changes in ERG wave form of the isolated bovine eye during long term perfu-sion.

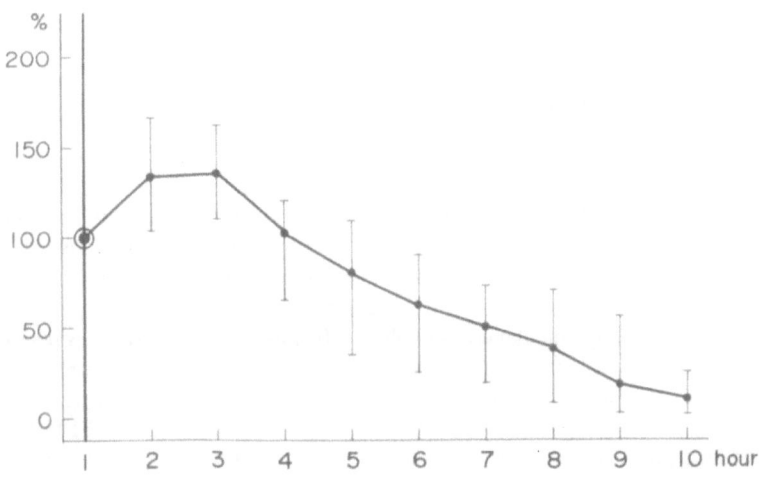

Fig. 2. Changes in amplitude of a-wave of the isolated bovine eyes during long term perfusion.

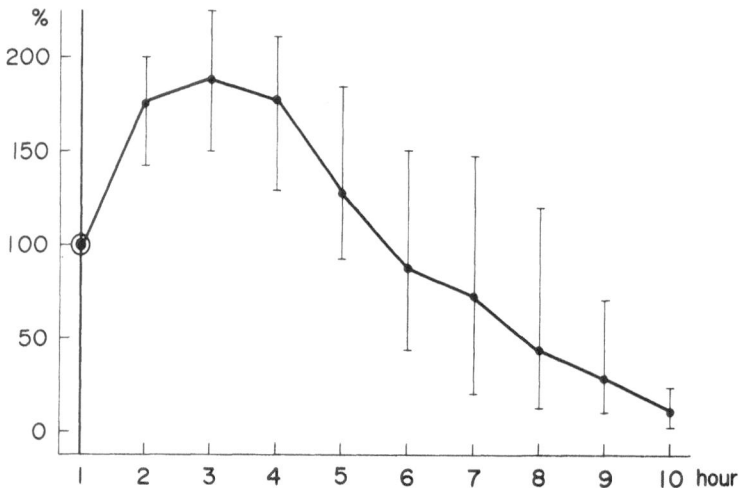

Fig. 3. Changes in amplitude of b-wave of the isolated bovine eyes during long term perfusion.

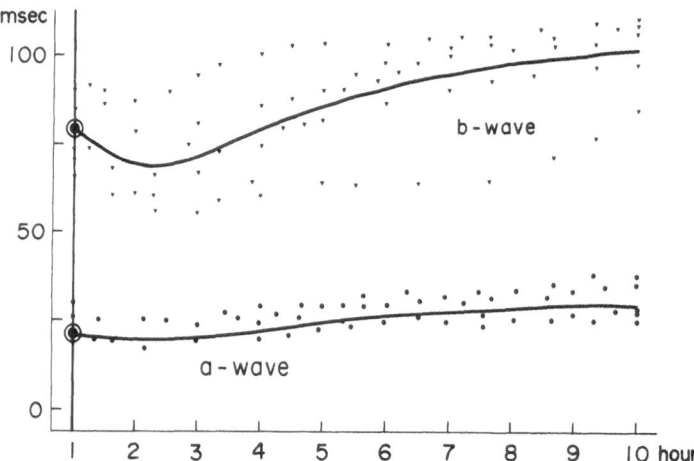

Fig. 4. Changes in peak times of a- and b-waves of the isolated bovine eyes during long term perfusion.

al., 1974) of the interrelation between the perfusion pressure and the amplitude of a- and b-waves of ERG of isolated bovine eyes had demonstrated reduction of amplitudes of both waves to about 70% of the control in 8 minutes at a perfusion pressure of 500 mmH₂O. This reduction of amplitudes was reversed by the elevation of the perfusion pressure to 650 mmH₂O, 20 minutes after maintaining the eye at the low perfusion pressure. The level of the decreased perfusion pressure to 550-600 mmH₂O, during transportation, was intermediate between the level facilitating a normal ERG and that causing low-amplitudes of a- and b-waves. This might possibly cause slight hypoxia to the isolated yee. However, Hoff & Gouras (1972) observed no evidence of such a transitory overshoot phenomenon in their experiments with isolated feline eye preparations, where a complete recovery of a- and b-waves of ERG as well as optic nerve response occurred by reperfusion even after 2 hours of complete anoxia. It would follow that the transient increase in amplitude observed in the present ERG might have little relation to the recovery process from slight hypoxia occurring during transportation. However, this remains to be further investigated.

There seem to be several interpretations for the delay in reaching maximum amplitude of the b-wave by about 30 minutes compared to the a-wave. Namely, the diminished perfusion pressure may exert a greater influence upon retinal circulation than choroidal circulation, or it may predominantly affect the metabolic process in the inner layers of the retina, or the retinal inner layers may recover more slowly from hypoxia. No conclusion can be drawn from the present findings in this respect.

The fact that the amplitudes of a- and b-waves were maintained at their maximum levels for about 1 hour seems to indicate that the conditions during this period are most favorable for the 'Living Extracorporeal Bovine Eye'. The ERG response during this 4-5 hour period after enucleation may be said to be analogous to the physiological state. All ERG activities diminished progressively with time from 5 hours after enucleation onward. In their study using isolated feline eye preparations. Hoff & Gouras (1972) reported that electrophysiological responses decreased after 8 to 10 hours of perfusion. The nonpulsating perfusion at a relatively constant pressure employed in the studies of Hoff & Gouras and of the present authors differs from physiological blood supply to the eye where the blood is being circulated by pulsation due to cardiac pumping action, and may affect metabolism of the ocular tissues.

A 10% reduction of peak time occurred for both a- and b-waves approximately 90 minutes after the initiation of ERG tracing, at which time both waves retained maximal amplitudes. This stage may, therefore, be regarded as a perfusing condition favorable for the enucleated eye when evaluated with respect to peak time changes.

Influence of prolonged perfusion on oscillatory potentials

Oscillatory potentials which were evident from the initial course of the experiment increased in amplitude during the period with increased amplitudes of a- and b-waves (Fig. 5). With time, oscillatory potentials gradually diminished in amplitude and eventually became obscure, although they persisted longer than a- and b-waves. The characteristic finding of oscillatory potentials is that neither the peak time nor interwavelet intervals showed any significant change throughout the ERG tracing unlike the situation with a- and b-waves (Fig. 6). The bipolar cell layer and adjacent areas are believed to be the most probable sites of origin of oscillatory potentials as suggested by the experimental studies of Tomita (1952), Brindley (1968), Yonemura (1962) and other investigators. The discrepancy in the time-course of peak time changes between the a- and b-waves pattern and oscillatory potential pattern observed in our study suggests that a- and b-waves

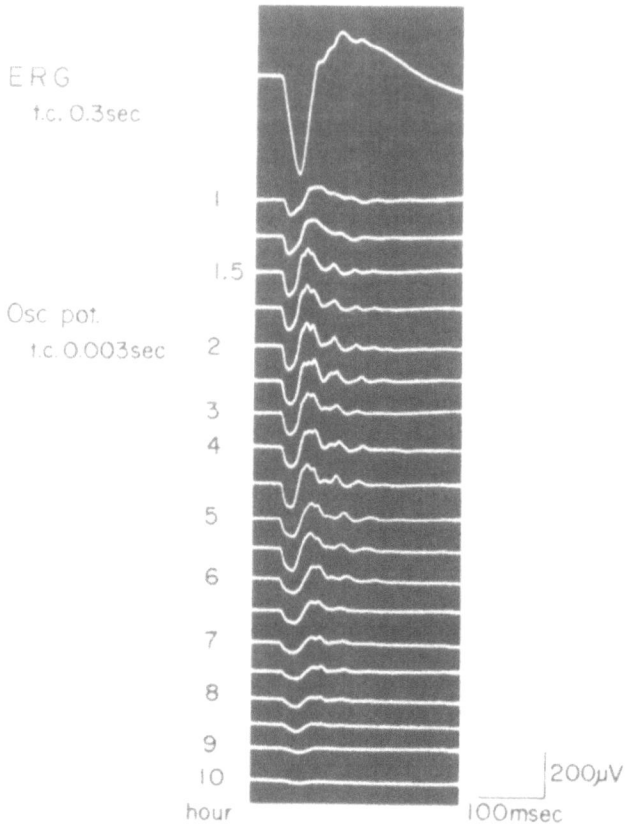

Fig. 5. Changes in wave form of oscillatory potentials of the isolated bovine eye during long term perfusion.

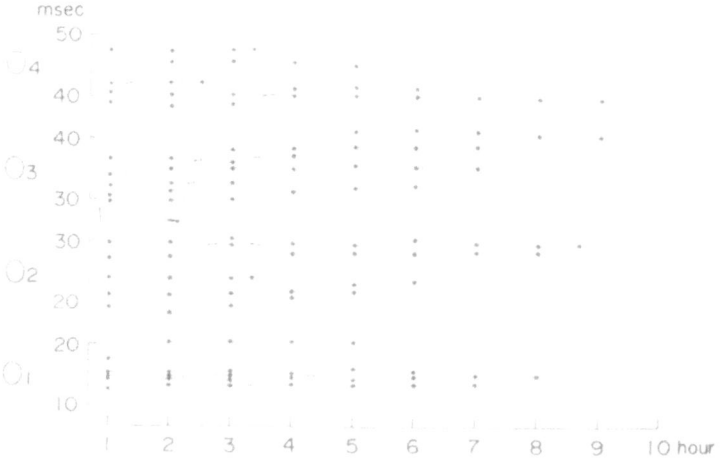

Fig. 6. Changes in peak time of oscillatory potentials of the isolated bovine eyes during long term perfusion.

248

may not share their site of origin in part with oscillatory potentials, and also provides evidence in support of the opinion of Yonemura (1962) that oscillatory potentials differ in site of origin from b-wave.

While this study represents an attempt to maintain ERG wave patterns of the isolated bovine eye perfused with blood at a constant pressure, further prolongation of the duration of extracorporeal ocular perfusion may be achieved by investigating effects of different perfusates, and perfusion flow rates on the ERG pattern.

SUMMARY

Prolonged continuous perfusion with heparinized bovine blood facilitated ERG recording of responses of the isolated whole bovine eye over a period of about 10 hours. The amplitude decline of a- and b-waves and behavior of oscillatory potentials indicate that favorable ERG responses to photic stimuli can be recorded for 4 to 5 hours of perfusion after eye enucleation by the above procedure.

REFERENCES

Brindley, G. B. The sources of slow electrical activity in the frog's retina. *J. Physiol.* 140: *247–261* (1968).

Hoff, M. & P. Gouras. Tolerance of ammalian retina to circulatory arrest. pp. 57–63 in: Proceedings Xth ISCERG Symposium, Docum. Ophthal. Proc. Series (1972).

Imaizumi, H. Influence of sodium ion concentration on electroretinogram of the living extracorporeal bovine eye. *Acta Soc. Ophthal. Jap.* 78: *831–843* (1974).

Imaizumi, K. et al. Electrophysiological application of the living extracorporeal bovine eyes. pp. 119–123 in: Advances in experimental medicine and biology, Vol. 24: The visual system. Neorphysiology, biophysics and their clinical applications. Plenum, New York (1972).

Imaizumi, K. et al. ERG and O_2-tension of the retina in the living extracorporeal eye. Fifth Afro-Asian Congr. Ophthal., pp. 420–425 (1972).

Imaizumi, K. et al. Recording the slow components of retinal electric responses of the living extracorporeal bovine eye. *Folia Ophthal. Jap.* 24: *544–545* (1973).

Imaizumi, K. et al. Effects of $[Na^+]$ in the blood on electroretinogram. *Folia Ophthal. Jap.* 25: *1134–1136* (1974).

Imaizumi, K. et al. Electroretinogram of the living extracorporeal bovine eye and blood flow. *Jap. J. Ophthal.* 18: *177–186* (1974).

Mera, H. Electroretinographic studies on the living extracorporeal eye perfused with high potassium- and sodium-blood. *Acta Soc. Ophthal. Jap.* 76: *921–929* (1972).

Otsuko, T. Erythrocytes substitute for perfusion of the living extracorporeal bovine eye. An electroretinographical study. *Acta Soc. Ophthal. Jap.* 77: *1102–1115* (1973).

Takahashi, Y. The minimum oxygen volume necessary for maintaing ERG of the living extracorporeal bovine eye. *Jap. J. Ophthal.* 18: *177–186* (1974).

Tazawa, Y. & A. J. Seaman. The electroretinogram of the living extracorporeal bovine eye. The influence of anoxia and hypothermia. *Invest. Ophthal.* 11: *691–698* (1972).

Tomita, T. Studies in interretinal action potential with low-resistance micro-electrode. *J. Neurophysiol.* 15: *75–84* (1952).

Yonemura, D. The oscillatory potential of the electroretinogram. *Acta Soc. Ophthal. Jap.* 66: *1566–1684* (1962).

Authors' address: Iwate Medical University
Department of Ophthalmology   Morioka
School of Medicine   Japan.

GABA AND TAURINE: IMPLICATION IN ORGANIZATION OF RECEPTIVE FIELDS OF GANGLION CELLS IN THE FROG RETINA

N. BONAVENTURE & N. WIOLAND

(Strasbourg, France)

Biochemical and physiological results strongly suggest that some amino-acids like taurine and GABA could be considered as inhibitory transmitters in the retina.

An intravitreal injection of Taurine or GABA induces a progressive reduction in the amplitude of the ERG b-wave (Scholes & Roberts, 1964; Kramer et al., 1967; Roberts & Kuriyama, 1968; Pasantes-Morales et al., 1973), the disappearance of tectal evoked responses (Bonaventure et al., 1974) and the suppression of retinal ganglion cell discharges (Kishida & Naka, 1967; Straschill & Perwein, 1969; Ames & Pollen, 1969).

The depressive action of these amino-acids on the ERG b-wave can be antagonized by specific substances: picrotoxin antagonizes the action of GABA but not that of taurine, while strychnine rapidly reverses the depressant effect of taurine but not that of GABA (Bonaventure et al., 1974).

The object of the present study is double:
1) to localize the site of fixation of these amino-acids in the retina;
2) to determine whether GABA and taurine are implicated in the organization of the receptive field of the ganglion cells in the retina.

Experiments were carried out on frogs.

Since the studies by Maturana et al. (1960) and by Grüsser et al (1968) it has been well known that at least three different classes of ganglion cells can be distinguished in the frog retina: sustained cells, ON-OFF cells, and OFF cells. All exhibit a spatial organization of their receptive field with an excitatory centre and an inhibitory surround. The receptive field of the ON-OFF cells only, was analysed in this study.

The inhibitory effect of GABA and taurine on the receptive field cannot be directly analysed, all cell activity being suppressed by these amino-acids; this inhibitory effect is better approached by analysing the effects of their specific antagonists, picrotoxin and strychnine, which selectively suppress the inhibitory effects of these putative neurotransmitters.

A historadiographic study was performed after intravitreal injection of these amino acids. Such a work has been already done on isolated retinae (Voaden et al., 1974; Marshall & Voaden, 1975; Kennedy & Voaden, 1976) but it was interesting to do it in vivo, and to take off the retina at the moment, when the depressive action on the ERG b-wave was maximal.

The frogs (*Rana temporaria*) were curarized with D-tubocurarine (0.9 mg per animal) and covered with moist cotton. Lids were cut and the pupil was dilated with atropine and Neosynephrine. Ganglion cell discharges were recorded on the superficial tectal layers where their axons terminate. Recordings were carried out with glass micropipettes (1 μ at the tip, 2−4 MΩ of resistance, filled with NaCl 2M). A cathode follower allows one to introduce the signal to an 'Alvar' amplifier. Experiments were done in mesopic illumination; the photic stimulus of different sizes and intensities can be moved on a screen with a system of two mirrors in order to delimit the receptive field area. Recordings were carried out before and after intraocular administration of 30 μl of either picrotoxin (0.005 M), or strychnine 0.001−0.01 M) or taurine (0.01 M).

In the histoautoradiographic study, 1 mCi of tritiated GABA or taurine was injected intravitreally. Eyes were taken out 60-90 min after injection, following an ERG record that checks the b-wave decrease. Eyes were fixed in glutaraldehyde and in osmic acid. Samples were then included in araldite after progressive dehydration with ethanol. Slices of 1 μ were covered with an 'Ilford L$_4$' emulsion and put in darkness for five weeks.

RESULTS

Study of the receptive field of ON-OFF ganglion cells before and after administration of drugs

The receptive field of the ON-OFF ganglion cell is of irregular shape, slightly oval, with a diameter of about twelve or thirteen degrees. Spontaneous discharges are never recorded, as already demonstrated by Maturana et al. (1960), and Grüsser et al. (1968).

After intravitreal injection of picrotoxin (0.005 M) the appearance of spontaneous discharges was observed, a decrease of the reactivity threshold, and especially, a marked increase of the receptive field area: from twelve at the start, it reached twenty four degrees under the effect of picrotoxin. At the same time, the amplitude of the ERG b-wave doubled: from 500 μV at the start, it reached 1000 μV after injection of picrotoxin.

Strychnine, which specifically antagonizes the depressive action of taurine, has a much more complicated effect, and its action depends on the concentration of the injected compound: for moderate doses (0.001 M) the size of the receptive field does not change; firing is recorded at ON and at OFF, but the threshold for the ON response is higher than that for the OFF response. The appearance of a periphery where only OFF responses can be elicited was observed. For doses ten times more concentrated (0.01 M) only OFF responses are recorded throughout the enlarged field.

Taurine itself, at high doses, suppresses the ERG b-wave and all activity of the ganglion cells; but very limited doses (0.01 M) which entail only a slight decrease of the ERG b-wave, do not act upon the size of the receptive field. However, contrary to strychnine, they provoke the total suppression of the

OFF discharges, without modifying the ON discharges of the ganglion cells. These results are summarized in Table 1.

Table 1

	SIZE OF THE RECEPTIVE FIELD (DEGREES)	ON	OFF
CONTROL GANGLION CELL	12	X	X
PICROTOXIN .005 (GABA ANTAGONIST)	24	X	X
STRYCHNINE .001 (TAURINE ANTAGONIST)	12	↘ INCREASE OF THE THRESHOLD	X
STRYCHNINE .01	24	—	X
TAURINE .01	12	X	—

Histoautoradiography of the frog retina after intravitreal injection of tritiated GABA or Taurine.

Both labelled GABA and taurine are found in the internal plexiform layer and in amacrine cells, but GABA alone is additionally fixed at the horizontal cell level. Radioactivity was found neither in photoreceptor nor in bipolar cell layers. Figure 1 shows the percentage of radioactivity fixed in the different retinal layers. The reference (R = 100) is the radioactivity found in

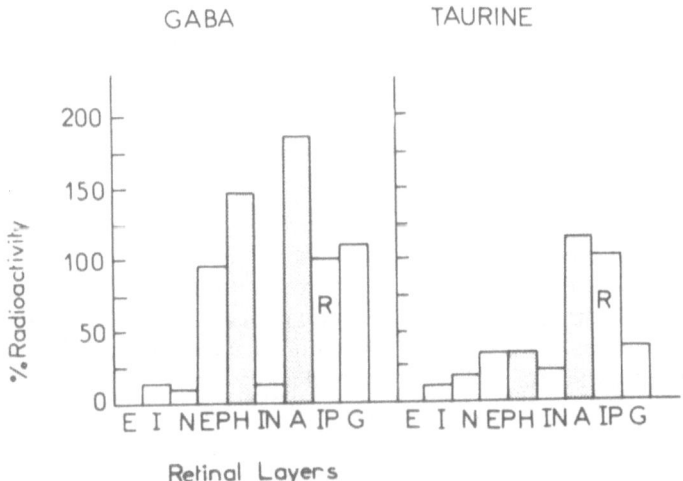

Fig. 1. Percentage of radioactivity in the different retinal layers after intravitreal injection of tritiated GABA or Taurine; the amount of radioactivity fixed in the inner plexiform layer is taken as a reference (R = 100). E = external segment of the photoreceptors; I = internal segment of the photoreceptors; N = nucleus of the photoreceptors; EP = external plexiform; H = horizontal cells; IN = inner nuclear; A = amacrine cells; IP = internal plexiform; G = ganglion cells.

the inner plexiform layer. This reuptake of GABA or taurine by amacrine and/or horizontal cells is in good agreement with the hypothesis that these putative inhibitory neurotransmitters would act in modulating the retinal sensitivity by processes of lateral inhibition.

DISCUSSION

Under the effect of picrotoxin, the area of the receptive field of the ON-OFF ganglion cell doubles. Thus, it seems that picrotoxin, which specifically antagonizes the inhibitory action of GABA, induces a spatial reorganization of the receptive field. GABA must then intervene in the bringing about of the centre-surround arrangement of the receptive field of ON-OFF ganglion cells in the frog retina. These results are in agreement with those of Kirby & Enroth Cugell (1976): in the ganglion Y-cell of the cat retina, picrotoxine modifies the balance between the centre and the surround to the detriment of the surround.

Strychnine and taurine can separate the ON and the OFF channels and have opposite compared effects. This was also noted by Cunningham & Miller (1976) in ganglion cells of the rabbit retina. Taurine must then be implicated in the temporal organixation of the receptive field of ganglion cells.

Histoautoradiographic studies have shown that after intravitreal injection, GABA and taurine are found in the internal plexiform layer and in amacrine cells, and GABA is additionally fixed at the horizontal cell level. These data have already been observed in the frog retina in vitro (Voaden et al., 1974; Lake et al., 1975; Kennedy et al., 1976). Voaden et al. have also found taurine in the photoreceptors, but at this level, it seems that this amino acid must play another role in retinal function. Our results are in agreement with the model proposed by Werblin (1974). In another amphibian, the mudpuppy, Werblin suggested that horizontal cells may be responsible for spatial organization of the receptive field of ganglion cells, whereas the internal plexiform layer and amacrine cells may be implicated in their dynamic or temporal organization.

The results obtained with picrotoxin, an antagonist of GABA, show that GABA may be implicated in bringing about the centre-surround arrangement of the receptive fields by way of the horizontal cells. The results obtained with strychnine, an antagonist of taurine, and with taurine itself, show that taurine may be involved in temporal organization of the receptive field separating the ON and OFF channels. Histoautoradiographic study suggests that this process must occur at the amacrine cell level.

REFERENCES

Ames, A. & D.A. Pollen. Neurotransmission in central nervous tissue: a study of isolated rabbit retina. *J. Neurophysiol.* 32: *424-442* (1969).

Bonaventure, N., N. Wioland & P. Mandel. Antagonists of the putative inhibitory transmitter effects of taurine and GABA in the retina. *Brain Res.* 80: *281-290* (1974).

Cunningham, R. & R.F. Miller. Taurine: its selective action on neuronal pathways in the rabbit retina. *Brain Res.* 117: *341-345* (1976).

Grüsser, O.J., D. Finkelstein & Ü Grüsser-Cornehls. The effect of stimulus velocity on the movement-sensitive neurons of the frog's retina. *Pflügers Arch.* 309: *49–66* (1968).

Kennedy, A.J. & M.J. Voaden. Studies on the uptake and release of radioactive taurine by the frog retina. *J. Neurochem.* 27: *131–138* (1976).

Kirby, A.W. & C. Enroth-Cugell. The involvement of gamma-aminobutyric acid in the organization of cat retinal ganglion cell receptive fields. A study with picrotoxin and bicuculline. *J. gen. Physiol.* 68: *465–484* (1976).

Kishida, K. & K.I. Naka. Interaction of excitatory and depressant aminoacids in the frog retina. *J. Neurochem.* 15: *833–841* (1968).

Kramer, S.Z., P.A. Sherman & J. Seifter. Effects of gamma-aminobutyric acid (GABA) and sodium glutamate (glutamate) on the visual system and EEG of chicks. *Int. J. Neuropharmacol.* 6: *463–472* (1967).

Lake, N., J. Marshall & M.J. Voaden. Studies on the uptake of taurine by the isolated neural retina and pigment epithelium of the frog. *Biochem. Soc. Trans.* 3: *524–525* (1975).

Marshall, J. & M. Voaden. Autoradiographic indentification of the cells accumulating 3H-γ-aminobutyric acid in mammalian retinae. A species comparison. *Vision Res.* 15: *459–461* (1975).

Maturana, H.R., HJ.Y. Lettvin, W.H. Pitss & W.S. McCullogh. Anatomy and physiology of vision in the frog (Rana pipiens). *J. gen. Physiol.* 43: *129–175* (1960).

Pasantes-Morales, H., N. Bonaventure, N. Wioland & P. Mandel. Effect of intravitreal injections of taurine and GABA on chicken electroretinogram. *Int. J. Neurosci.* 5: *235–241* (1973).

Roberts, E. & K. Kuriyama. Some correlations in studies of the GABA System. *Brain Res.* 8: *1–35* (1968).

Scholes, N.W. & E. Roberts. Pharmacological studies of the optic system of the chick: effect of γ aminobutyric acid and pentobarbital. *Biochem. Pharmacol.* 13: *1319–1329* (1964).

Straschill, M. & J. Perwein. The inhibition of retinal ganglion cells by catecholamines and γ aminobutyric acid. *Pflügers Arch.* 312: *45–54* (1969).

Voaden, M.J., J. Marshall & N. Murani. The uptake of [3H] glycine by the isolated retina of the frog. *Brain Res.* 67: *115–132* (1974).

Werblin, F.S. Control of retinal sensitivity. *J. gen. Physiol.* 63: *62–110* (1974).

Authors' address:
Laboratoire de Neurophysiologie
Centre de Neurochimie du C.N.R.S.
11 rue Humann
67000 Strasbourg
France

ELECTRORETINOGRAPHIC FINDINGS IN CHRONIC URAEMICS TREATED WITH PERIODIC HAEMODIALYSIS

M. PEROSSINI & G. TOTA

(Pisa, Italy)

Numerous eye alterations have been reported for uraemics treated with haemodialysis (Table 1).

Small white sub-epithelial spots may appear on the bulbar conjunctiva, while superficial opacity of a granulous structure is formed on the cornea near the limbus (Déodati et al., 1971; Ehlers et al., 1972; Porter, 1973; Hanselmayer et al., 1974; Demco et al., 1974).

Hypocalcaemia is probably also responsible for a subcapsular cataract (Mautner, 1972; Boudet et al., 1973), which is generally bilateral and of rapid evolution, while the osmotic variations, which appear on the blood-aqueous barrier (Galin et al., 1961; Galin, 1965) during haemodialysis determine transient modifications of the intraocular pressure (Sitprija & Holmes,

Table 1. Pathological changes in chronic uraemics treated with periodic haemodialysis.

Authors	Year	Pathological findings
Berlyne	1968	*Conjunctiva and cornea*
Déodati et al.	1971	Sub-epithelial white spots; corneal opacities of
Ehlers et al.	1972	granulous structure near the limbus
Porter	1973	
Hanselmayer et al.	1974	
Demco et al.	1974	
Mautner	1972	*Lens*
Boudet et al.	1973	Subcapsular cataract
Modugno et al.	1970	*Fundus*
Yamanouchi	1972	Small retinal haemorrhages, narrowing of the
Inomata & Oka	1972	lumen and thickening of the walls of the
Takahashi	1973	blood vessels
Sitprija & Holmes	1962	*Changes of intraocular pressure*
Sitprija et al.	1974	Decrease in intraocular pressure during the first
Biagini & Gloria	1967	two hours of dialysis and subsequently increase
Modugno et al.	1970	in the value of intraocular pressure.
Ramsell et al.	1971	(from +1.06 to 8.9)
Shimizu	1972	
Burn	1973	
Yamanaka et al.	1974	
Agzamova	1975	

Table 2. Voltage of the b-wave and electrolytic values before and after dialytic treatment.

No. of patients	Wave b: μV (average $\pm \sigma$) before after	Duration of dialysis mean average	Calcaemia (mg%) before after	Potassaemia (mg%) before after	Sodiaemia (mg%) before after	Osmolarity (mOs/KgH$_2$O) before after
26	208 ±79 206 ±62	1 year 6 months	9 ±1.16	21.3 ± 3.48	308 ±17.39	310 ±18.11
			9.9 ±0.07	16.2 ±2.06	284 ±20.96	279 ±12.92

Table 3. Voltage of the b-wave and electrolytic values in chronic uraemics treated with dietetic-pharmacological therapy

No of patients	Wave b, μV (average $\pm \sigma$)	Calcaemia (mg%)	Potassaemia (mg%)	Sodiaemia (mg%)	Osmolarity (mOs/KgH$_2$)	Azotemia (mg%)	Creatininemia (mg%)
11	270 ±4.9	8.7 ±2.83	19 ±3.87	311 ±7.32	302 ±12.56	192 ±47	8.6 ±2.12

1962; Sitprija et al., 1964; Watson & Greenwood, 1966; Biagini & Gloria, 1967; Modugno et al., 1970; Ramsell et al., 1971; Shimizu et al., 1972; Burn, 1973; Yamanaka et al., 1974; Agzamova, 1975).

Modugno, Romani & Signore (1970) observed small retinal haemorrhages in the fundus whereas narrowing of the lumen and thickening of the walls of the blood vessels were observed by Yamanouchi (1972), Inomata & Oka (1972) and Takahashi (1973).

We thought it would be interesting to study the ERG in chronic uraemics treated with haemodialysis, because the ionic variations of the intra and extracellular liquids produced by haemodialysis constitute a remarkably interesting field of study from some components of the electroretinogram.

Our research was carried out on 26 chronic uraemics (16 males and 10 females) between the ages of 16 and 60, treated periodically with haemo-dialysis by means of coil type filters. Haemodialysis was effected three times a week for a period which varied from 1 month to 9 years and 6 months. In all the patients we registered the electroretinogram, both before and after dialysis, adapted to the dark. Later, in order to evaluate the results obtained, we extended the electroretinographic research to a group of 11 chronic uraemics who were following an exclusively dietetic-pharmacological therapy. On the other hand, we were able to find in literature during the experience that the ERG is pathologically reduced in nephronophthisis' patients (Severin, 1975).

The results of our experiments are summarized in Tables 2 and 3 in which one finds the average values of the electroretinogram and of some electrolytic concentrations. From a comprehensive analysis of these data it is possible to draw the following conclusions (Table 3):

1) In patients treated with haemodialysis the voltage of the b-wave is considerably reduced; in two cases, however, this wave was paradoxically supernormal and in 4 patients we also found a negative b (Fig. 1).

2) In the above-mentioned patients, after a single dialysis, the voltage of the b-wave did not show appreciable variations with respect to predialysis values.

3) In chronic uraemics treated with conservative therapy (Table 3) the

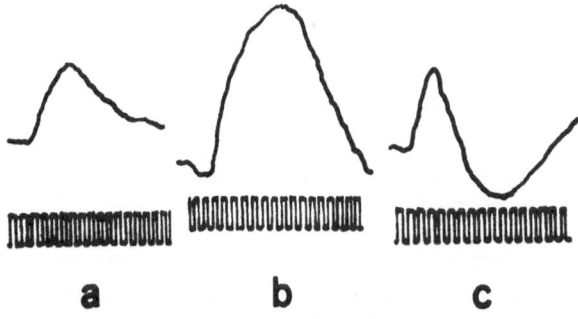

a   **b**   **c**

Fig. 1. ERG modifications in chronic uraemics treated with haemodialysis. Registration in full dark-adaptation, instantaneous energy of the stimulus 1 joule; time marking 50 cy/sec. The voltage of the b-wave is nearly always subnormal (a), but sometimes it is paradoxically supernormal (b); furthermore in 4 cases a negative b was found (c).

electroretinogram, though sub-normal, was only slightly reduced and shows a voltage which is clearly superior to that of the previous group (Fig. 2). 4) A statistical analysis made with Student's t showed the difference between the voltage of the b-wave of thé two groups to be significant at the P = 0.05.

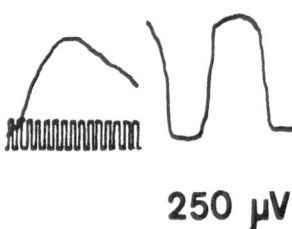

250 µV

Fig. 2. In chronic uraemics treated with conservative therapy the voltage of the b-wave is only slightly reduced.

DISCUSSION

The results of our experiments show that in chronic uraemics the voltage of the b-wave is nearly always reduced, but that in patients treated with haemodialysis the modifications of the electroretinogram are greater. In our opinion a correct interpretation of these data may be obtained by taking into consideration the following:

(a) the effect on the retina by the toxic substances retained in the uraemic syndrome;

(b) the electrolytic modifications produced by haemodialysis.

With regard to (a), i.e. the effects of uraemic intoxication on the retina, we may presume that there are retinal injuries comparable to those found in C.N.S. caused by chronic uraemia and which reveal themselves, clinically, with alterations in behaviour, disturbances of motility and electroencephalic modifications (Tyler, 1968; Teschan, 1970; Teschan, 1974; Ginn & Teschan, 1975).

From a strictly electrophysiological point of view (b), our problem is connected with that of the membrane potential which, as is known, is generated by the different ionic concentrations of the intra- and extracellular fluids.

In our case it is important to note that haemodialytic treatment interferes with the electrolytic equilibrium with complex mechanism which may be outlined as follows:

— the values of calcaemia in uraemies are slightly increased at the end of dialysis treatment;*

— the concentration of potassium in the blood, on the other hand, diminishes, but only insignificantly, since it tends to equilibrate with the potassium of the dialysis solution.**

* The ionized calcium in the dialysis bath has a higher concentration than that in the blood and therefore we have an increase of this ion due to passive diffusion connected with the different gradient of concentration.
** The potassium does not however reach the low values of this solution since, as the extracellular compartment becomes impoverished, there is a passage of the ion from the intra compartment to the extracellular one.

— at the beginning of dialysis the uraemics are hyposodiemic, with the haemodialysis there is a further reduction of sodiaemia, which becomes inferior to the sodium concentration present in the dialysis bath.***

Therefore, we believe that the ERG modifications found after dialysis are strictly connected with these electrolytic variations since the voltage of the b-wave is directly proportional to the logarithm of the concentration of extracellular sodium and inversely proportional to that of the external potassium (see Table 4), and that the functional activity of the retina is strictly correlated to the active transport of sodium, since by inhibiting ATP-ase Na+K the b-wave rapidly disappears (Frank & Goldsmith, 1967). Furthermore, we think it improbable that the ERG reduction depends on the toxic action of the catabolites retained in the uraemic syndrome, because the voltage of the b-wave is less compromised in uraemics who are not treated with haemodialysis, but in whom the various uraemic symptoms are more serious.

Table 4. Modifications of the ERG determined by electrolytic variations.

Author	Year	Effects produced on the ERG components by electrolytic variations	Animal used
Hamasaky	1963	Voltage of the b-wave proportional to the log of the Na present in the external medium	Isolated frog retina
Hanawa et al.	1967	Reduction of the ERG with low concentrations of Na or high concentrations of K	Isolated frog retina
Arden & Ernst	1969	Suppression of the b-wave by eliminating the Ca in the external medium	Isolated retinas of birds and mammals
Sillman et al.	1969a	Reduction of the PII and PIII by eliminating the Na in Ringer's liquid	Isolated frog retina
Sillman et al.	1969b	Voltage of the b-wave inversely proportional to the log of the external K; b-wave directly proportional to the log. of the external Na	Isolated frog retina
Arden & Ernst	1970	Directly proportional ratio between electric response and Na concentration and the Cl in the external medium	Isolated pigeon retina
Pautler et al.	1971	PIII inversely proportional to the Ca concentration	Isolated frog retina
Winckler	1963	Reduction of the ERG by diminishing the Na or Cl; biphasic effect with the variations in K; increase in the a and b-waves by eliminating the Ca	Isolated rat retina

*** This may be justified if we admit that the remarkable reduction of potassium in the extracellular liquid inhibits the pumping of sodium in the cells (Haddy, 1974) and therefore a lower plasmatic concentration of this ion.

SUMMARY

We have registered the ERG in 26 chronic uraemics treated with periodic haemodialysis, nearly always finding a subnormal b-wave. In 11 chronic uraemics treated only with dietetic-conservative therapy, the electroretinogram resulted only slightly reduced and with a voltage clearly superior to that of the previous group.

REFERENCES

Agzamova, H.S. Tonographic values in patients with chronic renal insufficiency. *Oftal. Zh.* 20: *32–34* (1975).

Berlyne, G.M. Microcrystalline conjunctival calcification in renal failure. *Lancet* II: *366–370* (1968).

Biagini, M. & E.M. Gloria. Comportamento della pressione intraoculare durante emodialisi in pazienti affetti da uremia cronica. *Ann. Ottal.* 93: *705–713* (1967).

Boudet, Ch., B. Arnaud & D. Pincemin. Cataracte au cours d'h'emodialyses (dans les insuffisances rénales chroniques). *Bull. Soc. Ophtal. France* 73: *199–205* (1973).

Burn, R.A. Intraocular pressure during haemodialysis. *Br. J. Ophthal.* 57: *511–513* (1973).

Cavallacci, G., G. Tota & A. Wirht. Studio sperimentale sull'effetto della difenilidantoina sull'Elettroretinogramma. *Ann. Ottal.* 100: *560–568* (1974).

Demco, T.A., A.Q. McCormick & J.S.F. Richards. Conjunctival and corneal changes in chronic renal failure. *Can. J. Ophthal.* 9: *208–213* (1974).

Deodati, F., P. Bec, M. Camezind & J.B. Labro. Les manifestations oculaires au cours de l'hémodialyse périodique. *Bull. Soc. Ophtal. France* 71: *87–92* (1971).

Ehlers, N., F. Kruse Hansen, H.E. Hansen & O.A. Jensen. Corneoconjunctival changes in uremia. *Acta Ophthal. Kbh.* 50: *83–94* (1972).

Frank, R.N. & T.H. Goldsmith. Effects of cardiac glycosides on electrical activity in the isolated retina of the frog. *J. Gen. Physiol.* 50: *1585–1606* (1967).

Galin, M.A. Hemodilution and intraocular pressure. *Arch. Ophthal.* 73: *25–31* (1967).

Galin, M.A., H. Nano & R. Davidson. Aqueous and blood urea nitrogen levels after intravenous urea administration. *Arch. Ophthal.* 65: *805–807* (1961).

Ginn, H.E. & P.E. Teschan. Neurotoxicity in uremia. Kidney Int. 7: *357–360* (1975).

Haddy, F.J. Local control of vascular resistance as related to hypertension. *Arch. Intern. Med.* 133: *916–931* (1974).

Hanselmayer, H., H. Pogglitsch & H. Schmidberger. Kalzifikationen in der bindehaut und hornhaut bei chronischer niereninsuffiziens und hamodialyse. *Klin. Mbl. Augenheilk.* 164: *98–105* (1974).

Inomata, H. & Y. Oka. Ultrastructure alterations of the retinal blood vessels in renal retinal retinopathy. Two cases which had undergone and not undergone hemodialysis. The pathogenesis of metastatic calcification in the vessel walls. *Acta Soc. Ophthal. Jap.* 76: *1079–1088* (1973).

Klaus, W. Spostamenti funzionali degli elettroliti nel miocardio. *Triangolo* 4: *152–160* (1972).

Mautner, W. Hämodialysebehandlung und Veränderungen am vorderen und mittleren Augenabschnitt. *Klin. Mbl. Augenheilk.* 160: *350–352* (1972).

Mihara, M. Studies on the eyes of patients with renal disease undergoing treatment by hemo and peritoneal dialysis: Report I. The correlations between the EOG and the number of times of dialysis. *Acta Soc. Ophthal. Jap.* 77: *119–128* (1973).

Modugno, G.C., E. Romani & L. Signore. Variazioni del fondo e della pressione oculare durante emodialisi. *Boll. Ocul.* 49: *108–117* (1970).

Porter, R. A.L. Crombie. Corneal and conjunctival calcification in chronic renal failure. *Br. J. Ophthal.* 57: *339–343* (1973).

Ramsell, J.T., P.P. Ellis & C.A. Paterson. Intraocular pressure changes during hemodialysis. *Am. J. Ophthal.* 72: *926–930* (1971).

Severin, M. Augenveränderungen bei familiarer juveniler nephronophthise. *Klin. Mbl. Augenheilk.* 166: *674–686* (1975).

Sitprija, V. & J.H. Holmes. Preliminar observations on the change in intracranial pressure during hemodialysis. *Trans. Am. Soc. Artif. Int. Organs* 8: *300–308* (1962).

Sitprija, V., J.H. Holmes & P.E. Ellis. Intraocular pressure changes during artificial kidney therapy. *Arch. Ophthal.* 72: *626–631* (1964).

Shimizu, Y., Y. Mihara & F. Nakamura. The effects of hemodialysis on intra-ocular pressure. *Rinsho Ganka* 26: *151–154* (1972).

Takahashi, M. Retinal changes in patients who had undergone a long term hemodialysis. *Folia Ophthal. Jap.* 24: *1148–1152* (1973).

Teschan, P.E. On the pathogenesis of uremia. *Am. J. Med.* 48: *671–677* (1970).

Teschan, P.E. Qualified functions of nervous system in uremic patients on maintenance hemodialysis. *Trans. Am. Soc. Artif. Int. Organs* 20A: *388–394* (1974).

Tyler, H.R. Neurological disorders in renal failure. *Am. J. Med.* 44: *734–748* (1968).

Watson, A.G. & W.R. Greenwood. Studies on the intraocular pressure during hemodialysis. *Can. J. Ophthal.* 1: *301–314* (1966).

Yamanaka, T., Y. Yoda & M. Mihara. Changes of intraocular pressure in a hemodialysed patient. *Folia Ophthal. Jap.* 25: *183–186* (1974).

Yamanouchi, U. Histopathological findings of the eye in patients undergoing a long term hemodialysis. *Folia Ophthal. Jap.* 23: *700–706* (1972).

Authors' address:
c/o Spagnoli
Viale Italia 289
57100 Livorno
Italy

CASE REPORT OF A FAMILY WITH SECTORAL RETINAL PIGMENTARY DYSTROPHY

Y. TAZAWA, R. TAKAHASHI, K. MITA & H. KURIHARA

(Morioka, Japan)

INTRODUCTION

Since the first report by Bietti in 1937, sectoral retinal pigmentary dystrophy has been investigated by many investigators from various viewpoints (see References). There is, as yet, no established theory concerning the essential nature of sectoral retinal pigmentary dystrophy. It is not known whether it represents one stage in the progress of typical retinitis pigmentosa or, otherwise, a non-progressive, independent form of retinal pigmentary degeneration localized in a portion of the retina.

This report presents the findings in a detailed ophthalmologic evaluation of a pedigree of sectoral retinal pigmentary dystrophy possibly inherited as a dominant trait.

SUBJECTS AND METHODS

The pedigree consisted of fifteen subjects in three consecutive generations, who could be interviewed. In the present study three patients were evaluated in detail: they were a 49 year old female (Case II-4, proband), a 45 year old male (Case II-5) in the second generation and a 16 year old male (Case III-10) in the third generation (Fig. 1).

The examinations included assessment of the visual acuity, visual field and dark adaptation threshold, ERG and EOG.

RESULTS

The results of ophthalmologic examinations performed on the three patients are summarized in Table 1.

Case II-4, a 49 year old female, was the propositus in the present study was referred here for detailed ophthalmologic workup. With the exception of slightly diminished vision at night since she was about 45 years of age, the patient had experienced no particular ophthalmological complaints in the past and the hemeralopia had not been progressed to any appreciable extent. The patient's visual acuity was normal, 1.0 on both sides and there were no abnormal findings for the outer portions or media of the eyes. Both optic discs appeared normal and the macular regions presented no abnormal

Pedigree of Family K

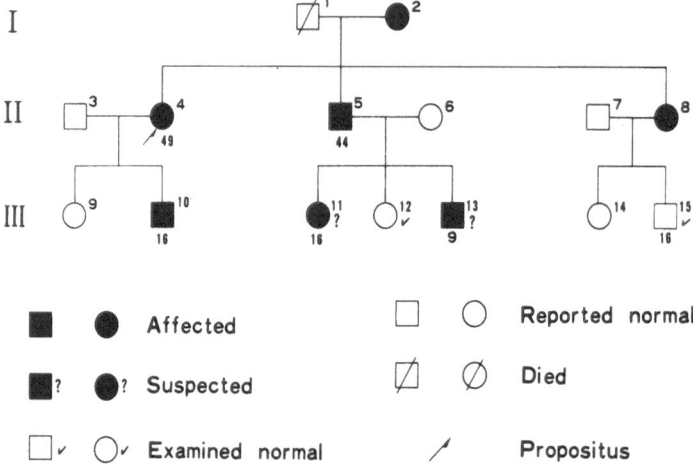

Affected ■ ●

Suspected ■? ●?

Examined normal □✓ ○✓

Reported normal □ ○

Died ▨ ⊘

Propositus ╱

Fig. 1. Pedigree of a family with sectoral retinal pigmentary dystrophy.

findings. The ophthalmoscopic examination, nevertheless, revealed bilaterally symmetrical degenerated areas extending from below the papilla toward the lower temporal region, associated with a circumscribed, pronounced greyish-blue haziness and various shapes of pigment deposits (Fig. 2 and 3). The retinal blood vessels in the degenerated area appeared slightly narrowed, as compared to those in other areas of the retina. Retinal degeneration was

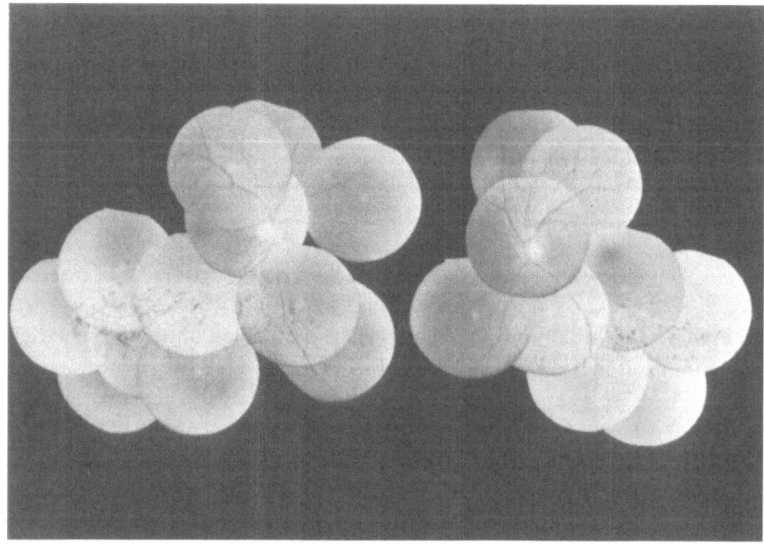

Fig. 2. Fundus pictures of Case II-4. Bilateral symmetrical degenerated areas are extending from below the papilla toward the lower temporal region.

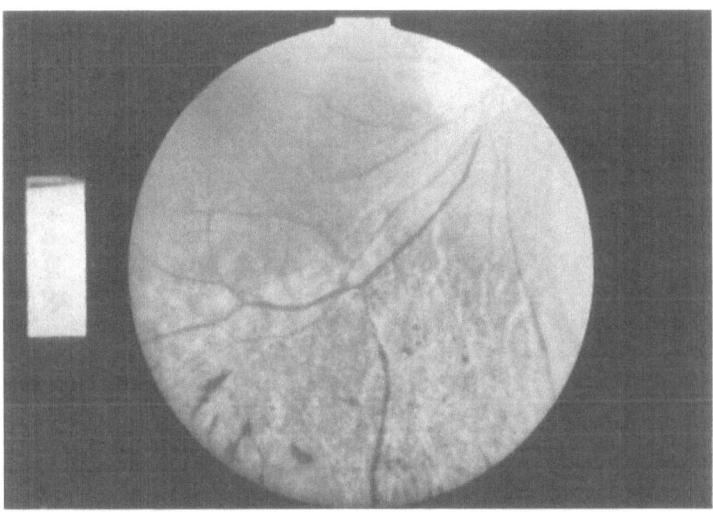

Fig. 3. Fundus picture of Case II-4 (right eye). A circumscribed haziness and various shapes of pigment deposit are seen. The retinal vessels in the degenerated area appear slightly narrowed.

limited to the vicinity of the equator, and there was no cloudiness. Blood vessels were normal in the retina peripheral to the lesion. As shown in Fig. 4, fluorescein fundus angiography disclosed an indiscrete abnormal background fluorescence forming a horizontal line below the macular area, de-

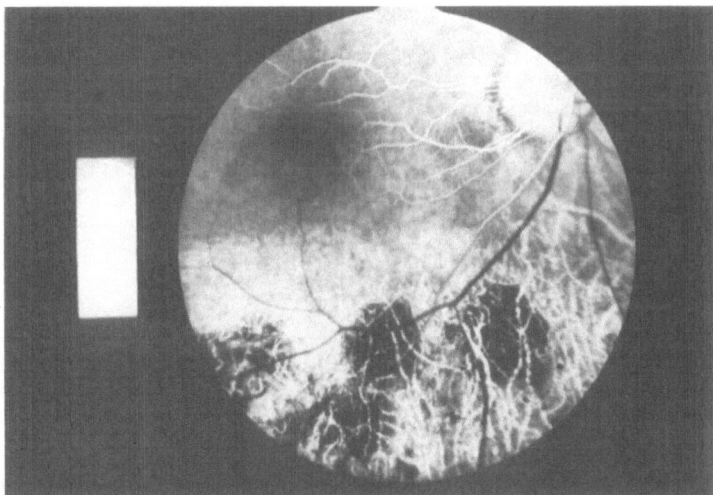

Fig. 4. Fluorescein fundus angiogram of Case II-4. Arterial phase. Abnormal background fluorescence, slightly more extensive than the area ophthalmoscopically demonstrated, forming a horizontal line below the macula. Areas suspected to be defective of the pigment epithelium, with loss of choriocapillaris are present in the degenerated region.

267

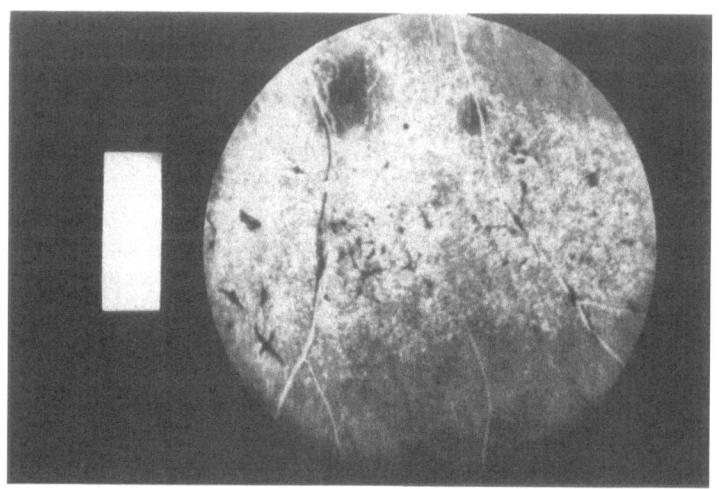

Fig. 5. Fluorescein fundus angiogram of Case II-4. Normal fluorescence pattern is seen at the periphery of the degenerated region.

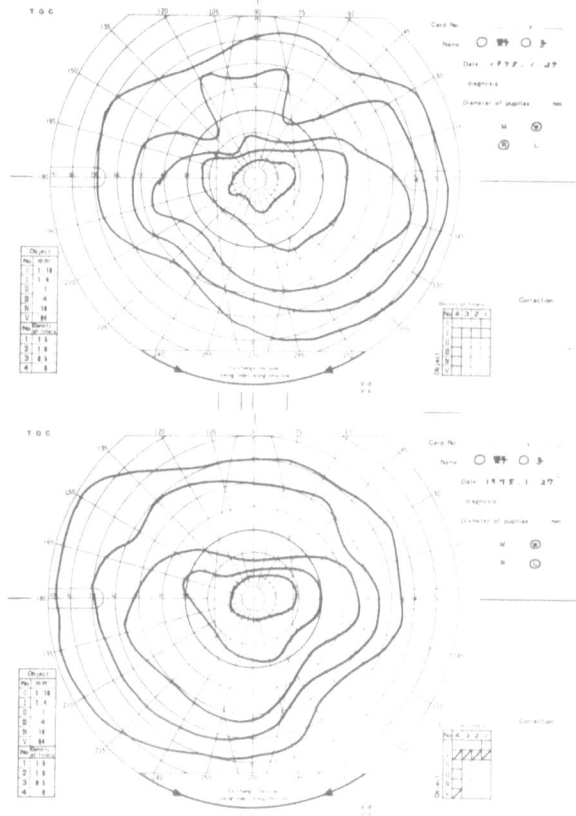

Fig. 6. Visual fields of Case II-4.

monstrable already at the early arterial phase. The abnormal fluorescence was noted to be slightly more extensive than the ophthalmoscopically demonstrable area of retinal degeneration, and there was an indication of somewhat prolonged circulation time in the blood vessels supplying the degenerated region. Possibly of greater importance is that sporadically distributed map-like areas suspected to be defective of the pigment epithelial layer, with loss of the underlying choriocapillaris, were present in the degenerated regions. The peripheral retina was completely free from such abnormal fluorescence; hence, fluorescein-angiographically demonstrable degeneration was circumscribed (Fig. 5). Quantitative visual field examination of the patient showed an upper depression, virtually corresponding to the localization of the fundus degeneration (Fig. 6). The threshold for dark adaptation was found to be slightly elevated to 2.6 at 30 minutes.

Electroretinograms were of a subnormal type, characterized by normal a-waves, abnormal oscillatory potentials and low-amplitude b-waves. In contrast to the modes abnormality in ERG, electro-oculograms revealed a remarkable low Q value and a normal base value, thus practically a flat type (Fig. 7).

Case II-5, a 45 year old natural brother of case II-4, had no ophthalmological subjective symptoms, except myopia. He visited this clinic for detailed ophthalmologic checkup on the advice of the proband. The patients's visual acuity was normal, 0.6 (1.2X-1.0D) on the right and 0.2 (1.2X-1.5D) on the left, and there was no abnormality with respect to the outer portions or media of eyes. Ophthalmoscopic findings noticeably resembling those in Case II-4 were noted, viz. as shown in Figs. 8 and 9: bilaterally symmetrical lesions characterized by dirty retinal clouding with pigment deposition localized below the optic disc and extending toward the lower temporal region. Fluorescein fundus angiography demonstrated a similar circumscribed fluorescence (Fig. 10 and 11) as in Case II-4. There was also upper depression of the peripheral visual field, as illustrated in Fig. 12, corresponding to the area of retinal degeneration. The patient's threshold for dark adaptation was al-

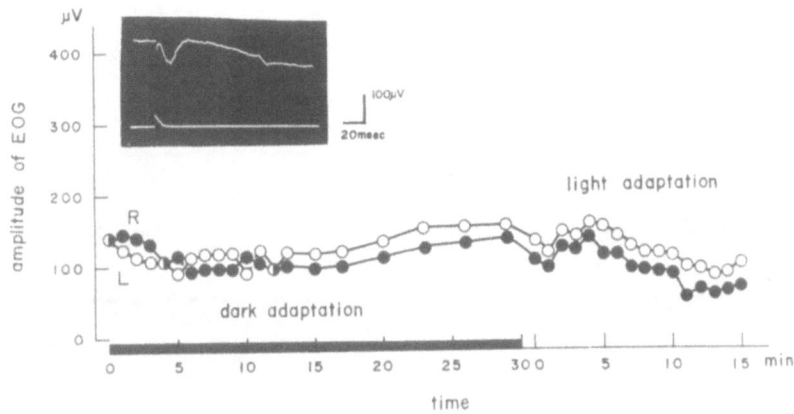

Fig. 7. ERG and EOG recorded from Case II-4.

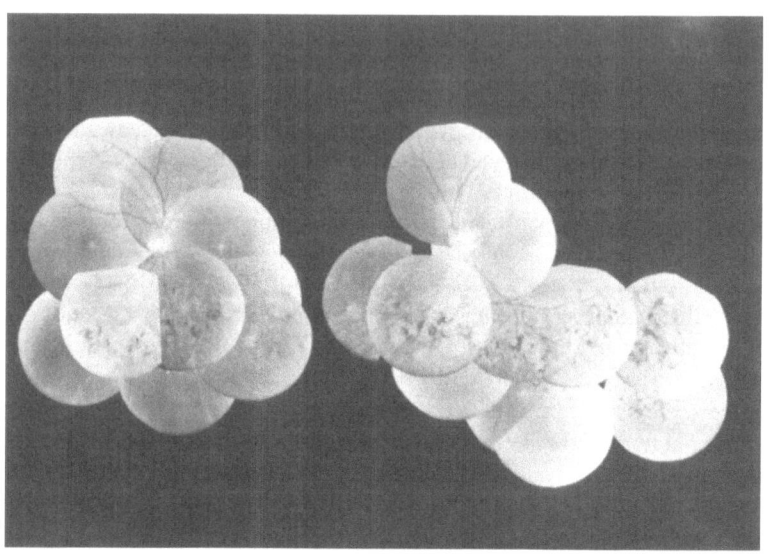

Fig. 8. Fundus pictures of Case II-5.

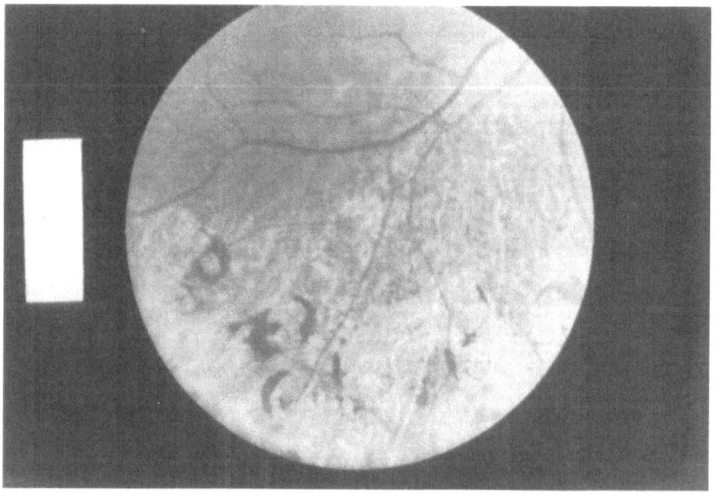

Fig. 9. Fundus picture of Case II-5. Degenerated area with depigmentation and pig-mentation of lower temporal region.

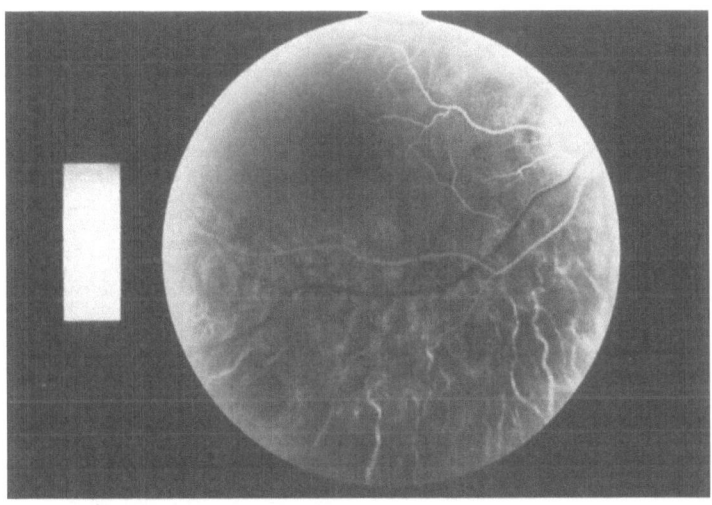

Fig. 10. Fluorescein fundus angiogram of Case II-5. Arterial phase. The retinal arteries toward the degenerated area are slightly narrower than those to the intact part of the fundus.

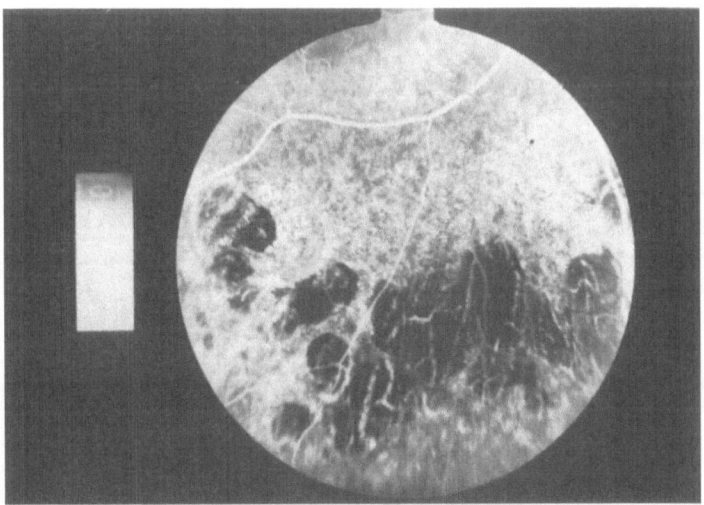

Fig. 11. Fluorescein fundus angiogram of Case II-5. Arteriovenous phase.

271

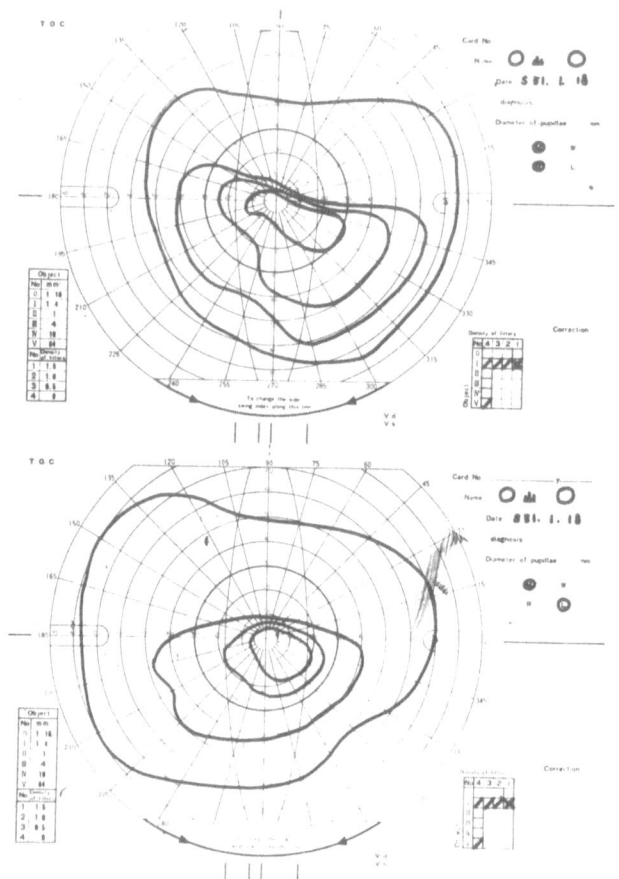

Fig. 12. Visual field of Case II-5.

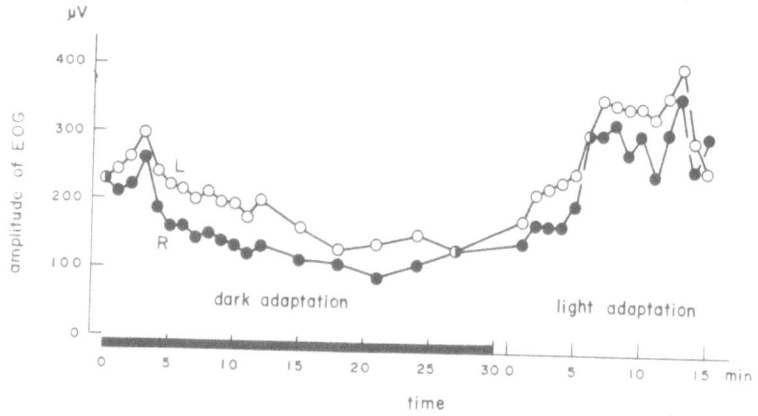

Fig. 13. EOG recorded from Case II-5.

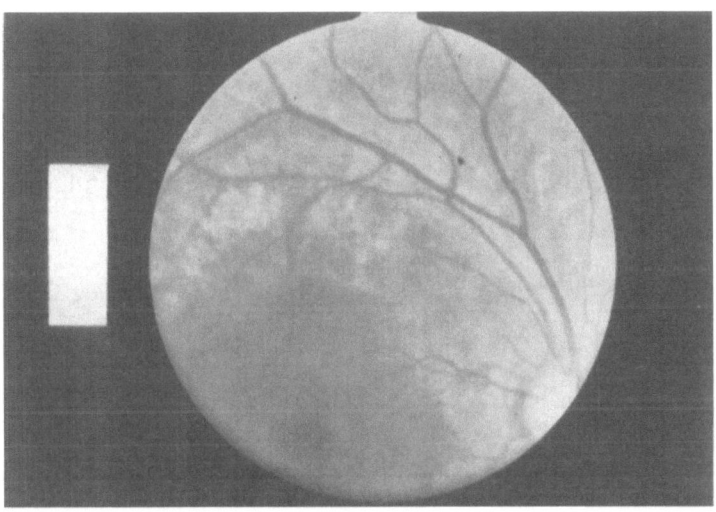

Fig. 14. Fundus picture of Case III-10 (right eye).

most normal, 2.2 at 30 minutes. ERG tracings were of the subnormal type and EOG showed normal type with a normal Q value of 2.5 (Fig. 13).

Case III-10, male, aged 16 years, is the oldest son of the proband, Case II-4. The patient also had no ophthalmological complaints in his life, except myopia, and was examined in detail on the advice of his mother. On ophthalmoscopic examination, retinal pigmentary dystrophy, apparently less severe than in the foregoing cases, was noted bilaterally as symmetrical lesions with modes pigmentation along the course of the upper temporal retinal vessel (Figs. 14 and 15). A characteristic abnormal fluorescence was revealed by fluorescein angiography in the upper temporal region of the fun-

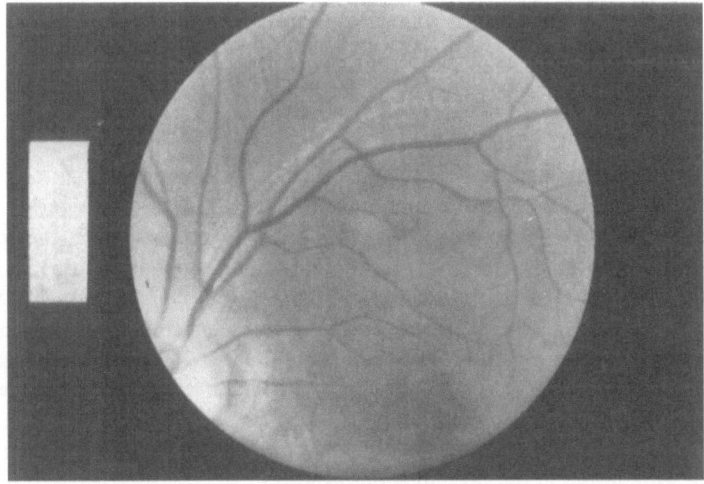

Fig. 15. Fundus picture of Case III-10 (left eye).

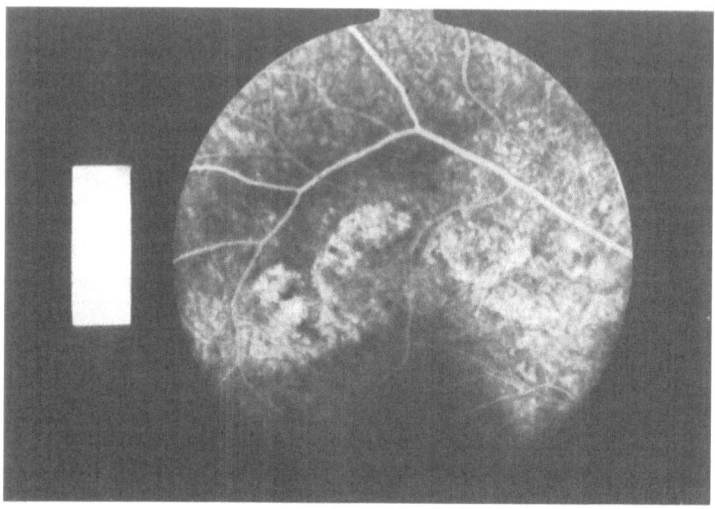

Fig. 16. Fluorescein fundus angiogram demonstrating retinal degeneration corresponding to the area noted ophthalmoscopically.

dus corresponding to the ophthalmolscopically demonstrated area of abnormality (Fig. 16). Within the area of retinal degeneration, leakage of the dye
suggested an abnormality of the choriocapillaris layer. Visual field examination did not reveal any significant changes necessarily corresponding to the
lesion of the fundus. The patient's threshold for dark adaptation was moderately impaired, 4.0 at 30 minutes, the degree being the most severe among
the three cases described. ERG tracings were of the subnormal type with
slightly diminished amplitude of the b-wave, whereas, in the EOG, considerable depression of the amplitude of light rise was noted in the course of
light adaptation despite a satisfactory base value (Fig. 18).

No typical case of retinitis pigmentosa has as yet been found in the pedigree, however.

DISCUSSION

Sectoral retinal pigmentary dystrophy is characterized, according to reports
by other investigators, by non-progressive degeneration of the retina localized in the lower quadrant of the fundus, with no changes in the retinal
vasculature, normal visual acuity with night blindness (Batra, 1966) contrac-
tion of the visual field, subnormal ERG and abnormal EOG (Hellner & Rickers, 1973). It has also been described that fluorescein fundus angiograms demonstrated abnormal fluorescence in the fundus slightly more extensive
than the degenerated region observed ophthalmoscopically (Krill et al.
1970).

Ophthalmological findings virtually consistent with these reported characteristics were noted in the present series as well.

However, the development of bilaterally symmetrical lesions of sectoral

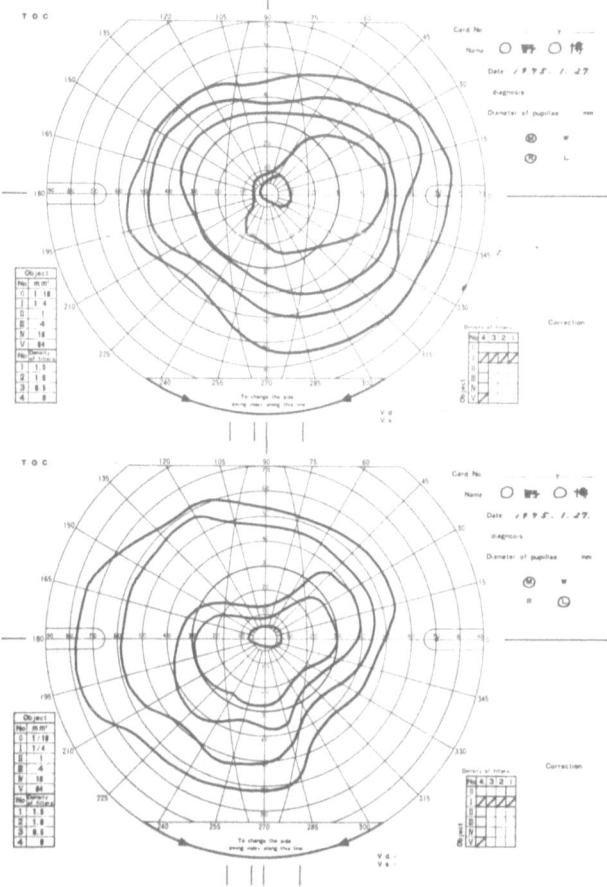

Fig. 17. Visual field of Case III-10.

degeneration localized in the upper temporal region found in Case III-10 seems to be rare in that no such development of sectoral degeneration has been previously reported, except the cases described by Jacobson (1961) and Straub (1961).

The EOG revealed a considerable depression of amplitude in our case, as compared with previously reported cases. This finding suggests that the outer layer of the retina might be more extensively affected than implied by fluorescein fundus angiography.

The following three characteristic findings in the fluorescein angiography are considered to be of particular note: First, the degenerated areas revealed by fluorescein angiography exceed in area the extent the ophthalmoscopically demonstrable retinal degeneration, as already pointed out by Krill et. al. (1970). Secondly, the blood vessels supplying the area of degeneration show a diminished flow rate, compared to those in normal portions of the retina. Third, prominent exposure of choroidal vessels with areas of possi-

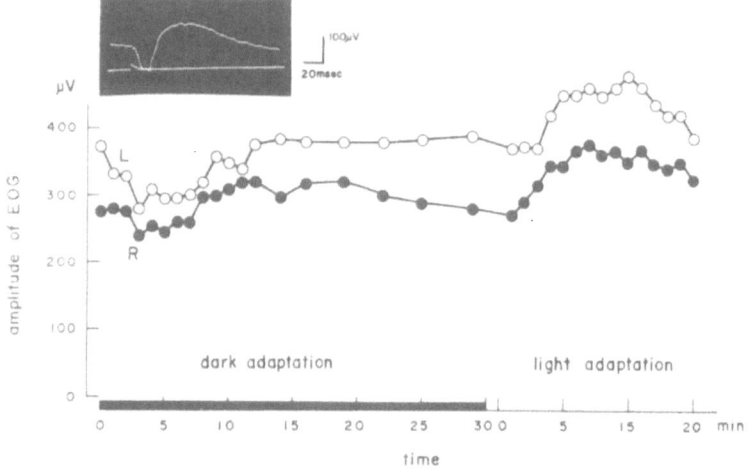

Fig. 18. ERG and EOG recorded from Case III-10.

ble defect of the pigment epithelium and loss of choriocapillary layer are seen within the region of retinal degeneration. This third angiographic feature seems to be of profound significance insofar as it not only suggests the possibility of further progress of degeneration within the localized lesion but also may provide some clue regarding the pathogenesis of this desease.

From the facts noted in the present study — the visual function did not differ significantly and the extent of retinal degenerative lesions were virtually comparable among all three patients irrespective of age — it has been suggested that the condition is relatively non-progressive and localized. This point, would have to be verified by further detailed investigations of the remaining members in this pedigree and by long-term follow-up of these patients.

SUMMARY

A pedigree with sectoral retinal pigmentary dystrophy, possibly transmitted by autosomal dominant inheritance, has been evaluated by detailed ophthalmologic examinations, with the following results obtained in three principal subjects:

1. Clinical findings virtually consistent with previously reported cases were noted in all three patients, of whom one (Case III-10) was found to have bilaterally symmetrical lesions of retinal degeneration localized in the upper temporal quadrant of the fundus.

2. Fluorescein fundus angiography revealed characteristic findings, viz.:

— Degeneration revealed by fluorescein angiography exceeded in area the ophthalmoscopically demonstrated lesion of retinal degeneration, thus confirming the findings of Krill et al. (1970).

— There was evidence of diminished circulatory rate for the retinal blood vessels supplying the degenerated area, as compared to those in the normal portions of the retina.

276

— Within the lesions of retinal degeneration, there were prominent choroidal vessels and areas possibly deficient in pigment epithelium with loss of the underlying choriocapillaris layers.

3. All three cases showed practically comparable degree of retinal degeneration, irrespective of age.

REFERENCES

Batra, D. V. Bilateral symmetrical sectoral retinal pigmentation. *Br. J. Ophthalmol.* 50: *734* (1966).

Berson, E. L. & J. Howard. Temporal aspects of the electroretinogram in sector retinitis pigmentosa. *Arch. Ophthal.* 86: *653* (1971).

Hellner, K. A. & J. Rickers. Familiary bilateral segmental retinopathia pigmentosa. *Ophthalmologica.* 166: *327* (1937).

Hommer, K. Das ERG bei sektorenförmiger Retinitis pigmentosa. *Graefes Arch. Ophthal.* 161: *16* (1959).

Jacobson, J. H. Clinical Electroretinography. Charles C. Thomas, Illinois (1961).

Krill, A. E., D. Archer & D. Martin. Sector retinitis pigmentosa. *Am. J. Ophthal.* 69: *977* (1970).

Küper, J. Familiäre sektorenförmige Retinitis pigmentosa. *Augenheilk.* 136: *97* (1960).

Ponte, F. Electroretinographic evaluation of the sectoral tapeto-retinal degenerations. *Jap. J. Ophthal.* Suppl. 282 (1966).

Straub, W. Das Electroretinogramm-Experimentelle und klinische Beobachtungen. Enke, Stuttgart, p. 118 (1961).

Vukovich, V. Das ERG bei Retinitis pigmentosa mit bitemporalen Gesichtesfeldausfall. *Graefes Arch. Ophthal.* 161: 27 (1959).

Authors' address:
Department of Ophthalmology
School of Medicine
Iwate Medical University
Morioka
Japan

STUDIES ON THE EARLY RECEPTOR POTENTIAL
IN THE HUMAN EYE

VI. ERP IN THE FELLOW EYES OF PATIENTS
WITH IDIOPATHIC RETINAL DETACHMENT

AKIHIKO TAMAI

(Yonago, Japan)

ABSTRACT

The early receptor potential (ERP) was measured and examined in 41 fellow eyes of 41 patients under 60 years of age with unilateral, idiopathic retinal detachment, who were free from myopia over -8 diopters and myopic chorioretinal atrophy. Eighty-six eyes of 50 normal subjects, comparable in age and in refractometric findings, served as normal controls. Mean ERP amplitudes in the group of 19 fellow eyes with some degenerative changes in the peripheral retina of the patients were, statistically, greatly decreased at the 1% level of significance, as compared with the normal controls. Even in the group of 22 fellow eyes with no appreciable retinal abnormalities, the mean ERP amplitude was significantly decreased at the 5% level, as compared with normal.

Based upon these ERP findings, the possibility of a "predisposition" to retinal detachment and the pathogenesis of this condition are discussed.

The present study investigated the fellow eyes of patients with idiopathic retinal detachment by taking as the parameter of observation, not the scotopic or photopic ERGs, but the early receptor potential (ERP) which is mainly generated in the outer segments of the visual cells (predominantly the cones) in the human eye. The technique reflects the functional and morphological integrity of the retinal pigment epithelium and the choroid (Goldstein & Berson, 1969; Tamai, 1972a,b, 1974a,b, 1976b).

MATERIALS AND METHODS

Forty-one fellow eyes of 41 patients, under 60 years of age with unilateral, idiopathic retinal detachment were examined. Considering the influence of aging and refractive errors on the ERP (Tamai, 1976b), the patients with refractive error over -8 diopters and with myopic chorioretinal atrophy were excluded. Fundi were examined by direct and binocular indirect ophthalmoscopy with scleral depression, and by means of the three-mirror contact lens when indicated.

Eighty-six eyes of 50 physically and ophthalmologically normal subjects, otherwise the same as the patients, served as normal controls.

The details of the apparatus for measuring the ERP and the method have been fully described in previous papers (Tamai, 1972a,b, 1974a,b, 1976b), and only the main points will be described below.

The initial test flash with a discharge energy of 80 joules was presented after 15 minutes of dark adaptation; the ERP elecited by this stimulus being called the first flash ERP. The second test flash was presented 2 minutes later, merely to ascertain the reliability of the first flash ERP in this study, since the initial ERP response must be higher than the second one, indicating a 2 minute recovery ERP response (Goldstein & Berson, 1969; Tamai, 1974a). The amplifier time constant was 0.01 sec and the high frequency cutoff was set at 10 kHz.

Fig. 1 shows the first flash ERP (lower trace) and the second flash ERP (upper trace) of a 38 year old normal female subject (right eye). Upward deflection indicates positivity of the corneal electrode. Although one can see a stimulus artifact (arrow) of approximately 0.1 msec duration simultaneously evoked by xenon discharge (Tamai, 1972a,b, 1974a), the initial cornea-positive phase (R_1) and the later cornea-negative phase (R_2) of the ERP followed by the distal a-wave (a_1) of the ERG are observed distinctly in both traces. Note that the second flash ERP amplitude was about 75% that of the first flash ERP amplitude (referred to hereinafter simply as the ERP amplitude), which was measured from the peak of the R_1 to the peak of the R_2.

RESULTS

In table 1, the mean ERP amplitude in the total fellow eyes of the patients was 74.6 ± 21.6 μV (one standard deviation), indicating, statistically, a

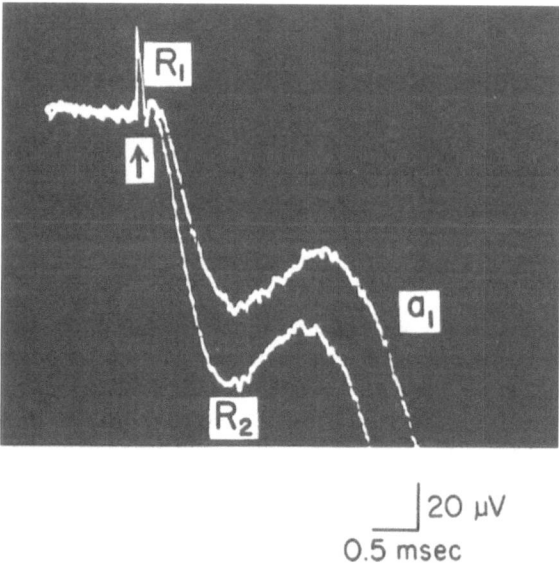

20 μV

0.5 msec

Fig. 1. ERPs of a 38 year old normal female subject. Positivity upwards. Arrow indicates stimulus artifact simultaneously evoked by xenon discharge. Upper trace: second flash ERP 2 minutes after the first flash ERP. Lower trace: first flash ERP. The initial cornea-positive phase (R_1) and the later cornea-negative phase (R_2) of the ERP followed by the distal a-wave (a_1) of the ERG are clearly observed in both traces.

Table 1. Changes of the ERP amplitude (μV) in the eyes of normal subjects and in the fellow eyes of patients with idiopathic retinal detachment.

	No. of eyes	ERP amplitude	t_S
Normal controls	86	87.2 $\pm$ 20.4*	
Fellow eyes	41	74.6 $\pm$ 21.6	0.001 $<$ p $<$ 0.01
Without abnormalities	22 (53.6%)	76.8 $\pm$ 22.2	0.02 $<$ p $<$ 0.05
With abnormalities	19 (46.4%)	72.2 $\pm$ 21.1	0.001 $<$ p $<$ 0.01

* Mean $\pm$ σ

t_S: Significance of the differences; 't' test

highly significant decreased amplitude at the 1% level, paired t-test, as compared with the mean ERP amplitude in the normal controls (87.2$\pm$ 20.4 μV).

Twenty-two out of the 41 fellow eyes of the patients (53.6%)showed no appreciable retinal abnormalities. The mean ERP amplitude was 76.8$\pm$22.2 μV, indicating, statistically, a significant decreased amplitude at the 5% level, as compared with the normal controls.

The other 19 fellow eyes (46.4%) showed some degenerative changes, including breaks in the peripheral region of the retina. The mean ERP amplitude was 72.2$\pm$21.1 μV, indicating, statistically, a highly significant decreased amplitude at the 1% level, as compared with normal.

DISCUSSION

The results obtained indicate, electrophysiologically, the presence of some functional and morphological changes in the outer layer of the retina, especially in the receptor outer segments, irrespective of the presence or absence of ophthalmoscopic retinal findings. Greater significance is attached to these results in cases where some degenerative changes are demonstrable in the fellow eye. Furthermore, because of the nature of the human ERP or the cone-cell predominant ERP (Goldstein & Berson, 1969; Tamai, 1972a, b, 1974a,b, 1976b), these significantly decreased ERP amplitudes may suggest more deteriorated conditions in the outer segments of the cone cells in the posterior polar region of the retina, than those in the rod cells in the peripheral retina.

Therefore, the results seem to support, from a different point of view, the possibility of a 'predisposition' to retinal detachment initially postulated by Karpe & Rendahl (1952), and successively by Rendahl (1957), Makabe (1969), Yonemura et al. (1972) and Tamai (1976a, 1977) on the basis of their scotopic or photopic ERG findings.

Furthermore, these ERP findings are of profound interest, even from the embryologic point of view, in that retinal detachment occurs between the visual cell layer and the retinal pigment epithelium, which, in turn, has an important bearing on the generation of the ERP (Goldstein & Berson, 1969; Tamai, 1972a,b, 1974a,b, 1976b).

Although the importance of pathological changes of the vitreous or vitreoretinal factors (Toyofuku & Hirose, 1975) must be considered concerning the mechanisms whereby degeneration and breaks of the retina develop, the findings bring up the problem that pathological alterations of a factor or factors on the retinal side (Toyofuku & Hirose, 1975), for example, fragility of the outer segments of the visual cells or changes in the acid mucopolysaccharide which is believed to function as a sort of gluing material between the visual cell layer and retinal pigment epithelium (Zimmerman & Eastham, 1959; Zauberman et al., 1972), cannot be disregarded. No hasty conclusion should be drawn from the present ERP findings. Prior work on the 30 Hz flicker ERG and the monochromatic flash ERG through a red Wratten filter No. 23A showed significantly abnormal photopic ERG changes (Tamai, 1976a), but also introduced the possibility of some pathological changes in the photopic system of the retina, especially in the outer segments of the cone cells, which may relate to the mechanisms whereby detachment and breaks of the retina develop in the macular area.

In conclusion, more discreet clinical examinations on the entire fundus and sufficient follow-ups should be undertaken on the fellow eyes of patients with idiopathic retinal detachment, as well as the affected eyes. There remains the possibility of a 'predisposition' to this condition as evidenced electrophysiologically, regardless of fundus appearance, especially in cases where some degenerative changes are demonstrable in the peripheral retina.

ACKNOWLEDGMENTS

The author is very grateful to Professor Yutaka Fujinaga for his constant interest and counsel in this investigation. The author also appreciates the help of Mr. Kazuhiro Uryu of the Nihon Kohden Kogyo Co., Ltd. in all practical aspects of the work.

REFERENCES

Goldstein, E. B. & E. L. Berson. Cone dominance of the human early receptor potential. *Nature* (Lond.) 222: *1272–1273* (1969).

Karpe, G. & I. Rendahl. The clinical electroretinogram. VI. The electroretinogram in detachment of the retina. *Acta Ophthal.* (Kbh.) 30: *303–316* (1952).

Makabe, R. Elektroretinogram bei zu Netzhautablösung disponierten *Klin. Mbl. Augenheilk.* 154: *450–452* (1969).

Rendahl, I. The electroretinogram in detachment of the retina. *Arch. Ophthal.* (Chicago) 57: *566–576* (1957).

Tamai, A. Studies on the early receptor potential in the human eye. I. Some clinical records. *Yonago Acta Med.* 16: *23–28* (1972a).

Tamai, A. Studies on the early receptor potential in the human eye. II. ERP in a case of ethambutol intoxication. *Yonago Acta Med.* 16: *97–104* (1972b).

Tamai, A. Studies on the early receptor potential in the human eye. III. ERP in primary retinitis pigmentosa. *Yonago Acta Med.* 18: *18–29* (1974a).

Tamai, A. Studies on the early receptor potential in the human eye. IV. ERP in patients with senile cataract. *Yonago Acta Med.* 18: *30–35* (1974b).

Tamai, A. Electrophysiological studies on the fellow eyes (so-called healthy eyes) of the patients with idiopathic detached retina. I. Findings of the averaged 30 Hz flicker ERG and the monochromatic flash ERG. *Acta Soc. Ophthal. Jap.* 80: *1055–1061* (1976a).

Tamai, A. Studies on the early receptor potential in the human eye. V. ERP in various types of uveitis. *Jap. J. Ophthal.* 20: *420–437* (1976b).

Tamai, A. Electrophysiological studies on the fellow eyes (so-called healthy eyes) of the patients with idiopathic detached retina. II. Scotopic ERG findings. *Folia Ophthal. Jap.* 28: *816–819* (1977).

Toyofuku, H. & T. Hirose. Current progress of retinal detachment. IV. Pathogenesis of rhegmatogenous retinal detachment. *Jap. Rev. Clin. Ophthal.* 60: *1–15* (1975).

Yonemura, D., K. Kawasaki, C. Kawasaki & H. Usukura. The oscillatory potential of the ERG in idiopathic detachment of the retina. *Acta Soc. Ophthal. Jap.* 76: *267–270* (1972).

Zauberman, H., H. de Guillebon & F. J. Holly. Retinal traction in vitro. Biophysical aspects. *Invest. Ophthal.* 11: 46–55 (1972).

Zimmerman, L. E. & A. B. Eastham. Acid mucopolysaccharide in the retinal pigment epithelium and visual cell layer of the developing mouse eye. *Am. J. Ophthal.* 47: *488–499* (1959).

Author's address:
Department of Ophthalmology
Tottori University School of Medicine
Yonago
Japan

FUNCTIONAL AND HISTOLOGICAL MEASURES OF
RETINAL DAMAGE IN CHRONIC LIGHT EXPOSURE*

THEODORE LAWWILL, S. CROCKETT & GLENNA CURRIER

(Louisville, Ky, USA)

When discussing effects of toxic agents on the retina one must not exclude the most common physical agent to which the eye is exposed, light.

There has been much discussion about the possibility that exposure to light might hasten the course of degeneration in retinitis pigmentosa (Johnson, 1901; Leber, 1916; Collins, 1919; Falls, 1948), but little is known of the effect exposure to light might have on normal retina. In 1966, Noell (Noell, 1966, 1966a) found that rats left under fluorescent lamps for one week had their retinas totally destroyed. His findings raised the question whether light, slightly above assumed physiological levels, might permanently injure the normal retina.

We have set out to find what level of light is definitely damaging to the retina for large exposure areas over periods of several hours. By determining the level of light necessary to cause damage and the characteristics of this damage, we hope to clarify the relationship between light exposure and retinal degeneration of several types.

We reported our data concerning rabbits in 1971 (Lawwill, 1973) and our preliminary data from rhesus monkeys in the 1974 ISCERG Symposium (Lawwill, 1972).

METHOD

We evaluate functional damage with the flash ERG, morphological damage with ophthalmoscopy and fluorescein angiography, and histological damage with light and electron microscopy.

We grade the damage on a $\emptyset$ to 4+ scale for each technique. Total or almost total destruction is graded 4+, and when damage is suspected but not certain, the grade ± is used.

In our study of rhesus monkeys, we have established the threshold for damage for four hour exposures to large fields of white light, and highly chromatic laser lines at 590, 514.5, 488 and 457.9 nm.

* Supported in part by Contract No. DAMD17-74-C-4026 from the Office of the Surgeon General, U.S. Army and Grant No. FD 00874 from HEW, Food and Drug Administration, Bureau of Radiological Health.

Monkey ERGs are recorded with Burian-Allen type contact lens electrodes which have been modified to include the indifferent electrode and to fit the curvature of the monkey eye and cornea. The monkey cornea has an eight to ten diopter steeper curvature than that of the human. The monkey is tranquilized with phencyclidine HCl, 1 mg/Kg injected intramuscularly, and the pupils are dilated. The animal is first light adapted to 100 ft-L for two minutes in a Ganzfeld; and then the ERG is recorded every three minutes for thirty minutes. The ERG stimulus is provided by a Grass PS2 bulb mounted in the Ganzfeld, flashed at I-16. The growth of the ERG during dark adaptation is thus recorded. As it turns out, the amplitude for the seventh flash which occurs at twenty-one minutes dark adaptation is about the most stable measure for following the ERG from day to day. Computer fit polynomial curves for each day's ERG dark adaptation curve, when used for comparison, only slightly decrease the variability of the daily measures of the a- and b-waves. As seen in Figure 1, the day-to-day variability for the seventh flash ERG is not great. The exposure to light can have a dramatic effect on the ERG amplitude, and there is evidence of some recovery over a two to four week period. The exposure does not cover all of the peripheral retina and so we do not expect to find the ERG totally destroyed.

After a suprathreshold exposure, a change in pigment in the pigment epithelium can be seen in the fluorescein angiogram (Figs. 2, 3). The distribution of the most severe damage is usually paramacular, as is the pigment epithelial disturbance shown. Fluorescein angiography highlights the pigment epithelial disturbances, but other vascular changes such as leakage or staining in the fluorescein angiogram are not prominent.

For exposures ten times threshold, histological examination shows severe damage to the pigment epithelial and receptor layers. Figure 4 shows almost total destruction of the pigment epithelium and receptor cells. Many pig-

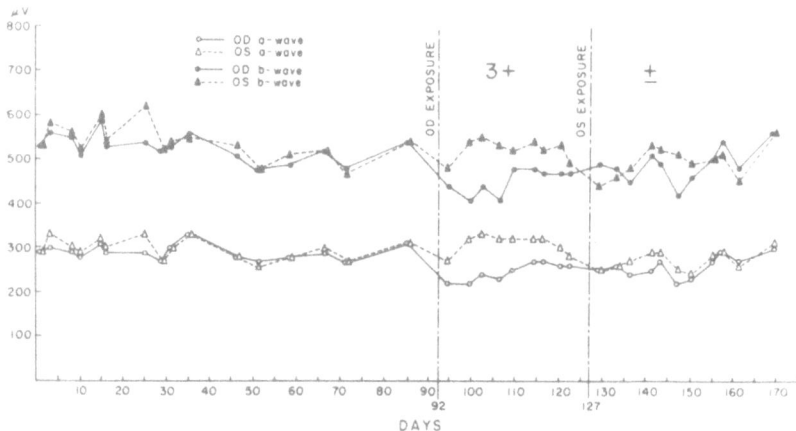

Fig. 1. Record of ERG a and b-wave amplitudes over a 170 day period during which single four-hour exposures were carried out in each eye. The fall in amplitude after exposure of the right eye is quite evident; after exposure of the left eye, the change is not as dramatic. The day-to-day variability in the amplitude is at an acceptable level for detecting functional damage after exposure.

286

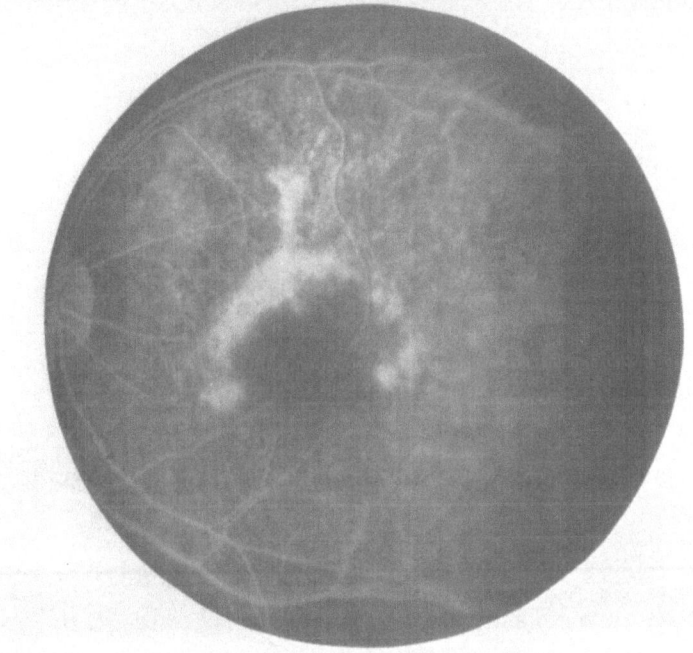

Fig. 2. Fluorescein angiogram of a light damaged monkey fundus. The pigment changes in the pigment epithelium are highlighted. The damage was less obvious on fundus photography.

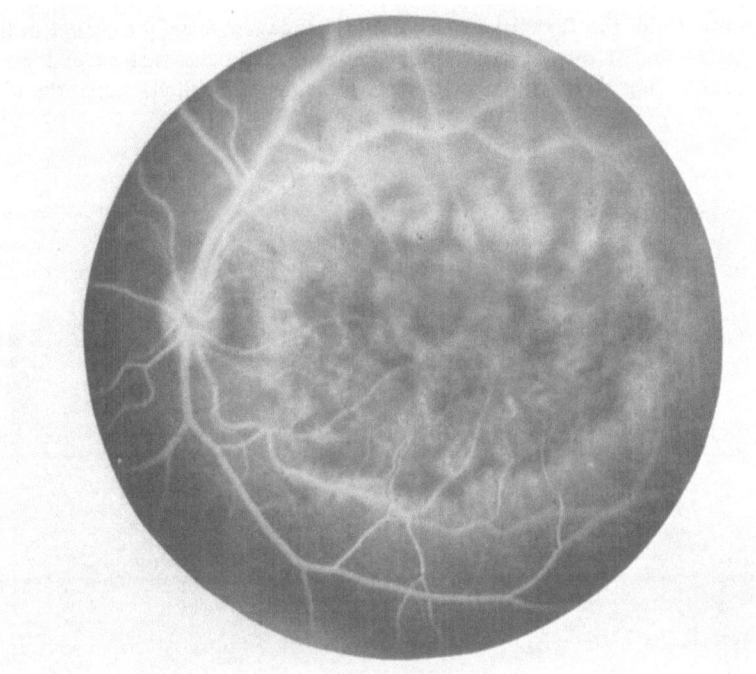

Fig. 3. Early fluorescein angiogram showing multiple defects in the pigment epithelium through the center area of the posterior pole.

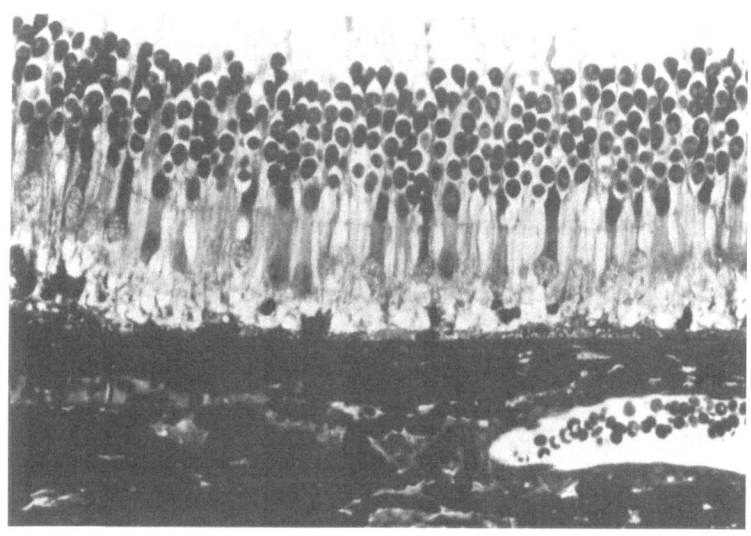

Fig. 4. Histologie section of a retina (x585) with severe light damage from a supra-threshold, four-hour exposure. The pigment epithelium is largely destroyed as are many receptor cells, but the outline of the architecture of the retina remains after two months.

ment epithelial cells are dead and most receptors do not look viable. At threshold, the first light microscopic changes are usually a change in the distribution of pigment in the pigment epithelial cells. Instead of the normal pallisading at the inner border of the pigment epithelial cells, the pigment

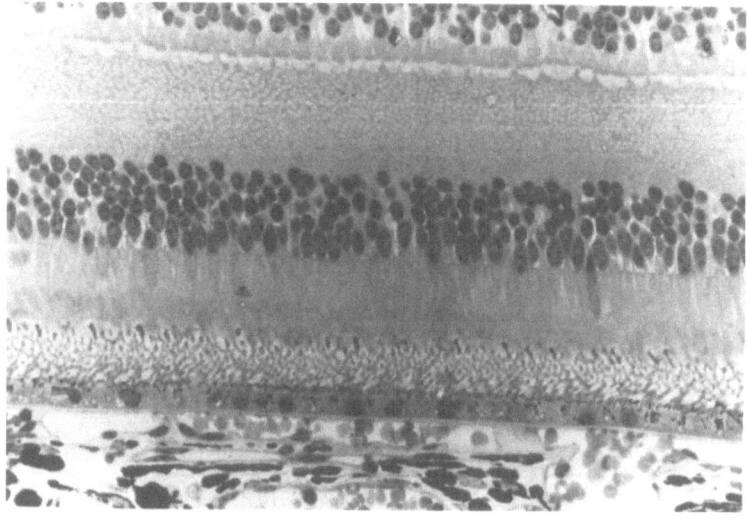

Fig. 5. Histologic section (x575) showing a change in the distribution of pigment within the pigment epithelial cells and swelling and distortion of the outer segments.

288

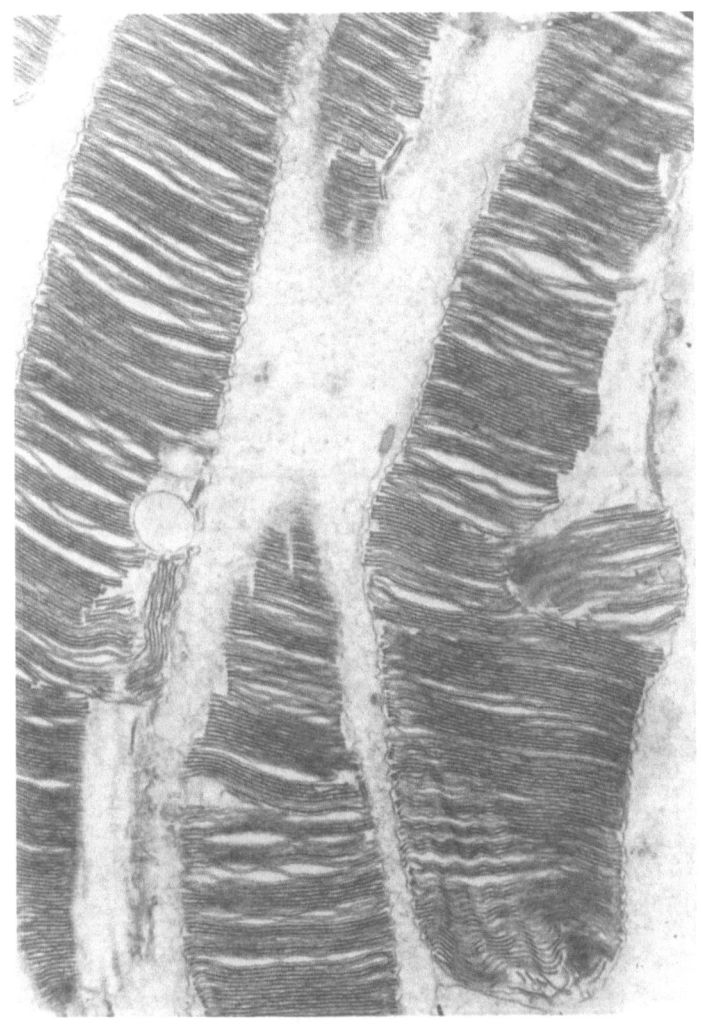

Fig. 6. Electron micrograph (x22,000) of ± changes in the outer segments. There is vesicle formation and distortion of the lamellae of the outer segments.

granules appear in the inner one-third of the cell more rounded and balled-up and less cigar shaped. (Figure 5). We suggest that this change is on two bases: one, the retraction back into the cell of the villi which normally contain the pigment and which normally run up between the outer segments; and two, the accumulation of greater than normal amounts of lipofucsin. A second change, seen in Figure 6, is the swelling of outer segments and the distortion of the individual discs within the outer segment. Here, there is distortion of the outer segments and vesicle formation in the lamellae. In the inner layers, three changes occur: swelling in the fiber layers, hyperchromasia of nuclei and pyknosis of the nuclei. In Figure 7 pyknosis can be

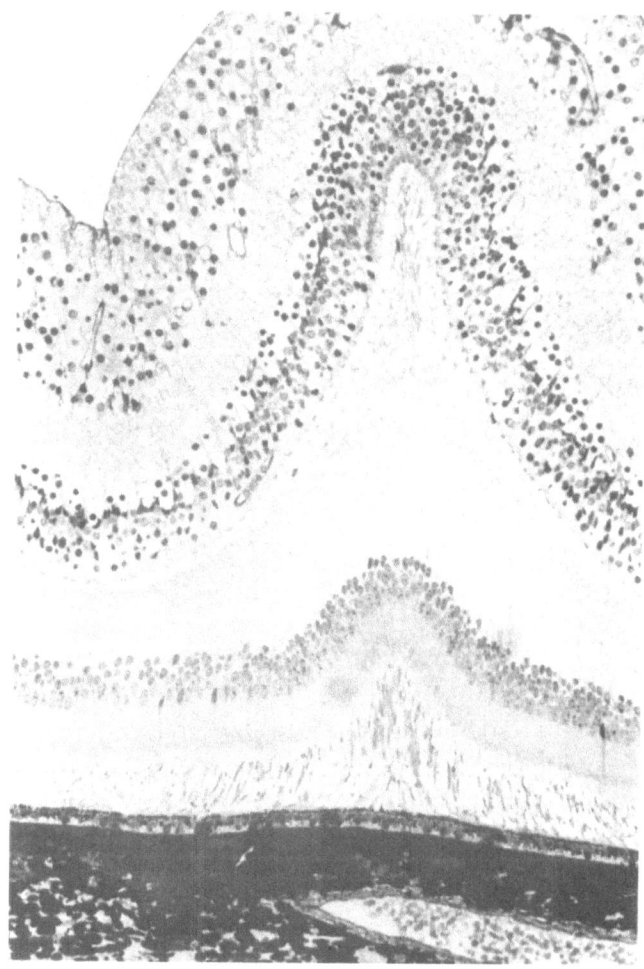

Fig. 7. Light micrograph of area near macula in light damaged eye. There is a fold secondary to slight swelling of the retina. Damage of inner layer is extensive while the outer layers are almost spared.

seen throughout the several nuclear layers, but the outer segments and the pigment epithelium are not severely disturbed.

In reporting threshold for light damage we plot the damage score for each technique for each eye against the level of the four hour exposure. The level reported is the total power entering the cornea in a Maxwellian view system divided by the area of retina exposed. Figure 8 shows the damage scores for white light. At 100 mw/cm^2, damage is consistent and severe. At 10 mw/cm^2, damage is less severe and less frequent but does occur occasionally. At 1 mw/cm^2, damage probably does not occur, but there is an occasional artifactual point above 1+ which probably does not represent damage.

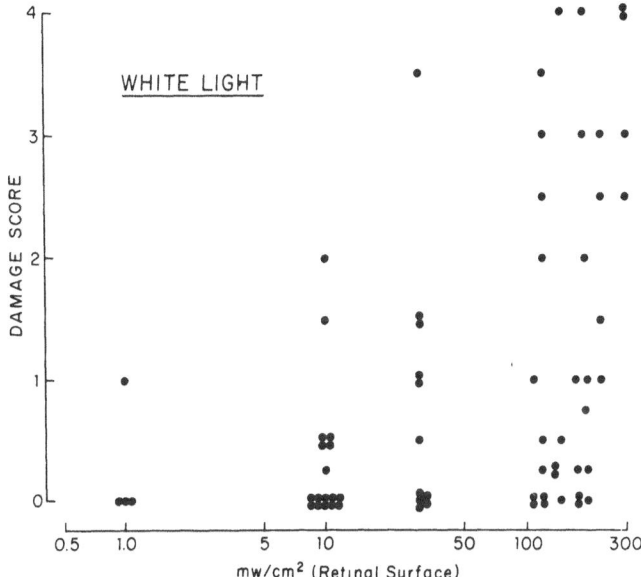

Fig. 8. This scattergram gives the damage grade for each technique for each eye plotted against the intensity of exposure for that eye. Damage is severe and consistent above 100 mw/cm². At 1.0 mw/cm², damage is unlikely. A minimal number of 1+ grades also occur in unexposed and lower exposure eyes in keeping with the intent of having the techniques sensitive enough to detect any damage that might be present.

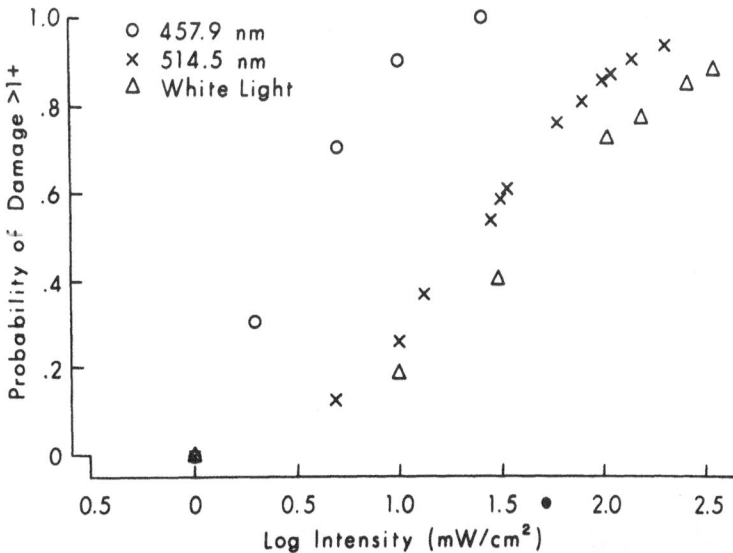

Fig 9. This graph depicts the cumulative probability of greater than 1+ damage for three wavelengths. The 457.9 nm line is approximately 0.8 log units more effective, on an intensity basis, in causing damage. The broad band white light and 514.5 nm exposures are about equally effective, except that the laser line causes more severe damage just above threshold.

The threshold for the highly chromatic 514.5 nm green line of the argon laser is not much different from the white light, except there is more severe damage immediately above threshold. There is a difference for the 457.9 nm line. When the cumulative probability for greater than 1+ damage is plotted for the three exposure wavelengths, it is noted that the 457.9 nm line threshold is about 0.8 log units lower than the other two (Fig. 9). This shift would be greater if the absorption of the ocular media were taken into account, and much greater if the units used were luminance units rather than intensity units.

Another spectral difference is shown by the difference in ERG and histological damage thresholds for the 514.5 and 457.9 nm lines of the argon laser (Figure 10). At 514.5 nm, there is very little difference in the thresholds for functional damage shown by ERG and cellular damage shown by histology. But, at 457.9 nm, the cellular damage is relatively greater than the functional damage (Figure 11). There is a hint in our 590 nm data that this relationship may reverse at the long wavelength end of the spectrum. These findings imply two mechanisms — one short wavelength mechanism effecting permanent cellular damage seen on histology, and second, a longer wavelength mechanism producing functional damage seen on ERG, which may be partially reversible.

The values for Table 1 were produced by human psychophysical matching between the exposure source and a carefully measured lighted surface and

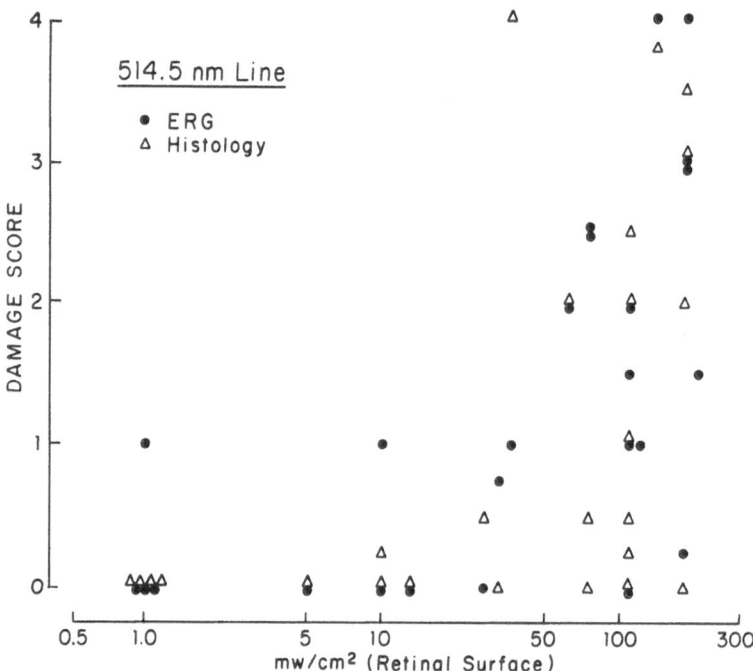

Fig. 10. Scattergram showing just ERG and histological damage scores for 514.5 nm exposures. The ERG and histological changes are about equal at this wavelength.

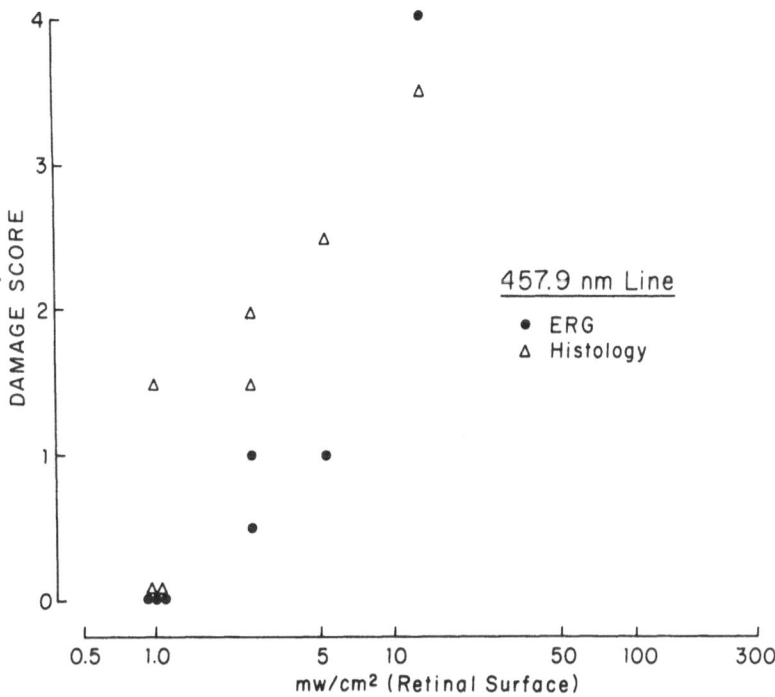

Fig. 11. Scattergram showing just ERG and histological damage scores for 457.9 nm exposures. The histological changes are greater than the ERG change at this wavelength.

monkey ERGs recorded in the exposure apparatus. The damage thresholds shown for the different wavelengths are similar in luminance to everyday light sources, except that the highly chromatic laser lines are not paralleled for concentrating a great deal of power into a small portion of the spectrum.

A recent finding raises many questions about the relationship of light damage to pathological processes in the human retina. Initial data implies that the damage threshold is the same whether the eye is exposed in a single four hour exposure or in four one hour exposures, each separated by twenty-four hours, If this additive effect occurs for even shorter periods separated by even longer times, one might suggest that light exposure will influence certain types of macular degeneration in susceptible individuals.

SUMMARY

The toxic effect of light upon the retina is shown to be significant at luminance levels which are present in the normal environment. When the highly chromatic lines of the argon laser are used for long term wide field exposure of the retina, the blue line at 457.9 nm is more effective in producing damage than the longer wavelength lines and white light. Histological changes are greater with the 457.9 nm and more significant than functional

293

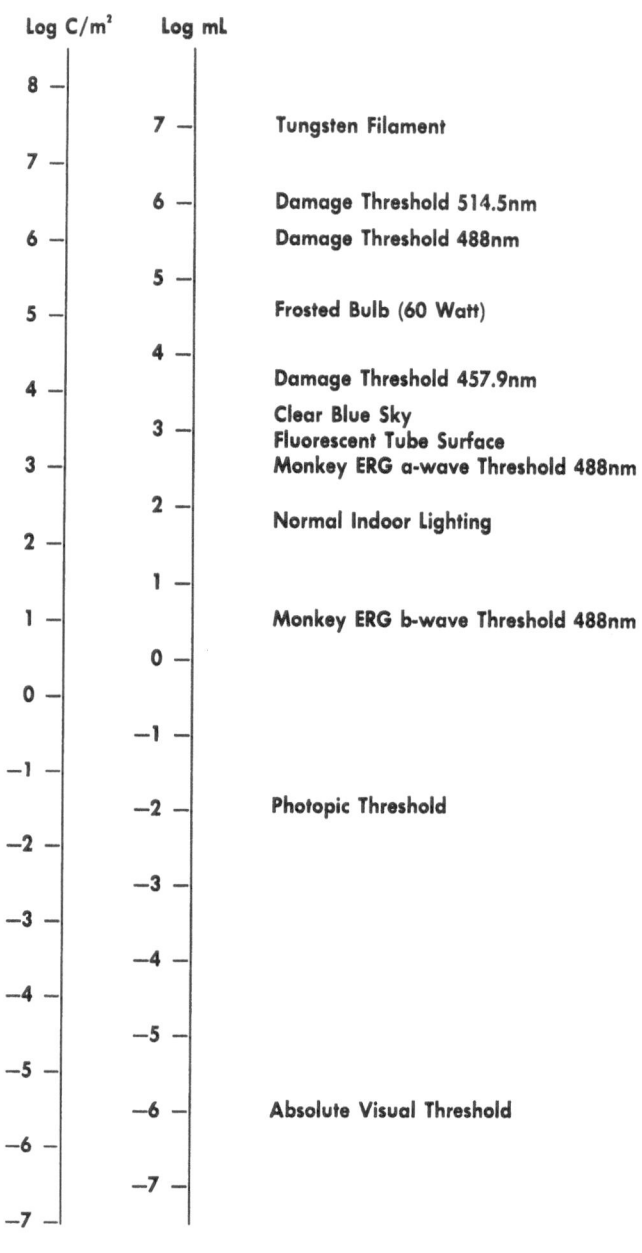

Log C/m²	Log mL	
8		
	7	Tungsten Filament
7		
	6	Damage Threshold 514.5nm
6		Damage Threshold 488nm
	5	
5		Frosted Bulb (60 Watt)
	4	
4		Damage Threshold 457.9nm
	3	Clear Blue Sky
		Fluorescent Tube Surface
3		Monkey ERG a-wave Threshold 488nm
	2	Normal Indoor Lighting
2		
	1	
1		Monkey ERG b-wave Threshold 488nm
	0	
0		
	−1	
−1		
	−2	Photopic Threshold
−2		
	−3	
−3		
	−4	
−4		
	−5	
−5		
	−6	Absolute Visual Threshold
−6		
	−7	
−7		

Table 1. Values for exposure damage and everyday light sources given in luminance units. The values on this table were determined by binocular human psychophysical matching of the exposure source and a surface illuminated by a portion of the same laser beam. The exposure source was measured in intensity units in our usual manner for exposures and the illuminated surface was measured by a photometer giving the luminance units. A correction factor was used to equate for eye size the human and monkey retinal levels for the Maxwellian view system.

changes recorded by ERG. The two are equally affected at 514.5 n.m. Recent data suggest that chronic light damage can be additive at least over a twenty-four hour period.

REFERENCES

Colins, ιE.T. Abiotrophy of the retinal neuroepithelium or 'retinitis pigmentosa'. *Trans. Ophthal. Soc. UK* 39: *165–196* (1919).

Falls, H.F. & C.W. Cotterman. Choroidoretinal degeneration: A sex-linked form in which heterozygous women exhibit a tepetal-like retinal reflex. *Arch. Ophthal.* 40: *685–703* (1948).

Johnson, G.L. Contributions to the comparative anatomy of the mammalian eye chiefly based on ophthalmoscopic examination (plates 1–30). *Phil. Trans. Roy. Soc. London* 194: *1–82* (1901).

Lawwill, T. The ERG and its correlation with damage caused by chronic exposure to light. Documenta Ophthalmologica Proceedings Series 2, Xth ISCERG Symposium, Los Angeles, 1972, August 20–23.

Lawwill, T. Effects of prolonged exposure of rabbit retina to low intensity light. *Invest. Ophthal.* 12: *45–51* (1973).

Leber, T. Die Pigment degeneration der Netzhaut and mit ihr Verwandte Erkrankungen, in Graefe Saemisch-Hess (ed): Handbuch der Gesamten Augenheilkunde, ed 2. Leipzig, Germany, W. Engelmann, 1916, vol. 7, pp. 1076–1225.

Noell, W.K. et al. Retinal damage by light in rats. *Invest. Ophthal.* 5: *450–473* (1966).

Noell, W.K. et al. Functional and structural manifestation of a damaging effect of light upon the rat retina. *Fed. Proc.* 25: *329* (1966).

Authors' address:
Department of Ophthalmology
University of Louisville
School of Medicine
301 E. Walnut Street
Louisville, Kentucky 40202
USA

PHOTOCOAGULATION AND THE ELECTRORETINOGRAM

R.P. SCHUURMANS, G.H.M. VAN LITH & J.A. OOSTERHUIS

(Leyden, The Netherlands)

INTRODUCTION

By means of the electroretinogram, the retinal function can be assessed objectively (Armington, 1974). The interest in the electroretinogram (ERG) for the clinical study of diabetic retinopathy has greatly increased since Yonemura (1962) found abnormal oscillatory potentials in diabetics, and Simonsen (1962) established that this was the case even in the absence of ophthalmoscopic evidence of a retinopathy.

Treatment of diabetic retinopathy by means of photocoagulation, as clinically introduced by Meyer-Schwickerath, is now generally in use. The alteration of the ERG after photocoagulation according to the DRS protocol (Collaborative Diabetic Retinopathy Study), in which a standard area of peripheral retina is destroyed, varies greatly among patients (Frank, 1975; Ogden, 1976). Both the photocoagulation itself and the retinopathy may lower the ERG. This is why the assessment of the retinal function by means of the ERG becomes difficult in diabetic retinopathy when photocoagulation has been applied. The effect of photocoagulation itself on the ERG should at least be known (Schmöger, 1974).

For this purpose we examined a group of rabbits before and after photocoagulation, comparing the decrease in height of the electrical responses with the extent and localization of the coagulated area.

METHODS

Before and after photocoagulation the scotopic and photopic ERGs were recorded. Photocoagulation was always carried out on the right eye, leaving the left eye intact for comparison. The image diameter of the coagulating xenon lamp was $3°$; coagulation was performed until the retina became white. This is not an objective, but a clinically used measure. In some cases the coagulated area was enlarged several times, the ERG being determined after each enlargement. Finally, the animals were sacrificed. After immediate enucleation and Bouin fixation (Romeis, 1948), the eyes were dehydrated and embedded in nitrocellulose 20%. The material was serially cross-sectioned at $8\ \mu$ and every 10th section was stained with haematoxilin-eosin.

The non-circumscript boundaries of the lesions in the serially sectioned material were arbitrarily chosen to be in the region showing any disorganization of the retina.

RESULTS

The serried field coagulations were applied in the 'visual streak' of the retina (Hughes, 1971). The extent of the area to be coagulated was determined by means of a hand-held Kowa fundus camera, the illumination of which covers a $30°$ retinal area. First, a $20°$ area was coagulated, which was successively extended to $30°$, $60°$ and $90°$. The histological appearance of the serried field coagulations showed that the retina outside the coagulated area remained intact. The percentages of the destroyed retinal areas were 3, 12, 30 and 44%, respectively, for the $20°$, $30°$, $60°$ and $90°$ coagulated areas. In the scotopic recordings of Figure 1 they are labelled as A, B, C and D. N represents the value of the non-coagulated eye. The reduction of the ERG after the various coagulations are surveyed in Table 1. It appeared that the decrease of the amplitude of the scotopic and photopic ERG is about the same. Furthermore, after coagulation of a $20°$ retinal area no decrease of the ERG could be observed.

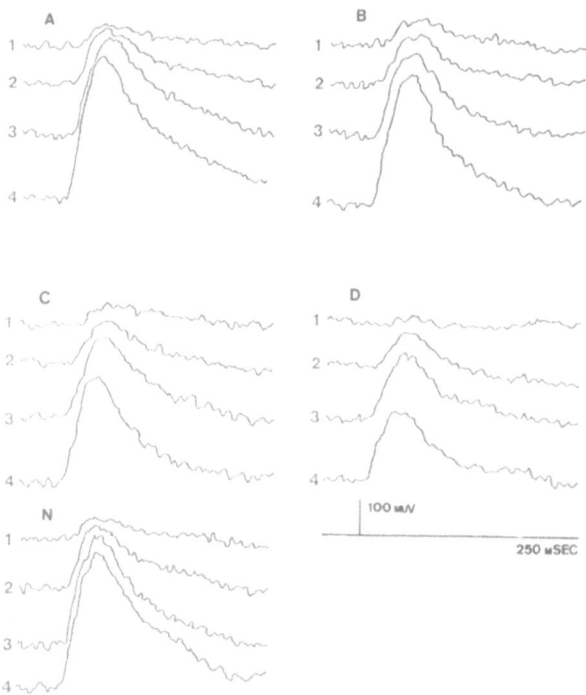

Fig. 1. Scotopic ERGs of the non-coagulated eye (N), and after 3% (A), 12% (B), 30% (C) and 44% (D) destruction of the retinal surface. The numbers on the left indicate the relative light intensity used.

	COAGULATED RETINA	SCOTOPIC ERG	PHOTOPIC ERG
K 76	0 %	100 %	100 %
	3	100	90
	12	90	80
	30	75	75
	44	40	35
K 77	2	100	100
	12	90	80
	25	80	75

Table 1. The scotopic and photopic ERG after a serried field coagulation in the posterior pole of the retina, covering 20, 30, 60 and 90 degrees areas.

This is in agreement with the results obtained by François & De Rouck (1964) who found that macular lesions showed no modification of ERG activity up to lesions with a diameter of 3 optic discs. After photocoagulation of 3 to 30% of the retinal surface (i.e. within a 60° area) the decrease of the ERG is proportionally related to the size of the destroyed part of the retina. The decrease of the ERG after destruction of a larger part of the retina is greater than the enlargement of the coagulated part.

The scotopic ERGs in Figure 1 were obtained four weeks after photo-

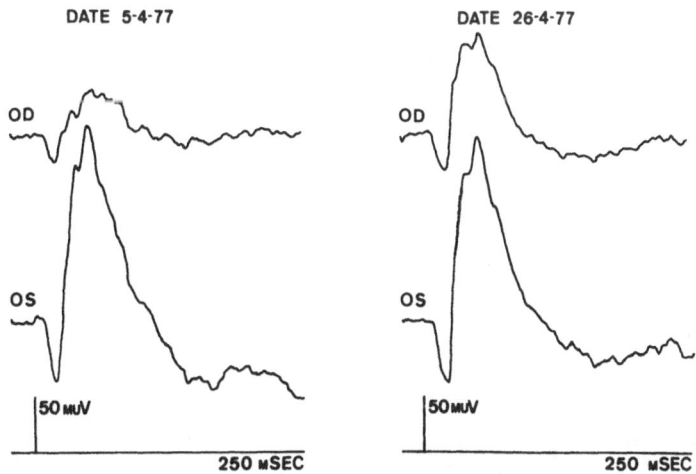

Fig. 2. Two recordings of the photopic ERG of both eyes; one immediately after photocoagulation (5-4-'77) and one three weeks thereafter (26-4-'77). OD represents the recordings of the right coagulated eye; OS those of the left untreated eye.

coagulation, when the white coagulations had become pigmented. In Figure 2, two recordings of the photopic ERG of both eyes are shown; one immediately after photocoagulation according to a checkerboard pattern and one three weeks thereafter. Immediately after photocoagulation there is an apparent loss of amplitude of the b-wave and, to a lesser extent, of the a-wave. After this initial decrease the amplitudes increase again, no increase being observed after four weeks. These findings also hold for the scotopic b-wave and are shown in Figure 3.

The photocoagulations which were carried out in a checkerboard pattern covered a 60° retinal area. Ophthalmoscopically, no degeneration could be observed between the coagulations. Histologically, however, it appeared that between the ophthalmoscopically visible coagulations – which are totally necrotic – the receptor layer and the outer nuclear layer degenerated. Therefore, this area cannot contribute to the ERG either, which implies that the destroyed area is larger than could be expected from the ophthalmoscopic appearance and equals that of a serried field coagulation, covering a 60° retinal area. This is in agreement with the findings of Figure 3 and Table 1, in which the final decrease of the ERG is related to a destruction of a 60° retinal area.

DISCUSSION

The decrease in the responses after checkerboard coagulation is more than one would expect in view of the ophthalmoscopic appearance. Ogden et al. (1976) did not find such extensive degeneration of the retina between co-

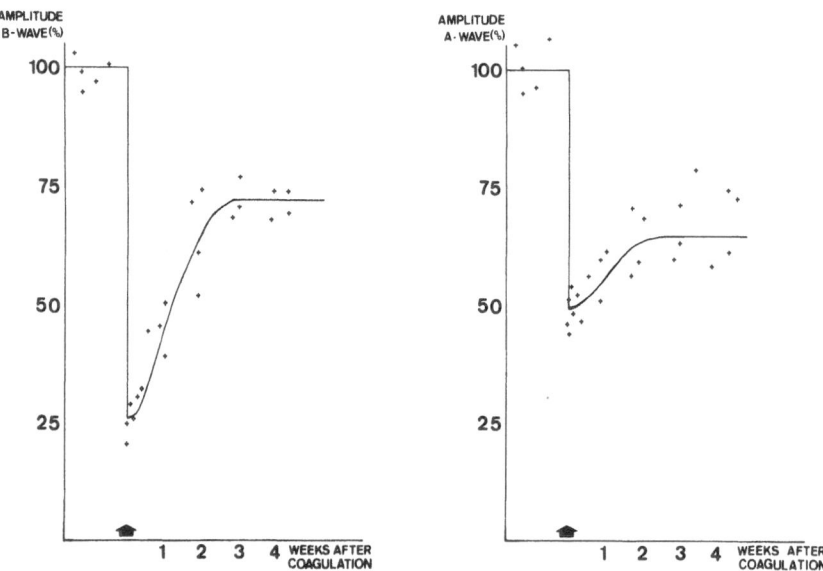

Fig. 3. Two graphs representing the initial decrease of the a- and b-wave immediately after photocoagulation (indicated by the arrow) and the recovery of the amplitudes during the next three weeks.

agulations. This may be attributed to the difference in thermal effect of xenon coagulation as compared with argon laser coagulation and with the species differences between rabbits' and monkeys' eyes. Lesions, clinically similar in magnitude in the two species, result in a disrupture of the internal limiting membrane of the retina in the rabbit, whereas the membrane of the monkey retina remained intact (Wallow, 1973).

The reason for the initial decrease of the ERG could be a partial impairment of enzyme activity within the retinal cell layers, due to the sensitivity of the enzymes to thermal injury (Geeraets, 1969). This implicates that the staining technique used (haematoxilin-eosin staining, which only visualizes morphological changes in the retinal cell layers) does not suffice to determine the amount of destruction during the first weeks.

SUMMARY

If the posterior pole of the rabbit retina is photocoagulated, the destruction of a $20°$ area or less reveals no measurable changes in the amplitudes of the scotopic and photopic ERGs. Between $20°$ and $60°$, the decreases are proportionally related to the destructed area. Immediately after photocoagulation, a much stronger effect on the ERG-amplitudes is found.

REFERENCES

Armington, J.C. The electroretinogram. Academic Press, New York (1974).

François, J. & A. De Rouck. Behavior of ERG and EOG in localized retinal destruction by photocoagulation. Clinical Electroretinography. Proc. Third Intern. Symp., 1964. Pergamon Press, Oxford/New York, pp. 191–202 (1966).

Frank, R.N. Visual fields and electroretinography following extensive photocoagulation. *Arch. Ophthal.* 93: *591–598* (1975).

Geeraets, W.J. Enzyme activity in the coagulated retina. *Acta Ophthal.,* Suppl. 76: *79–94* (1969).

Hughes, A. Topographical relationships between the anatomy and physiology of the rabbit visual system. *Docum. Ophthal.* 30: *33–159* (1971).

Ogden, T.E., et al. The electroretinogram after peripheral retinal ablation in diabetic retinopathy. *Am. J. Ophthal.* 81: *397–402* (1976).

Ogden, T.E., et al. Correlation of histologic and electroretinographic changes in peripheral retinal ablation in the rhesus monkey. *Am. J. Ophthal.* 81: *272–279* (1976).

Romeis, B. Mikroskopische Technik. Leibniz, München, p. 69 (1948).

Schmöger, E., et al. ERG in cases of therapeutic light coagulation. pp. 329–332, in: Proceedings XIIth ISCERG Symp., Clermont Ferrand, 1974. Docum. Ophthal. Proc. Series, Vol. 10 (1976).

Simonsen, S.E. ERG in diabetics. The clinical value of electroretinography. pp. 403–412 in: Proceedings ISCERG Symp., Ghent, 1966. Karger, Basel/New York (1968).

Wallow, I.H.L., et al. Retinal repair after experimental xenon arc photocoagulation. *Am. J. Ophthal.* 75: *32–52* (1973).

Yonemura, D., et al. Clinical importance of the oscillatory potential in the human ERG. *Acta Ophthal.* (Kbh.) Suppl. 70: *115–123* (1962).

Authors' address:
Department of Ophthalmology
University Hospital
Leyden
The Netherlands

Docum. Ophthal. Proc. Series, Vol. 15

ELECTROPHYSIOLOGICAL STUDIES BEFORE AND AFTER
ARGON LASER PHOTOCOAGULATION IN DIABETIC RETINOPATHY

J. FRANÇOIS, A. DE ROUCK, E' CAMBIE
& A. CASTANHEIRA-DINIS

(Ghent, Belgium)

Electrophysiological tests, fluorescein angiography and psycho-physiological dark adaptation curves, were performed in 50 eyes with diabetic retinopathy, before and after Argon laser photocoagulation. These eyes belonged to 31 patients (16 men and 15 women), their ages ranging from 24–64 years. The duration of the diabetes was from 2 to 30 years, from the time of the first examination.

TECHNIQUE

For the ERG recording, a Xenon stroboscope Van Gogh was placed 10 cm in front of the eye. Neutral filters were used in order to attenuate the flash intensities up to 3 log units. Direct inscription of the records was made on an Elema ink-jet mingograph (time-constant: 1.2 sec and 0.006 sec; Filter-Band: 70 and 700 H).

The photopic ERG was performed in the light adapted state (300 lux): single flashes of increasing intensities (from 3.0 to 0.0 rel. log units); flicker ERG from 1 to 15 cycles/sec; CFF and off-effect (cone responses).

The scotopic ERG was performed in the fully dark adapted state: responses to single xenon flashes of increasing intensities; responses to inter-ferential filters: red (658 nm) and blue (381 nm).

The following data were taken into consideration:

a) Amplitudes and peak times of the various components (a- and b-waves, first wavelet of the late photopic oscillating potential, off-effect).

b) Relative values (1) relation between the maximal a-wave and maximal b-wave in the photopic light adapted ERG (a/b p); (2) relation between the maximal a- and maximal b-wave in the scotopic dark adapted ERG (a/b s); (3) relation between the maximal photopic b-wave and the maximal scotopic b-wave (bp/bs); and (4) relation between the amplitude of the first late oscillating potential (LO/bp) and the maximal amplitude of the photopic b-wave (intensity 1.0: flicker 6–8 c/s).

For the EOG we used the technique of François et al. (1966). We have mainly taken into account Arden's L/D ratio, which is normally greater than 180%, although values between 180 and 165% may occasionally be found in normal subjects. The classification of the EOG records was made in the following way: (1) normal: > 180%; (2) borderline values: 180–

165%, (3) subnormal: 165–130%; (4) abnormal: 130–110%; and (5) extinguished: below 110%.

The psycho-physiological dark adaptation was done with the Goldmann-Weekers adaptometer: after 5′ light adaptation at 2000 asb, the threshold was determined after 15′, the normal threshold being $\overline{5}$.0 with an upper limit of $\overline{5}$.7.

The treatment was performed according to the technique described by François & Cambie (1977).

RESULTS AND DISCUSSION

Our electrophysiological data showed some characteristic findings which were not always in agreement with the classical findings described in the literature.

Recordings before Argon laser treatment

In our cases we found:
1. A severe and early involvement of the EOG (L/D ratio) and this at a time when the ERG was still normal. Most authors agree that the EOG decreases only when the ERG has already decreased (Kris, 1965; Arden et al., 1962; Henkes & Hautmüller, 1964).
2. The first alteration of the ERG consisted of the reduction and disappearance of the fast wavelets, as already mentioned by numerous authors (Yonemura et al., 1962; Simonsen, 1966; and others). In some of our cases with absent oscillatory potentials, double a-waves with normal peak-times could be recorded with some stimulus intensities. In other cases, especially when the ERG amplitude became smaller, this duplication could no longer be observed. This fact supports, however, the hypothesis that the duplication of the a-wave with a light stimulus of well defined intensities is not only the consequence of the appearance of the oscillatory potentials, but also the result of an interaction between two negative a-waves.
3. The ERG records remained normal in the first stages of the diabetic retinopathy. The mean-amplitudes were even higher than in a normal population. A decrease in the ERG amplitude started only with the development of large ischemic and avascular zones, while the EOG (L/D ratio) was already involved by the appearance of these zones.

In our experience, the scotopic b-wave is more sensitive to this process than the photopic b-wave. This is not in agreement with the findings of other authors, who have claimed a precocious involvement of the photopic response (Nagata et al., 1962; Garnier, 1967; Gliem et al., 1971) or found no difference between both b-waves (Tassy et al., 1971).

On the contrary, we found a gradual decrease of the scotopic b-wave, first in blue light, later also in white light, and this at a stage when the photopic b-wave was still within normal limits. The peak-time of the photopic b-wave was, however, often increased beyond normal values. A decrease of the photopic b-wave occurred at a later stage and a decrease of the negative waves in the terminal stages of the diabetic retinopathy.

Changes in the ERG induced by argon laser photocoagulation consisted mainly of a decrease in amplitude. This phenomenon was much more evident when the ERG was normal at the beginning. Cases already demonstrating a severely reduced ERG before the treatment, scarcely showed a decrease of ERG amplitudes. This fact seems evident because in less severe diabetic retinopathy the avascular zones are less extensive than in more severe cases.

The a-wave was less involved than the b-wave and the photopic b-wave less than the scotopic b-wave, at least in the cicatricial stage. This difference was statistically significant. In the oedematous stage, two days after treatment, both b-waves were reduced in the same way. This difference in behaviour could be explained by the retinal oedema.

There was no relation between the number of coagulation spots and the decrease in amplitude of the ERG, but there was a relation between the number of coagulation spots in the perfused areas. This is in agreement with the findings of Schuurmans et al. (1976) who, after checkerboard coagulation of less than 30% of the retina, found a decrease in the ERG response proportionally to the destroyed area. When more than 30% of the retinal surface was destroyed, the decrease in the responses was greater than could be expected.

Eventually remaining oscillatory po.entials disappeared after treatment by photocoagulation. The duplication of the a-wave was no longer seen. The late photopic oscillation seemed more depressed that the photopic wave. This phenomenon is, perhaps, due to an enlargement of the b-wave itself.

The peak-times of the responses, which in many cases were already increased before the photocoagulation, were generally not, or only slightly, modified, if the visual functions were not modified.

An important increase of the peak-times, associated with a decrease of the amplitude, was the consequence of the progress of the retinopathy and not of the photocoagulation itself.

The L/D ratio of the EOG was always severely reduced. In the oedematous stage it was nearly always extinguished. Occasionally an L/D ratio of 125% was obtained. In the cicatricial stage, a slight recovery seemed to be possible, but the L/D ratio still remained abnormal.

The dark adaptation curves, which were often subnormal before treatment, were not modified by photocoagulation. This confirms the findings of Wepman et al. (1976).

SUMMARY

Fifty eyes with diabetic retinopathy were studied before and after treatment with Argon laser coagulation. A decrease of the L/D ratio of the EOG and of the amplitude of all the components of the ERG were found. The scotopic b-wave was more involved than the photopic b-wave. The peak times were hardly modified. The dark adaptation curves were not altered. It was interesting that the EOG was involved before the ERG in the pre-treatment state. The L/D ratio decrease started when avascular and ischemic zones were seen on fluorescein angiography.

REFERENCES

Arden, S.D., A. Barrada & J.H. Kelsey. New clinical test of retinal function based upon the standing potential of the eye. *Br. J. Ophthal.* 46: *449–467* 1962).

François, J. & E. Cambie. Argon laser photocoagulation in diabetic retinopathy. A comparative study of three different methods of treatment. *Metabolic Ophthal.* 1: *125–130* (1977).

François, J., A. De Rouck, G. Verriest & M. Szmigielski. An extended clinical test of the ocular standing potential and its results in cases of retinal degeneration. pp. 257–268 in: Proc. IVth ISCERG Symp., Hakone, 1965. *Jap. J. Ophthal.* 10 Suppl. (1966).

Garnier, J.P. L'électrorétinographie dans le diabète. Thesis, Rennes (1967).

Gliem, H., C.E. Möller & S. Kietzmann. Die bioelektrische Aktivität der Netzhaut bei der diabetischen Retinopathie. *Acta Ophthal.* (Kbh) 49: *353–363* (1971).

Henkes, H.E. & A.J. Houtsmüller. Fundus diabeticus. An evaluation of the preretinopathic stage. *Am. J. Ophthal.* 60: *662–670* (1965).

Kris, E.C. Cyclic cornea-fundal potential EOG variations. pp. 88–89 in: Proc. IVth ISCERG Symp., Hakone, 1965. *Jap. J. Ophthal.* 10, Suppl. (1966).

Nagata, M., T. Yamane, H. Takata, T. Jono & A. Hoshino. Studies on photopic ERG of the human eye. *Acta Soc. Ophthal. Jap.* 66: *1614–1673* (1962).

Schuurmans, R.P., W.A. de Lege, G.H.M. van Lith & J.A. Oosterhuis. The influence of photocoagulation of the retina on the electroretinogram. pp. 191–195 in: Proc. 170th Meeting of the Netherlands Ophthal. Society. Junk, The Hague (1976).

Simonsen, S.E. ERG in diabetics. pp. 403–411 in: Proc. XXth Int. Congr. Ophthal., ISCERG Symp. Ghent: The clinical value of electroretinography. Karger, Basel (1968).

Tassy, A.F., G.E. Jayle & M. Gastaut-Maysou. Electrorétinographie classique et potentiel oscillatoire dans le diabète et dans la cataracte du sujet diabétique. *Arch. Ophtal.* (Paris) 31: *413–426* (1971).

Wepman, S., J. Sokol & J. Price. The electroretinogram and dark adaptation during the course of photocoagulation: changes in retinal function in diabetic retinopathy. pp. 139–147 in: Proc. 14th ISCERG Symp., Louisville, 1976. Docum. Ophthal. Proc. Series, Vol. 13. Junk, The Hague (1977).

Yonemura, D., T. Aoki & K. Tsuzuki. Electroretinogram in diabetic retinopathy. *Arch. Ophthal.* (Chic.) 68: *19–24* (1962).

Authors' address:
Department of Ophthalmology
University Hospital
135 De Pintelaan
9000 Ghent
Belgium

ELECTRODIAGNOSIS IN DOUBTFUL PHOTIC INJURY TO THE RETINA

HAROLD E. HENKES

(Rotterdam, The Netherlands)

ABSTRACT

The EOG and ERG were recorded in two patients clinically diagnosed as acute posterior multifocal placoid pigment epitheliopathy (A.P.M.P.P.E.). The EOG and ERG findings, however, were not in conformity with the electrodiagnostic data reported in the acute phase of A.P.M.P.P.E.

The hypothesis is posed that sub-threshold photic injury may have cleared the way for the manifestation of a fundus disorder resembling A.P.M.P.P.E.

Although photic injury attributable to retinal over-exposure has not yet been reported in humans, it seems unreasonable to assume that certain pathologic conditions might render the human retina more prone to photic damage. Findings in retinas of rats suggest that there is a correlation between the pathological process of certain hereditary dystrophic diseases and the impact of light on the retina (Kuwabara & Funahashi, 1976). The claimed beneficial effect of light exclusion on retinitis pigmentosa patients is still under study (Berson, 1971).

Viewed in this light, it seems justifiable to consider photic injury as a possible cause in acute bilateral blinding conditions of unknown origin, involving particularly those parts of the fundus oculi that are predominantly exposed to light, viz. the posterior pole.

Elsewhere (Henkes 1977a,b), we have reported case histories in which the question was raised whether photic injury can be held responsible for the appearance of a bilateral symmetric maculopathy, closely resembling A.P.-M.P.P.E.

In the present publication the role of electro-oculography and electro-retinography is underlined, in an attempt to establish the diagnosis through depth localization of the affected layers.

Case No. 1 concerns a 21 year old driver who had adjusted the broken-down fitting of a bumper light on his truck with both hands. During this manipulation, he looked into the light beam. The lamp lit up and went out again several times. Afterwards he felt blinded and was unable to drive. Vision in both eyes was found to be reduced to fingers counting at 5 meters.

The posterior pole of the eyes showed symmetric greyish-white areas of edema with blurred margins, closely resembling the fundus in A.P.M.P.P.E.

8° CENTRAL STIMULUS

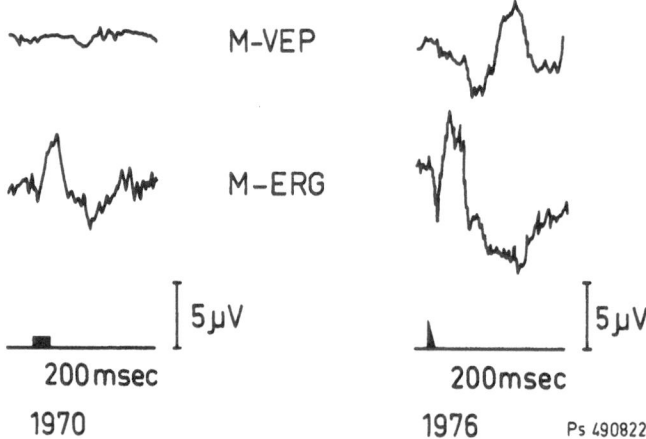

M–VEP

M–ERG

⌈5μV

200msec

1970

⌈5μV

200msec

1976   Ps 490822

Fig. 1. Patient No. 1. Local retinal stimulation of the right eye revealed reduced retinal and absent cortical activity. Six year later: normal responses are recorded after local retinal stimulation.

The electro-ophthalmological examination revealed a normal light-rise in the EOG and normal ERG responses to diffuse light stimuli. Local retinal stimulation (8° field), however, showed reduced retinal and absent cortical responses, giving rise to the assumption that the lesion was restricted to the superficial layers of the retina, predominantly to the macular area (Fig. 1).

The edema disappeared within a few days, leaving behind a moderate pigment dispersion. Vision returned to 1.0 in the right eye and 0.7 in the left eye.

Six years later, psychophysics and ophthalmoscopy showed very little changes. Apart from a normal EOG and normal ERG on diffuse stimulation, local retinal stimulation revealed a normal ERG and, correspondingly, normal VEP's (Fig. 1).

Case No. 2 concerns a 29 year old physician who noticed loss of central vision in both eyes after a day's sailing in bright sunshine off the coast of East Africa. He was admitted to the hospital 5 days after the onset of the disease.

Visual acuity was 0.1 in the right and counting fingers at 2 meters in the left eye. Ophthalmoscopy revealed a diffuse symmetric retinal edema in the posterior pole of both eyes, again resembling closely the initial phase of A.P.M.P.P.E. Electroretinography performed 10 days after the onset of the disorder, revealed a much reduced and broadened macular response and reduced VEP's in both eyes. The ERG-curve resembled the responses found in macular edema of various origin (Fig. 2). Unfortunately, the EOG was not recorded. In the course of the following weeks the retinal edema subsided

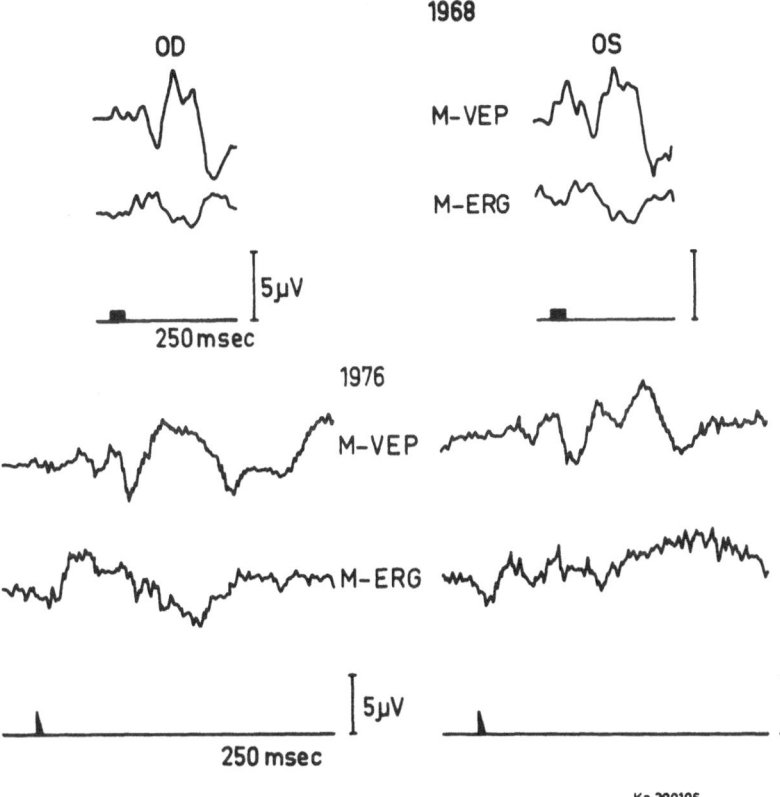

Fig. 2. Patient No. 2. Local retinal stimulation revealed a much reduced and broadened macular ERG and a reduced VEP in both eyes. Eight years later: more or less comparable recordings show identical results.

leaving behind a diffuse pigmentation located in the deep layers of the retina.

Vision improved to 0.6 in the right eye and 0.15 in the left. Eight years later, neither vision, nor fundus picture had changed essentially.

Diffuse retinal stimulation revealed normal ERG responses with a normal b/a-ratio. The macular ERG and VEP's, however, were still markedly reduced in size, although a comparison to the 1968-data is difficult due to changes made over the years in the recording technique.

DISCUSSION

The edematous lesions found in both cases resemble strongly the coagulating effects obtained with modest intensity light coagulation. The same holds for the acute phase of A.P.M.P.P.E. According to Bernard et al. (1976), fluorescence angiography is unable to distinguish between these two conditions, and thus seems of little importance in the differential diagnosis. Electrodiagnostic procedures, on the other hand, are of help.

Up to 1976, in only 6 cases of A.P.M.P.P.E., electro-oculography and electroretinography has been performed (Deutman et al., 1972; Ryan & Maumenee, 1972; Fishman et al., 1974). In only two of the 6 patients, electroretinography and electro-oculography was performed within 3 weeks from the onset of the disease; and only in one patient was the ERG recorded within this period of three weeks.

From the scarce data available in the literature, one may conclude that in the acute phase the EOG light-rise and the ERG b-wave and OP's are markedly reduced. In the scar phase, the EOG and the ERG values are normal, except in one case in literature, in which the EOG light-rise was still barely visible.

The severely affected EOG light-rise found in the acute phase of A.P.M.-P.E. points towards a strongly disturbed function of the retinal pigment epithelium, whereas the disturbed ERG is suggestive for a dysfunction of the photoreceptors and more superficial retinal layers.

In our first patient, the EOG light-rise recorded within the first few days was essentially normal, but the macular ERG was severely affected, as was the macular ERG in the second patient. These findings are suggestive for a superficially located retinal affection, and renders the diagnosis: A.P.M.-P.P.E. less probable.

Thus, a photic retinopathy?

However, in both of our patients the light impact on the retina seemed clearly insufficient to bring out a coagulating effect of the retina. In our first patient, measurement of the light output of the bumper light performed at the Institute for Sense Physiology in Soesterberg (Vos, 1976) revealed that a coagulating effect could only have been expected, if the light source had been viewed at arm's length for at least one full minute.

As to the conditions in our second case, it is generally accepted that the reflecting light from the sun on the sea surface as experienced by patient no. two, does not affect the normal retinal structures to a visible extent — even after hours and hours of exposure —, neither brings about functional defects.

However, the two diagnoses may be reconciled if one accepts the assumption that subthreshold photic injury is able to clear the way for the manifestation of fundus disorders resembling A.P.M.P.P.E. In this respect, it seems worthwhile to study patients suffering from unclassifiable edematous maculopathies in the light of this assumption.

REFERENCES

Bernard, J.A., J. Dureuil, A. Coscas, A. Gaudric & J. Haut. Acute multifocal posterior placoid pigment epitheliopathy and Argon laser photocoagulation, an angiographic comparison. pp. 371–375 in: Int. Symp. on Fluorescein Angiography, Ghent, 1976. Docum. Ophthal. Proc. Ser. Vol. 9. (1976).

Berson, E.L. Light deprivation for early retinitis pigmentosa. *Arch. Ophthal.* 86: *521–529* (1971).

Deutman, A.F., J.A. Oosterhuis, T.N. Boen Tan & A.L. Aan de Kerk. Acute posterior multifocal placoid pigment epitheliopathy. Pigment epitheliopathy or choriocapillaritis. *Br. J. Ophthal.* 56: *863–874* (1972).

Fishman, G.A., M.F. Rabb & J. Kaplan. Aucte posterior multifocal placoid pigment epitheliopathy. *Arch. Ophthal.* 92: *173–177* (1974).

Henkes, H.E. Lichtschädigung der Netzhaut und die Manifestation einer akuten hinteren multifokalen plazoiden Pigmentepitheliopathie. *Klin. Mbl. Augenheilk.* 170: *813–818* (1977a).

Henkes, H.E. Photic injury to the retina and the manifestation of acute posterior multifocal placoid pigment epitheliopathy. 171th Meeting Netherlands Ophthal. Soc., Amsterdam 1977. *Docum. Ophthal.* 44: *113–120* (1977b).

Kuwabara, T. & M. Funahashi. Light damage in the developing rat retina. *Arch. Ophthal.* 94: *1369–1374* (1976).

Ryan, S.J. & A.E. Maumenee. Acute posterior multifocal placoid pigment epitheliopathy. *Am. J. Ophthal.* 74: *1066–1074* (1972).

Vos, J.J. Personal communication (1976).

Author's address:
Department of Ophthalmology
Eye Hospital
Erasmus University
180 Schiedamse Vest
Rotterdam
The Netherlands

MACULAR RECOVERY FROM DAZZLE (PHOTOSTRESS)
IN NORMAL WOMEN ON BIRTH CONTROL PILLS (BCP)

J.R. HECKENLIVELY, J.T. PEARLMAN, L. SHAVER,
M. BRICKMAN & PAUL HENKIND (by invitation)

(Los Angeles, Ca./Bronx, N.Y., USA)

The ocular effects of chronic use of birth control pills (BCP) has been debated in the literature for the last decade. Numerous case reports of vascular occlusive phenomena, optic neuritis, pseudotumor cerebri, and migraine (Nicholson, 1969; Salmon, 1968; Collaborative Group, 1973; Walsh, 1965) are historically implicated with the use of oral contraceptives. Recently, Bos & Deutman (1975) reported four cases of maculopathy associated with long-term BCP use. Other reports, both in human and animal investigations (Drill, 1975a,b; Davidorf, 1972; Faust, 1966) suggest that there is no difference in ocular changes between control and female subjects receiving oral contraceptives.

Birth control pills create a physiologic state of 'false' pregnancy by inhibiting ovulation. The retinal physiologic effects of chronic BCP use are of interest, because female retinitis pigmentosa patients have reported a marked visual deterioration during or shortly following pregnancy (Pearlman, 1975). The photostress recovery time (PSRT) test has been used by several investigators (Severin, 1967; Carr, 1968) as a quantitative, reproducible method of testing regeneration of photosensitive pigments and, thus, the physiologic status of the macular cones and retinal pigment epithelium. Glaser et al. (1977), extending this concept to differentiate macular from optic nerve deficiencies in cases of unexplained central visual loss, found normal (PSRT) in the cases of optic nerve disease.

In view of the reports of deleterious effects of BCP in female patients, the macular PSRT was studied in normal young women taking the pill for varying lengths of time. Normal, age-matched women who had never taken the BCP served as controls. In addition, dark adaptometry and electro-oculograms were performed on smaller groups of subjects and controls.

MATERIALS AND METHODS

A Medin scotometer (Henkind, 1967) was used to measure the macular PSRT of 147 young women, ranging in age from 17 to 25 years. Of the subjects, 91 were on five brands of BCP and 56 had never taken oral contraceptives.

The subjects were instructed to look into the instrument through a viewing tube. A reduced Snellen chart within the instrument at optical infinity was internally illuminated. The women were asked to read the smallest line possible, and this line was noted. The dazzle (glare) light, measured at 10,000 foot-lamberts at the ocular, was turned on, and subjects were directed to look directly at it for 10 seconds. The dazzle light was turned off, and using a stop watch we recorded the time it took subjects to read the same line (20/20).

A group of seven subjects on the BCP and seven controls had EOGs and dark adaptometry tests performed.

RESULTS

The initial data were analyzed with individual evaluation of each eye. The average PSRT of the combined group was OD = 34.97 sec, OS = 35.08 sec. These averages are not significantly different. The PSRT values from both eyes, therefore, were averaged together for subsequent calculations. The mean age of the 56 controls was 19.16 years, compared to 20.31 years for the 91 subjects on BCP. This difference, using separate or pooled t tests is not significantly different.

The PSRT of the control group was 32.01 sec, while that of the overall BCP group was 36.87 sec. This difference was significant ($p < 0.038$). The data were further broken down by duration of BCP usage (Table 1). Subjects continuously on contraceptive medication less than 1 year averaged a PSRT of 31.94 sec; 1 to 2 years, 43 sec; and more than 2 years, 39.12 sec. There was no significant difference between the control group and those taking BCP for less than 1 year. However, there is a significant difference between the control group and the 1 to 2 year group ($p < 0.0046$) and the more than 2 year group ($p < 0.0076$).

Table 1. Relation of photostress recovery time test values to length of birth control pill usage.

Subjects	No.	PSRT*(sec)	Level of significance
Control group	56	32.01	–
BCP** 1 yr	36	31.94	0.97
BCP 1 to 2 yr	14	43.00	0.0046
BCP 2 yr	41	39.12	0.0076

* PSRT = photostress recovery time. Test values were analyzed by the student's t-test, using a two-tail test.
** BCP = birth control pill.

Five different brands of BCP were used by the subjects. None showed a significant difference in PSRT from the others. Electro-oculography and dark adaptometry performed on a control group and a BCP group of seven persons each showed no difference.

DISCUSSION

There is some variability between the PSRT in our control group with 32 seconds and in normal groups of other studies. The control group of Glaser et al. (1977) was 26 seconds; Carr and co-workers' (1968) normal group (of less than 40 years of age) averaged 29 seconds. These differences may be attributed to different dazzle intensities and to whether the subject was required, at recovery, to read the 20/20 or the next larger line. Severin et al. (1967) showed a significant difference in recovery time in normal subjects over and under 40 years of age.

The macular PSRT test would appear to be a sensitive quantitative method for detecting subclinical alterations in macular function that are not apparent on routine electrophysiologic testing. Carr et al. (1968) were able to demonstrate remarkable prolongation of recovery time in a group of patients on long term chloroquine therapy. Severin (1963) found prolongation of the PSRT in central serous retinopathy, macular degeneration, and choroidal sclerosis.

Our findings are indirectly supported by work (Marre, 1974) in which BCP users were tested with the panel D-15/Roth 28 hue test. Their control group had a 5% color vision deficiency; the users of BCP for less than 5 years, a 13% deficiency; and the 5 or more year group, a 49% color vision deficiency.

The exact changes in the receptors or retinal pigment epithelial cells causing the prolongation of the PSRT are unknown. Estrogens are known to cause a breakdown of the lysosome membrane (Dingle, 1969) with resultant metabolic complications.

From the above findings, it is reasonable to speculate that there may be a harmful effect with long term use of BCP in female retinitis pigmentosa patients of child bearing age. If the retinal pigment epithelium is already compromised by genetic errors of metabolism, additional BCP therapy could cause further decompensation and an unnecessary acceleration of the clinical disease. The long term ocular effects of BCP in normal women will have to be evaluated further, particularly now that definite retinal psychophysiological abnormalities have been found.

In summary, an evaluation of macular function as reflected by the photostress recovery time test, was made in normal young women on BCP. Significant differences in recovery time were found in those who had used birth control pills for over 1 year.

ACKNOWLEDGEMENTS

The authors wish to thank James Thomas, Ph.D., Department of Psychology, UCLA, who measured the luminance of the scotometer dazzle light; Betsy Carnahan, Health Sciences Computing Facility, UCLA (supported by NIH Special Research Resources Grant RR-3), who provided computing assistance; and Verona Pettyjohn for editorial assistance.

Information on the Medin scotometer can be obtained from: Medin Corp., 29 Main Avenue, Wallington, N.Y. 17055, USA.

REFERENCES

Bos, P.J.M. & A.F. Deutman. Acute macular neuroretinopathy. *Am. J. Ophthal.* 80: *573–584* (1975).

Carr, R.E., P. Henkind, N. Rothfield & I.M. Siegel. Ocular toxicity of antimalarial drugs: long-term follow up. *Am. J. Ophthal.* 66: *738–744* (1968).

Collaborative Group for the Study of Stroke in Young Women: Oral contraception and increased risk of cerebral ischemia or thrombosis. *N. Engl. J. Med.* 288: *871–877* (1973).

Davidorf, F.H. Ocular toxicity of systemic drugs. *Ohio State Med. J.* 68: *1022–1026* (1972).

Dingle, J.T. & H.B. Fell. The effects of steroids and drugs on lysosomes. In: Lysosomes in Biology and Pathology, Chapter 12. Elsevier, New York (1969).

Drill, V.A., K.S. Rao, R.G. McConnell & E.N. Souri. Ocular effects of oral contraceptives. I. Studies in the dog. *Fertil. Steril.* 26: *908–913* (1975a).

Drill, V.A., D.P. Martin, P.L. Golway & E.R. Hart. Ocular effects of oral contraceptives. II. Studies in the rhesus monkey. *Fertil. Steril.* 26: *914–918* (1975b).

Faust, J.M. & E.T. Tyler. Ophthalmologic findings in patients using oral contraception. *Fertil. Steril.* 17: *1–6* (1966).

Glaser, J.S., P.J. Savino, K.D. Sumers, S.A. McDonald & R.W. Knighton. The photostress recovery test in the clinical assessment of visual function. *Am. J. Ophthal.* 83: *255–260* (1977).

Henkind, P. & I.M. Siegel. The scotometer. A device for measuring macular recovery time. *Am. J. Ophthal.* 64: *314–315* (1967).

Marre, M., O. Neubauer & U. Nemetz. Colour vision and the 'pill'. *Mod. Probl. Ophthal.* 13: *345–348* (1974).

Nicholson, D.H. & F.B. Walsh. Oral contraceptives and neuro-ophthalmologic disorders. *J. Reprod. Med.* 3: *73–79* (1969).

Pearlman, J.T. & J. Saxton. Retinitis pigmentosa and birth control pills. *JAMA* 231: *810* (1975).

Salmon, M.L., J.Z. Winkilman & A.J. Gay. Neuro-ophthalmic sequelae in users of oral contraceptives. *JAMA* 206: *85–91* (1968).

Severin, S.L., J.Y. Harper & J.F. Culver. Photostress test for the evaluation of macular function. *Arch. Ophthal.* 70: *593–597* (1963).

Severin, S.L., R.L. Tour & R.H. Kershaw. Macular function and the photostress test 1. *Arch. Ophthal.* 77: *2–7* (1967).

Walsh, F.B., D.B. Clark, R.S. Thompson & D.H. Nicholson. Oral contraceptives and neuro-ophthalmologic interest. *Arch. Ophthal.* 74: *628–640* (1965).

Authors' addresses:
Department of Ophthalmology
Jules Stein Eye Institute
UCLA School of Medicine
800 Westwood Plaza
Los Angeles, California 90024
USA

Paul Henkind
Department of Ophthalmology
Montefiore Hospital and Medical Center
Bronx, N.Y. 10 467
USA

Reprint requests to Dr J.T. Pearlman at the California address.

STANDARDIZED ELECTRO-OPHTHALMOGRAPHY
BY USING SELF-CALIBRATING EQUIPMENT

W.J.M. BRAAKHUIS & J.M. THIJSSEN
(Nijmegen, The Netherlands)

Standardization in clinical electro-ophthalmography may greatly enhance the interpretability of the data and it will produce the conditions for a meaningful exchange of information between clinics. The aspects of the examination to be standardized are: the examination procedure, the equipment and the registration of the results. Moreover, it is necessary to perform adequate calibration procedures from both the stimulation and the measuring equipment.

The Netherlands' Group on Physical Methods in Ophthalmology recently formulated a proposal (cf. Thijssen et al., 1976) for a basic set-up for Electroretinography (ERG) and Electro-oculography (EOG). The measuring procedure of the ERG is sketched in Fig. 1; the aim is to achieve optimal separation of rod and cone contributions to the ERG. The stimulator is based on a previously described design (cf. Thijssen et al., 1974) which consisted of an adaptometer sphere mounted on a normal examination couch by means of a rotary arm. The details of the light conditions are listed below:

	Stimulation	*Adaptation*
ERG: Energy/Intensity:	max.: 5 luxsec min.: 2.5 x 10^{-4} luxsec	10 lux dark
Light distribution:	Ganzfeld	Ganzfeld
Calibration:	single flash, automatic	automatic
Inaccuracy:	$\leqslant 5\%$	$\leqslant 5\%$

EOG: Adaptation: max.: 2500 lux
min.: dark

Fixation lamps: 40° mutual distance

Rhythmic command: auditive

Amplifiers: Time constant: $\geqslant 1$ sec; High frequency cut-off: $\geqslant 70$ Hz.

A prototype of the equipment, meeting these requirements, has been built at our laboratory. The ERG stimulation is produced by a Xenon flashing tube, the light output of which is measured per flash and automatically calibrated by an electronic system. The light energy can be manually adjusted by the electronic control system from 5% to 100% and by additional neutral

electro retinography procedure

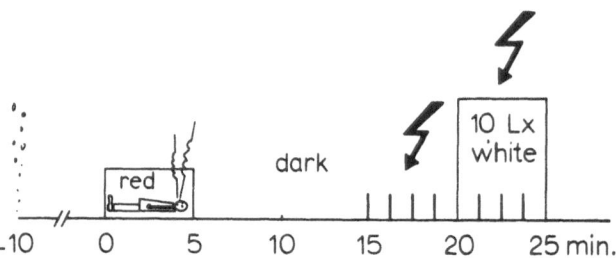

Fig. 1. The ERG procedure: mydriatics at − 10 min. preparation of the patient in red room light from 0−5 min, dark adaptation from 5−15 min, scotopic examination (5 different stimulation intensities) from 15−20 min. photopic examination at 10 lux light adaptation (again 5 different flash levels).

density filters (from photopic to scotopic levels). The adaptation light intensity is also monitored by a photodiode and again automatically kept at a selectable level.

The notation of the stimulation conditions is proposed as follows:

2 N 20.

From left to right: 2 indicates 2 log units attenuation; N means neutral density filter; 20 stands for 20% (with respect to the maximum of 5 luxsec).

The EOG examination is performed with the same equipment, the design of which was adapted to meet the requirements of the procedure proposed by Arden and Kelsey.

REFERENCES

Thijssen, J.M., A. Pinckers & A.J. Otto. A multipurpose optical system for Ophthalmic electrodiagnosis. *Ophthalmologica* (Basel) 168: *308−314* (1974).

Thijssen, J.M., W. Braakhuis, A. Pinckers & G. van Lith. Standardized electro-ophthalmography. Pp. 185−186 in: Proc. 170th Meeting of the Netherlands Ophthal. Soc. Junk, The Hague (1976).

Authors' address:
Dept. of Ophthalmology
University of Nijmegen
15, Philips van Leydenlaan
Nijmegen
The Netherlands

TESTING IN ELECTROPHYSIOLOGY

I. WILMANNS & R. STODTMEISTER
(Bonn, Fed. Rep. of Germany)

Routine testing of measuring and recording systems in electrophysiology is usually limited to the electronic instrumentation, e.g. preamplifiers, filters, and the like. The components of the complete system are easily accessible in a double sense: the input impedance of such components of an instrumentation system is already indicated by the manufacturer, and under normal conditions it is invariable. If the input impedance and the total amplification, also given by the manufacturer, are known for the system, then the test signal level to be fed into the input for testing the performance of the system is also known. This reasoning is based on the tacit assumption that the system is sufficiently specified, if the amplitude response of the electronic part of the system is known.

In reality, things are not quite that simple: the signal source and all other components serving the transfer of the signals from the source to the electronic system – in the classical sense – also influence the information processing of the biological signals. In electrophysiological measuring and recording systems it is important that the electrodes are properly applied to the tissue from which signals are to be picked up, and that the transition resistance between the electrode and the tissue is minimized. The classical test method (Cooper et al., 1974; Neher, 1974; Regan, 1972) gives no clear indication of the status of the input circuit. The test signal is usually fed into the input of the amplifying system while the input circuit is disconnected. In other words, the test signal, instead of the biological signal, is fed into the amplifier. We have, thus, only an indication that the electronic system – in the classical sense – is working properly as far as amplitude behaviour is concerned.

To overcome this limitation of testing, we used a different approach: the input impedance of a typical amplifier for electrophysiological measurements is of the order of 100 MOhms. Typical electrode impedances, as we found them for our system, are of the order of 10 kOhms. We have, therefore, inserted a small resistor of 2 Ohms in series with one of the connecting cables between one of the electrodes and the input of the amplifier. This method does not change the transfer properties of the input circuit in a measurable way. In addition, we connected this resistance with a pulse generator which feeds square wave current pulses through this resistance. Due to the voltage drop across this resistance it behaves like a voltage source.

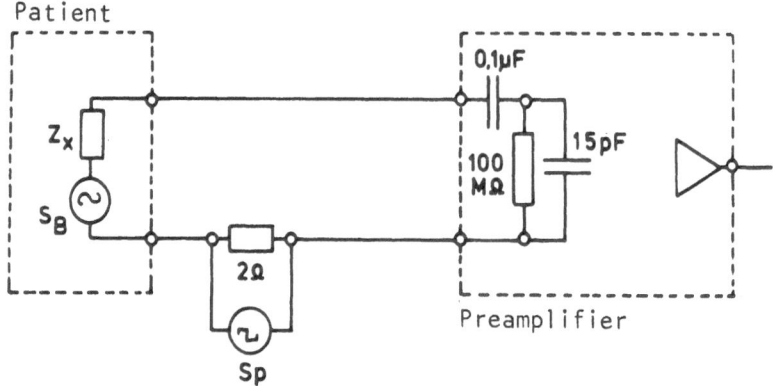

Fig. 1. Circuit diagram.

The current pulses are symmetrical about zero to avoid any action caused by unbalanced potentials. If a signal passes through, this is a clear indication that the electrodes are applied anc cables conducting. It also indicates whether the coupling of the electrodes to the tissue is satisfactory. The test signal has a composite waveform which contains high frequency components. Small spikes at the leading edges of the test pulses, after their passage through the system, indicate that the coupling of the electrodes to the tissue is no longer purely resistive but also capacitive, which favours the transfer of the high frequency components. We found that we can measure the electrode resistance by connecting a resistance of the same order of magnitude in parallel to the input of the amplifier. This causes a drop in the amplitude of the test signal as it appears at the output of the electronic system. If the amplitude is exactly halved, the two resistances of the electrodes and the parallel resistance are of the same magnitude. A simple curve avoids all calculations for the determination of the electrode resistance, if the signal does not drop to exactly one half of the original value. It is also possible to assess the transfer function of the complete system, including the electrodes, by checking the test signal form and detecting possible changes which may occur while the signal passes through the system.

We have shown that by a new way of feeding the test voltage in series with components of the input circuit of the complete operational measuring system, connected with the biological signal source, we can assess the important parameters of the operational system by examining the shape and the amplitude of the test signal at the output of the system. Adding a simple resistance in series permits one to determine the electrode resistance in situ for the operational system. Thus, it has become possible to compare measurements taken at different times by different methods, and to check all components whenever necessary or desirable, even during an operation, as the small test signal feed resistor can be left permanently in the circuit.

REFERENCES

Cooper, R., J.W. Osselton & J.C. Shaw. Elektroencephalographie. Fischer, Stuttgart (1974).
Neher, F. Elektronische Meßtechnik in der Physiologie. Springer, Berlin (1974).
Regan, D. Evoked Potentials. Chapman and Hall, London (1972).

Authors' addresses:
I. Wilmanns
Klinisches Institut für experimentelle
Ophthalmologie der Universität Bonn
5300 Bonn-Venusberg
Fed. Rep. of Germany

R. Stodtmeister
Universitats–Augenklinik
5300 Bonn-Venusberg
Fed. Rep. of Germany

Docum. Ophthal. Proc. Series, Vol. 15

A NEW INSTRUMENTATION FOR ERG AND VER RECORDING
UNDER CLINICAL CONDITIONS

RENE TRAU, CHÁRLES LIBERT, GEORGETTE LAHAYE
& PAUL SALU

(Brussels, Belgium)

INTRODUCTION

In a preceding publication (Neetens et al., 1975) we presented a first version of this new type of averager, as well as the first results obtained in hospital centres for the measuring of averaged ERGs and of evoked visual potentials.

In the face of the encouraging results obtained we perfected this averager, in order to evolve an apparatus that is complete in itself, homogeneous and specifically designed for the collection and recording of averaged ERGs and, simultaneously, of evoked visual potentials.

We are describing here, in succession, the various components of this integrated unit: preamplifier and amplifier, averager and photostimulator. The installations were designed and built in Belgium, by SAIT Electronics as regards the electronic equipment* and by the firm Ch. Libert** as regards the stimulation equipment, and this in close cooperation with our electrophysiology department (Figs. 1–4).

Pre-amplifier (Fig. 3)

The preamplifier is separated from the main amplifier so that it can be placed close to the patient when fixed on a stand, thus making it possible to use connecting cables of as short a length as possible; this simplifies handling procedures and avoids the appearance of secondary phenomena due to possible inducted currents.

Amplifier (Fig. 1)

The amplifier is compact in size and can thus be housed in a mobile trolley (for bedside-examination) with the averager, display, CRT and the synchrotimer.

It is suitable for operation, according to choice, on either AC or DC. The interest of measurements made on DC is stressed by various recent publications (Taümer, 1976; Knave et al., 1973), because such measurements permit the study of slow phenomena, for instance of c- and d-waves which have

---

* Recording averager, preamplifier and synchro-timer.
** Marketed by SAIT Electronics.

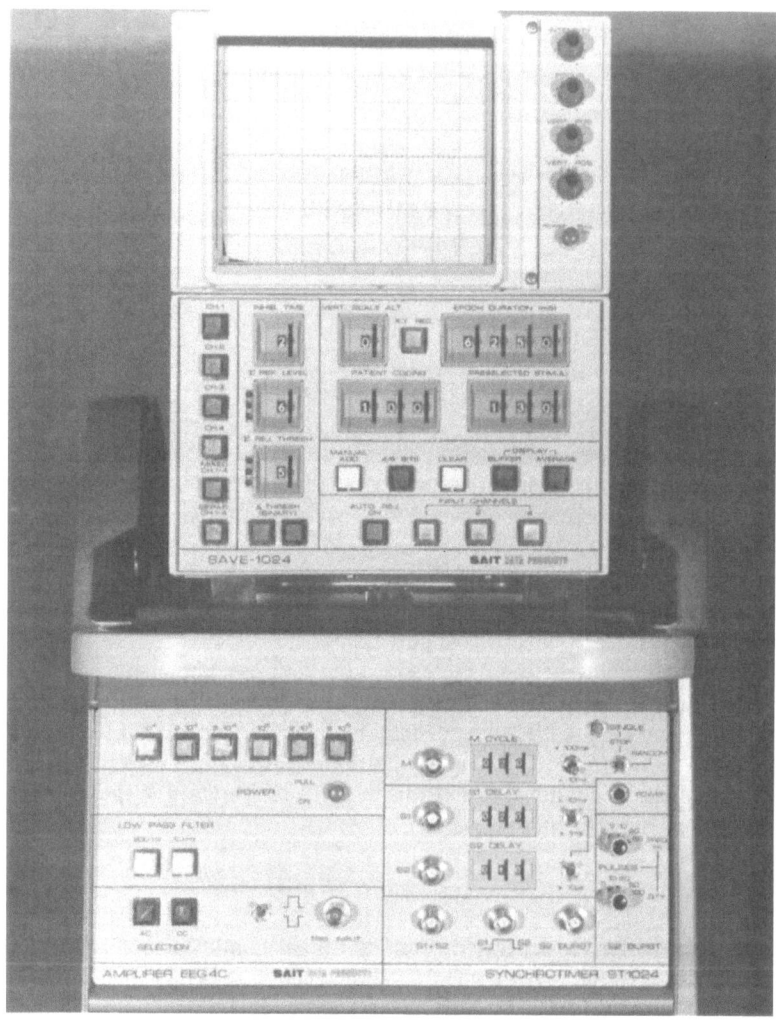

Fig. 1. View of the control panel of averager, amplifier and synchro-timer and CRT screen.

been neglected in earlier research on the ERG and to which the averaging process and the use of long-lasting stimuli shall certainly give fresh impetus in the clinical field; they are also more impervious to the after effects of stimulation.

Averager and display unit (Fig. 1)

Principle of the averager

The averager which we are here describing is capable of accepting 4 analogical signals emanating from four independent amplification channels. The

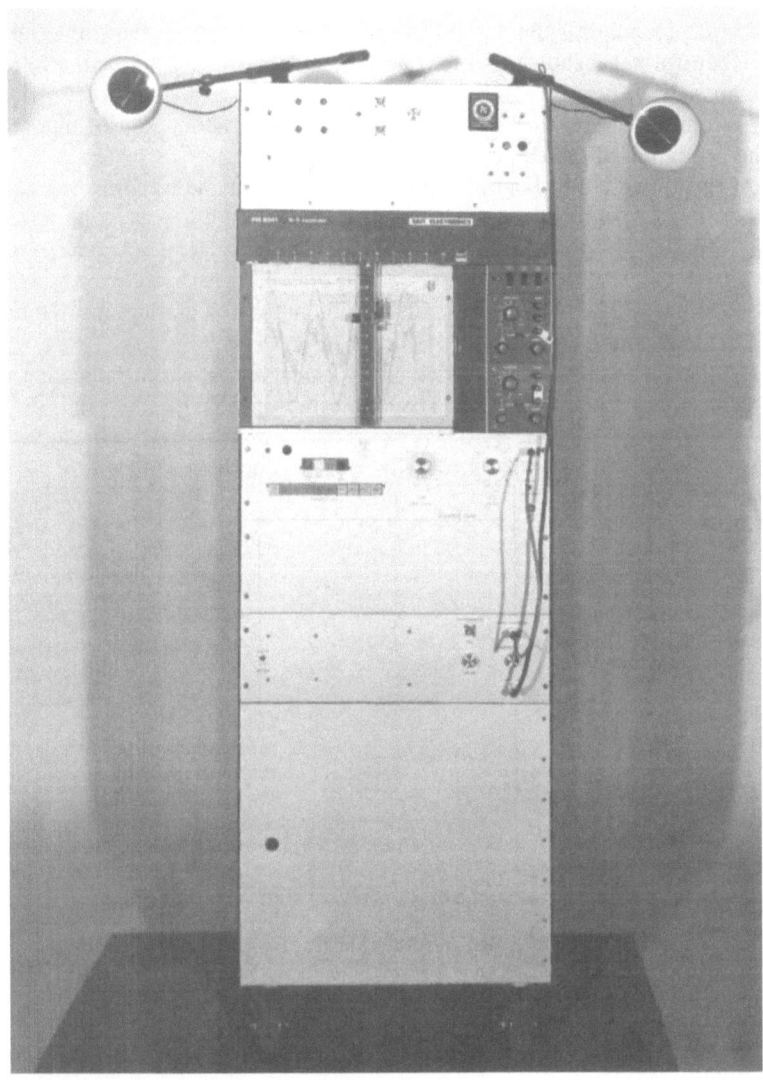

Fig. 2. Stimulator (rear view). Controls and XY plotter.

content of the eight most significant binary positions is continually con-
verted into analogic values for display on the cathodic screen. The examiner
can constantly follow the contents of the buffer storage or of the accumu-
lator on the screen, and thus follow each particular answer of the averaged
curve obtained at any given time during the test; he can follow simultaneously either 1, 2 or the tracings.

All the numeral data of the test are also displayed on the screen. The latter
may be photographed by means of a Polaroid camera adapted for this purpose; the data may also be transcribed on an XY plotter.

In order to simplify the description of the unit, we shall arbitrarily look at the control panel shown on Fig. 1 and then successively describe the various components, their use and the part of the averager to which they belong. This will enable us to describe at the same time the method of operation and utilisation of the equipment.

At the upper half of the unit is the cathodic screen and its controls.

Cathodic screen

Dimensions: 125 x 100 mm, divided by incorporated gratings into 10 horizontal parts and 8 vertical parts.

On the cathodic screen a series of 14 characters appears, indicating the parameters of the examination. They indicate respectively:

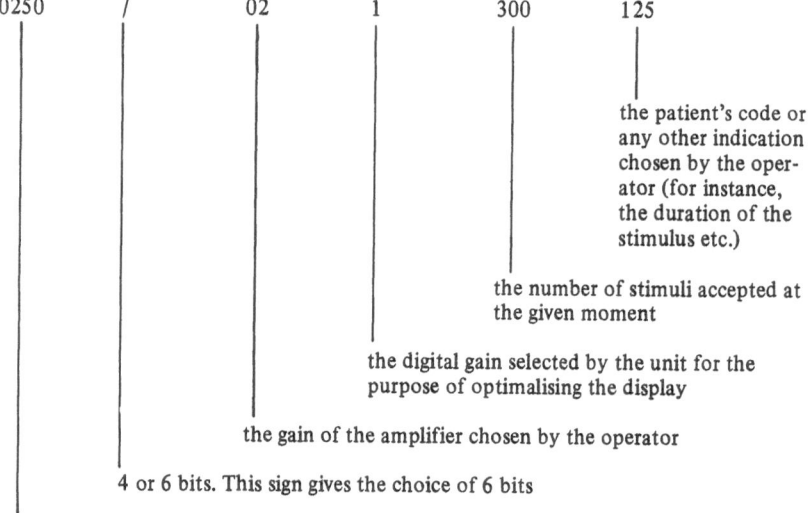

0250   /   02   1   300   125

the patient's code or any other indication chosen by the operator (for instance, the duration of the stimulus etc.)

the number of stimuli accepted at the given moment

the digital gain selected by the unit for the purpose of optimalising the display

the gain of the amplifier chosen by the operator

4 or 6 bits. This sign gives the choice of 6 bits

the epoch duration (to be determined by the operator).

The epoch duration makes it possible to determine the value, in terms of ms, of a division of the X axis of the screen.

The digital gain and the amplifier gain permit the determination of the value, in terms of μV, of the Y axis of the screen, and by dividing by the numer of stimuli accepted, to determine quantitatively the main value of an isolated response, with the help of the tables which are furnished with the equipment.

At the right hand side of the screen are the various controls (Fig. 1).

Under the screen, at the extreme left: CH_1 ... SEP. CH. 1–4. These luminous push-buttons permit the selection of the various ways in which the curves are liable to be presented: isolated, separately or superimposed.

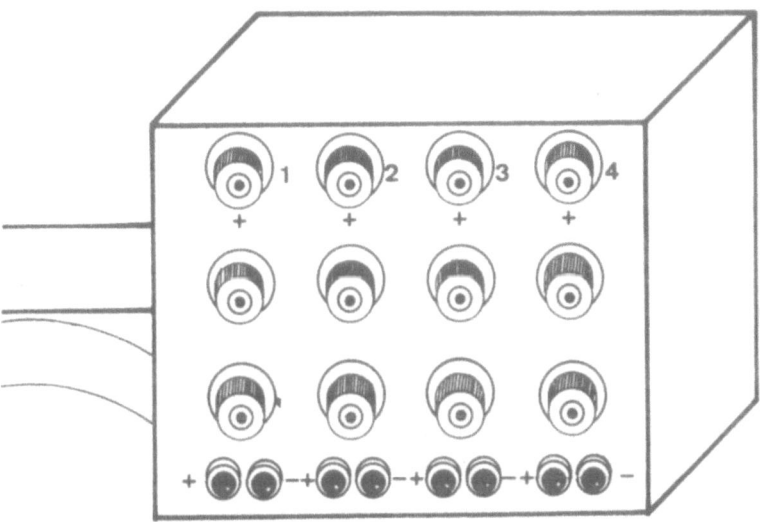

Fig. 3. Pre-amplifier.

Adjustable parameters

On the lower part of the apparatus, under the CRT (Fig. 1) are grouped all the controls which permit the selection of the parameters used for the examination.

At the left hand side is located the control for the adjustment of the rejection parameters, which we are examining more thoroughly further on. From the right to left, and from the top downwards, we find:

Vert. scale alt.

The indication of the gain selected either by hand or automatically is, at any rate, achieved on the screen.

XY rec.

Engages the listing of the tracing on the XY plotter (Fig. 2).

Epoch duration

This thumb-wheel control determines the duration of the scan period; it can go up to 999 ms. in steps of 1 ms.

Patient coding

Three figures chosen by the examiner for the purpose of identifying the patient, or any other information.

Preselected stimuli

Number of non-rejected responses desired by the examiner, at the end of which the examination comes automatically to an end.

Manual add.

Permits the addition, by hand, of tracing initially rejected by the automatic tests; the use of this control is optional.

4/6 bits

Choice of the word content at the input of the averager.

Clear

This button clears the content of the memories.

$Display\begin{cases}buffer\\average\end{cases}$

This control permits the comparison during the examination of each isolated response with the average obtained at any given moment. The examination may be terminated when neither the isolated response nor the averaged response do no longer change, and that their respective appearances are consistent.

Auto rejection

This button engages the operation of the automatic rejection process.

Input channels 1-2-4

Choice of the number of channels; with one channel the curve comprises 1024 points; in 2 channels 512 points, and in 4 channels 256 points. It behoves the examiner to decide whether he desires a curve that is more precise, or desires to cut down the duration of the test by examining simultaneously the 2 ERG, or the 2 ERG and the 2 PEV.

It should, however, be noted that in ordinary cases the standard of 256 points is sufficient (Fig. 4).

Automatic rejection (principle)

It is known that in summation the signal-to-noise ratio increases as the square root of the number n of stimuli $\left(\text{signal/noise ratio} = \dfrac{\frac{signal}{noise}}{\sqrt{n}}\right)$

If, therefore, the signal is ± equal to the noise, as happens to be the case both as regards the ERG and the VER (in the worst cases: children, nervous patients, etc....) after 100 stimuli the signal (ERG or VER) will be 10 times as great as the noise, and therefore sufficiently perceptible in most cases.

On the other hand, and inversely, if in the course of the test there occurs some interference or artifact the amplitude of which is 10 times that of the

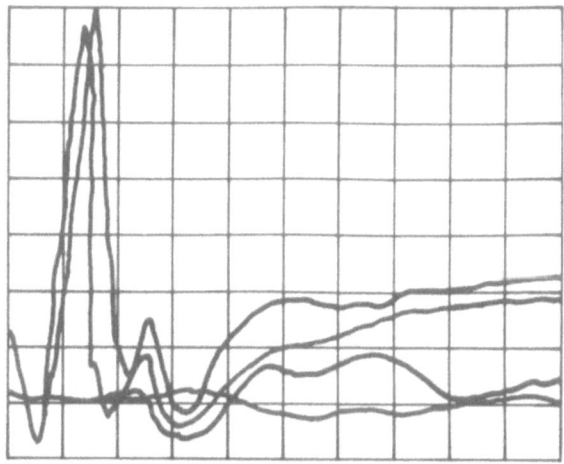

Fig. 4a. Simultaneous ERG-VER registration (photopic). Case: left hemianopsia. – absence VER right; synchronism between VER and late oscillatory potentials of ERG.

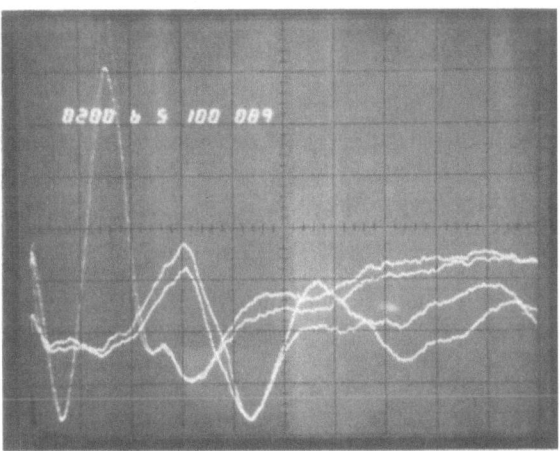

Fig. 4b. Polaroid photograph of screen. Simultaneous registration ERG-VER (photopic). Normal aspect.

response sought after, 100 additional stimuli will be required to reduce the interference to the level of the response, and a further 100 additional stimuli to reduce it to one-tenth of the amplitude of the response sought after; even at this level the interference is still liable to give rise to confusion, for instance if it falls at the place of the oscillatory potentials. It is needless to point out that these additional 200 stimuli will make the examination more unpleasant for the patient, and will increase by the same token the risk of various motions and consequently of fresh interferences, thus initiating a kind of vicious circle. On the contrary, the fact of suppressing that one parasited response only adds one more stimulus, and improves the appearance and reliability of the final curve.

There are, of course, manual means of eliminating the stray responses, but they either lengthen the duration of the test for the patient if the choice is made at the time of the test, or else demand additional equipment and additional time after the recording (magnetic tape recording of the res-ponses, and selection and rejection 'a posteriori').

Our mechanisms incorporate automatic rejection tests, based on the works of Colin, which obviate the drawbacks mentioned above as follows:

a) responses of unduly great magnitude are rejected;

b) responses affected with too many interferences are rejected;

c) responses presenting a too sudden shifting of the tracing are rejected.

PRACTICAL OPERATION

Rejection of responses of unduly great magnitude (Fig. 5)

This test does not call for the intervention of the observer. If the tracing ex-ceeds, during a fraction of the measuring time (14 points), the visualisation area of the screen, it is rejected.

Test of the sum of the absolute differences

Controls: Ref. level, rej. thresh. (Fig. 1.)

In this test one compares the sum of the absolute differences between the

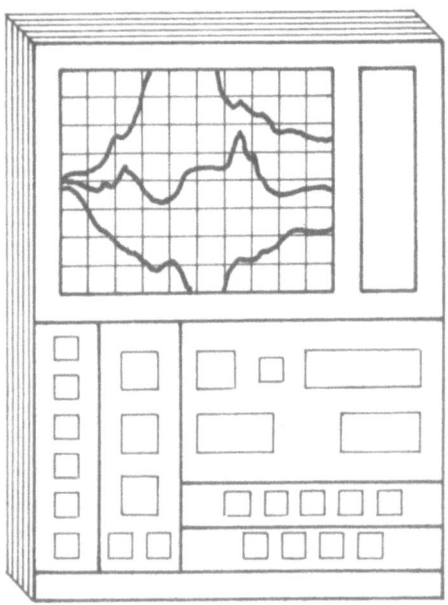

Fig. 5. Rejection. Criterion 1: amplitude too high.

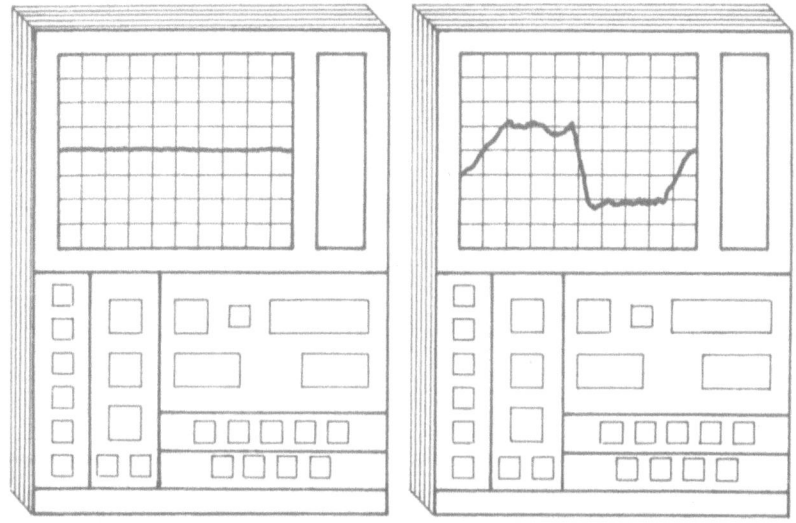

Fig 6. Rejection. Criterion 2: a. Σ too small (flat); b. Σ too big (artifact).

values indicated by the various successive points of the curve (digital values) and this same sum measured on a satisfying calibration curve chosen by the observer.

If this sum is either too small ('flat' curve) (Fig. 6) or too large (muscular phenomena, external phenomena (50 cycles)) the response is rejected.

Test of the difference between two successive points of the tracing

Control: Thresh. (binary). (Fig. 1)

This test calculates the difference between two successive points: if this difference is too pronounced: sudden shifting of the tracing, 'spikes' (Fig. 7), the response is eliminated. This anomaly, is frequent in clinical examinations.

Choice of the calibration curve

The sum of the absolute differences between the points of a curve is equal in value to a binary number of 12 figures (maximum) stored in the memory, for example:

000 1 0 0 1 1 1 0 0 1

a mobile window of three figures explores this binary number, made up of 3 lights (LED)

alight – 1
extinct – 0

a control by thumb-wheel displaces the 3-figure window from position 1 to 9, thus exploring 12 figures (Fig. 1).

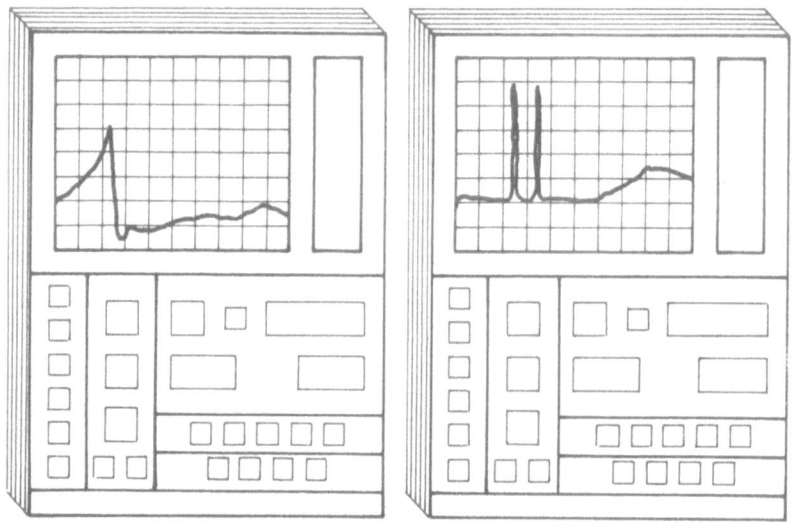

Fig. 7. Rejection. Criterion 3: a. Δ too big; b. 'spikes'.

The curve chosen for calibration is scanned in the manner described above: once that the value fixed as a rejection criterion has been obtained, for instance, that the sum obtained does not exceed the double of the reference sum (Σ ref. level) chosen. Therefore, one fixes the value indicated as the rejection threshold at the double of this figure, a fact which in a binary system is tantamount to a displacement of a decimal towards the left, and thus to a displacement of one notch of the exploration 3-figure window put in motion by the corresponding thumb-wheel.

Choice of the difference between two successive points

Control: A. thresh. (binary) (Fig. 1).

Is controlled by two luminous push-buttons which represent a binary number: alight = 1; extinct = 0. We have thus the choice between

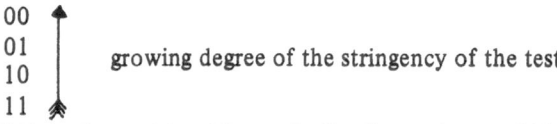

00
01
10   growing degree of the stringency of the test
11

(N.B. in the position 00 practically all samples would be rejected).

Inhibition of the rejection tests (Fig. 1)

A control permits the inhibition of these tests during a variable initial period in order to avoid, should the occasion arise, the rejection brought about by the after effects of stimulation.

332

TECHNICAL DESCRIPTION AND OPERATING PROCEDURE

Light source

The light is supplied by a halogen lamp with reflector which concentrates the light, through an infra-red filter, on an area of 8 mm in diameter. At this point is fixed the end of a flexible lead made of optical fibres, the other end of the lead being provided with a lens that diffuses the light at an angle of 30°, and fixed at the rear of a shutter.

Shutter

Made up of two aluminium masks 0.1 mm thick, each activated by an electromagnetic device with mobile frame; the masks are placed in such a way as to close the shutter when the apparatus is not plugged in. When the machine is switched on, the first mask closes the shutter, the second one being opened immediately behind the shutter. Two slides are provided for the fixing of grey or colour filters. It is thus possible to equalise the energies of each colour and to vary with precision the light intensity.

Electronic control

Two fully separated circuits produce rectangular impulses adjustable to durations of 10 - 30 - 100 - 300 - 1000 milliseconds. Each circuit controls a power amplifier which activates the two shutter masks. The synchro-timer, connected by means of optical couplers will send out the release impulses. Several working procedures can be adopted:

A single impulse is used towards the amplifier of the first mask. Thus light flashed of the chosen duration will be obtained (10 - 30 - 100 - 300 - 1000 ms), the second mask remaining always open.

Two separate impulses are used. The first opens the shutter; the second, after a delay selected by the synchro-timer, will close the second mask. It is, therefore, possible to obtain flashes, the duration of which may be chosen between 0 to 1 second.

The position of the selector will be chosen in relation with the frequency, the positions 10 and 30 m. sec. permitting frequencies op up to 40 Hertz maximum for the mechanical device of the shutter. A manual control opens the shutter, a lux-meter is placed at the level of the patient's eyes and the light intensity is determined with precision.

A device keeps the head at an unvarying distance from the light source. The intensity at the output of the optic fibre is of 15.10^6 lux.

Synchro-timer (Fig. 1)

We have previously used a system in which the same impulse engages the light stimulus and initiated the measuring of the response. This system does not permit a clear visualisation of the beginning of the response. The synchro-timer which we have perfected gives the possibility of spreading out clearly, timewise, the various processes.

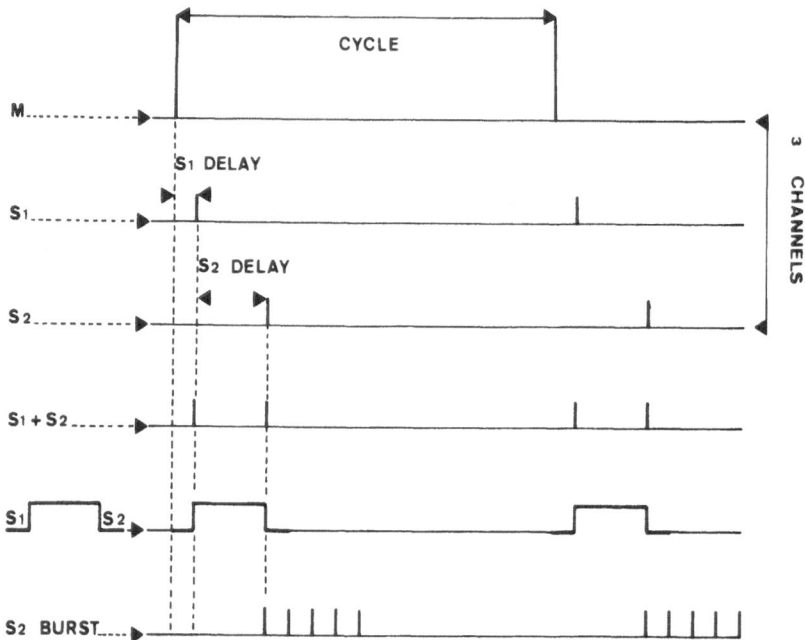

Fig. 8. Functions of synchro-timer.

Description and operating procedure

We shall describe the control panel of the synchro-timer, and the functions which correspond to the various controls, a course which will enable us to describe at the same time the operating procedure of the given equipment.

Channel M

This refers to the master impulse which determines the cycle (S_1 and S_2 are the slave impulses). We are here specifically concerned with the cycle of the synchro-timer, which is therefore quite distinct from the scanning duration of SAVE (averager) which can be independently adjusted by the control marked EPOCH DURATION. This cycle is adjustable from 10 ms to 10 s by steps of 10 ms, or from 100 ms to 100 s by steps of 100 ms.

There is also the possibility of controlling one cycle only (control marked SINGLE) or several cycles of aleatory frequency (control marked RANDOM), the recurrence period varying between 0.55 and 5.5 s.

Channel S_1

Lag with respect to M (S_1 Delay) adjustable from 1 ms to 999 ms by steps of 1 ms, or from 10 ms to 9.99 sec by steps of 10 ms. This lag makes it possible to start the scanning before the start of the stimulus and thus to have:
1. a basic line clearly perceptible as isoelectric reference;
2. an initial phase of the response which is perfectly visible;
3. the precise measurement of the various latency and culmination times, the importance of which has again been recently stressed (Babel et al., 1977;

334

Michiels et al., 1975) for the interpretation of the clinical signification of the ERG.

Channel S_2

Lag with respect to S_1 (S_2 Delay) adjustable in the same way as for S_1. Permits the issue of an impulse for the closing of the shutter of the photostimulator (S_1 having issued the opening impulse).

The duration of the stimulus may be adjusted from 1 ms to 9.99 s, a range which is sufficient for clinical needs and which permits the study not only on the initial deflections of the ERG (a, b, OP waves) but also of the late phases (c and d) and, in any case, of dividing clearly the on and off effects and also to observe the variations of the ERG (and of the VER) as dependent on the duration of the stimulus (a factor studied as early as 1903 by Broca-Sulzen, and more recently by numerous others).

CONCLUSION

The new equipment, compact and mobile, permits the measuring of the ERG and of the PEV, simultaneously, and in customary clinical conditions.

Automatic rejection tests permit the shortening of the examination and increase the reliability of the results. A new type of photo-stimulator makes it possible to use stimuli of variable duration. A synchro-timer makes it possible to regulate with precision and independently the stimulation cycle, the duration of the scan, the lag of the stimulus with respect of the start of the measuring process, the duration of the stimulus.

The first clinical results obtained in one hundred cases are satisfying. A larger series, as well as the study of pathological cases, will be the subject of a following paper.

Further developments foreseen (Fig. 2), are the inclusion of generators of accoustic and somesthesic stimuli in the stimulation unit, to allow simultaneous measures of ERG, and visual, accoustic and somesthesic evoked responses.

REFERENCES

Aiba, T.S. & S.S. Stevens. Relation of brightness to duration and luminance under light and dark adaptation. *Vision Res.* 4: *391–401* (1964).

Alpern, M. & J.J. Paris. Luminance-duration relationship in the electronic response of the human retina. *J. Optic. Soc. Am.* 46: *846–850* (1956).

Babel, J., N. Stangos, S. Korol & M. Spiritus. Ocular electrophysiology. A clinical and experimental study of electroretinogram, electro-oculogram, visual evoked response. Thieme, Stuttgart (1977).

Biersdorf, W.R. Luminance-duration relationships in the light-adapted electro-retinogram. *J. Optic. Soc. Am.* 48: *412–417* (1958).

Biersdorf, W.R. & A.M. Granda. Effects of stimulus duration upon spectral sensitivity of the human electroretinogram. *J. Optic Soc. Am.* 52: *1402–1406* (1962).

Bornschein, H. The response of the human eye to red stimuli with different temporal gradients of luminance. *Acta Ophthal.* Suppl. 70: *142–155* (1962).

Burian, H.M. The effect of variations of the stimulus rise time on the human electroretinogram. A contribution to its temporal aspects. *Invest. Ophthal.* 9: *410–417* (1970).

Butler, T.W. Luminance-duration relationships in the photopic ERG and the apparent brightness of flashes. *Vision Res.* 15: *693–698* (1975).

Colin. Personal communication.

François, J., A. De Rouck, E. Cambie & A. Zanen. L'électrodiagnostic des affectations rétiniennes (Etude des potentiels de repos et d'action rétiniens). *Bull. Soc. belge d'Ophtal.* 166 (1) (1974).

Howarth, C.I. On-off interaction in the human electroretinogram. *J. Optic. Soc. Am.* 51: *345–352* (1961).

Johnson, E.P. & N.R. Bartlette. Effect of stimulus duration on electrical responses of the human retina. *J. Optic. Soc. Am.* 46: *167–170* (1956).

Knave, B., S. Nilsson & T. Lunt. The human electroretinogram: DC recordings at low and conventional stimulus intensities. Description of a new method for clinical use. *Acta Ophthal.* 51: *716–726* (1973).

Long, G.E. The effect of duration of onset and cessation of light flash on the intensity-time relation in the peripheral retina. *J. Optic Soc. Am.* 41: *743–747* (1951).

Neetens, A., R. Trau & H. Schneider. Averaging in ERG and VER first clinical results. *Bull. Soc. belge d'Ophtal.* 170: *659–673* (1975).

Ronchi, L. On the electrical response of the human eye to red stimuli of different time distribution of luminance. *J. Optic. Soc. Am.* 48: *437–438* (1958).

Stanescu, B. & J. Michiels. Le 'temps implicite'; aspects théoriques et pratiques. *Arch. Ophthal.* 35: *527–532* (1975).

Stevens, J.C. & J.W. Hall. Brightness and loudness as functions of stimulus duration. *Percept. Psychophys.* 1: *319–327* (1966).

Tassi. Thèse, Marseille.

Taumer, R., N. Rohde, W. Wichmann & J. Rover. Experiments concerning the human c-wave. *A. v. Graefes Arch. klin. exp. Ophthal.* 198: *139–153* (1976).

Wachtmeister, L. Stimulus duration and the oscillatory potentials of the human electroretinogram. *Acta Ophthal.* 52: *729–739* (1974).

Authors' address:
Department of Electrophysiology
Ophthalmological Clinic
Vrije Universiteit Brussel
Brussels
Belgium

Docum. Ophthal. Proc. Series, Vol. 15

A NEW ELECTRODE FOR 'GANZFELD' ERG

LUC MISSOTTEN & BIANCA STANESCU

(Louvain/Brussels, Belgium)

This ERG contact lens has two silver electrodes positioned in the same way as on the Echte-Papst (echte & Papst, 1962) lens; one surrounding the cornea and the other at the external face, touching the palpebra (Fig. 1). Both electrodes are cut from the same piece of metal, ensuring an indentical voltaic potential difference at each contact. The corneal area, however, is free.

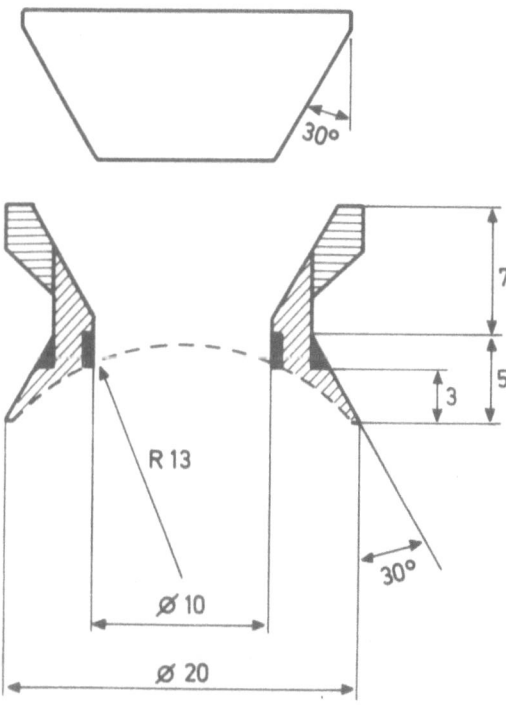

Fig. 1. The contact lens for ERG with local and Ganzfeld stimulation. The cross section shows the two electrodes (black) mounted on a plexiglass contactlens. On top the removable diffusor.

In order to elicit a 'Ganzfeld' stimulation, a translucent lid of acrylic plastic, is placed in the central hole. The lid is a truncated cone, with two translucent sides separated by an optically clear space (Fig. 1). This diffusor insures a perfect homogeneous scattering of the light over the whole retina, as may be appreciated subjectively by wearing the contact lens: all sense of direction of the illuminating light disappears. The idea is based on the concept introduced by Cone (1963) who used half a ping-pong ball as diffusing surface, when recording ERG in small mammals, and used by Weinstein and al. (1970) for 'Ganzfeld' ERG in Man.

Removal of the diffusor permits focal light stimulation of the retina.

The electrode presents several advantages:

1. The fixed electrodes eliminate the variations of the ERG due to the positions of the electrodes. The amplitude is some 10% lower than obtained with conventional lenses and electrodes on the skin, but the background noise is markely reduced.

2. The diffusor is the least cumbersome way to record ERG in perfect 'Ganzfeld' conditions, and its removal allows immediate transformation for focal illumination.

REFERENCES

Cone, R.A. Quantum relations of the rat electroretinogram. *J. Gen. Physiol.* 46: *1267* (1962).

Echte, K. & W. Papst. Vorteile der Linsen-Haftschale für die Registrierung des Elektroretinogramms. *Acta Ophthal.* (Kbh) Suppl. 70: *176* (1962).

Weinstein, G.W., R.S. Weinberg & R.R. Hobson. Constant amplitude electroretinography for the determination of retinal sensitivity in normal and abnormal subjects. *Am. J. Ophthal.* 69: *836* (1970).

Authors' addresses:
Prof. L. Missotten
University Eye Clinic
K.U. University
3000 Louvain
Belgium

B. Stanescu
University Eye Clinic
U.C.L.
10, Avenue Hippocrate
1200 Brussels
Belgium

GOLD-COATED MYLAR^{TM} (GCM) ELECTRODE
FOR ELECTRORETINOGRAPHY

R.P. BORDA, R.M. GILLIAM & A.C. COATS

(Houston, Texas, USA)

Since electroretinography first came to be regarded as a clinical test procedure, there has been a continuing quest for the ideal ERG electrode. Because the retinal response is recorded at maximal amplitude over the cornea, most electrodes represent a modification of a contact lens.

Each type of electrode currently in use has its merits, but most share the objectionable qualities of causing some degree of corneal irritation and discomfort to the patient. In addition, most contact lens electrodes provide a poor fit to the patient's cornea and subsequent inconsistent electrode contact, introducing considerable optical distortion. A recent report by Chase et al. (1976) described a new type of ERG electrode, which seemed to solve some of the problems inherent in the use of a contact lens. This electrode consisted of a thin strip of Mylar^{TM}, coated on one side with aluminum, and bent into a 'J' shape. The short leg of the 'J' was inserted into the lower cul-de-sac, and electrical contact with the globe was achieved through the aluminum-coated outside surface of the plastic strip. It was reported that electrical recordings of high quality were obtained with this electrode and that no topical anesthesia of the cornea was required.

We obtained samples of these electrodes for evaluation. Initial tests on the electrical properties of the aluminized Mylar indicated that the aluminum was only loosely bound to the plastic and could be freed by surprisingly low levels of alternating current in the range of $10 \mu A$. Since some amplification systems produce electrode leakage currents well in excess of this, it was felt that this property of the aluminized Mylar might pose a health hazard, that is, there was risk of introducing aluminum particles onto the surface of the globe. Also, the electrical properties of aluminum make it a less than ideal electrode for relatively low frequency bioelectric signals.

Samples of gold-coated Mylar were obtained from the manufacturer (Sheldahl Advanced Products, Northfield, Minnesota) and the electrical properties compared with those of the aluminum-coated strips. To insure that the original sample did not represent a manufacturing defect or that the 'unbonding' property was not a result of the heat process used to bend the plastic, unformed aluminized Mylar from a different manufacturer was tested also. The aluminum consistently exhibited the tendency to flake from the Mylar substrate, whereas the gold did not, at least at the low current levels applied.

Electrodes similar to those described by Chase and his coworkers (Chase et al., 1976) were then constructed of the gold-coated Mylar, the overall thickness being 1 mil (0.001 inch) or half that used by Chase (Fig. 1). For recording the ERG, these electrodes were inserted into the lower cul-de-sac and taped to the skin over the infraorbital ridge (Fig. 2).

Electrical contact with the GCM strip was made through a small alligator clip. To make objective evaluation of this new electrode, recordings were obtained from a series of eleven volunteer subjects with a standard contact lens electrode (scleral lens, Life-Tech Instruments, Houston, Texas) in one eye and the GCM electrode in the other. Before the electrodes were inserted, each subject had a slit-lamp examination of the cornea of each eye; this exam was repeated following the recording. The subjects were also asked to compare the two types of electrodes for (1) discomfort during insertion and during the recording and (2) residual discomfort following the recording. Topical anesthesia was necessary only with the contact lens electrode, but was employed bilaterally in two subjects to assess the effects on the cornea of the anesthetic (Ophthaine ®) itself.

Both single-flash and flicker ERGs could be recorded with the GCM electrode, but commonly were contaminated with eye movement artifacts (Fig. 3). Amplitudes of the responses recorded with the GCM electrode were consistently lower (by 34–44%) than those recorded with the contact lens, but, surprisingly, evidenced a lower variability. These lower amplitudes could be explained by the fact that the GCM electrode makes electrical contact with the sclera as well as the cornea, the GCM strip partially blocks the stimulus, and/or the contact lens diffuses the light stimulus slightly.

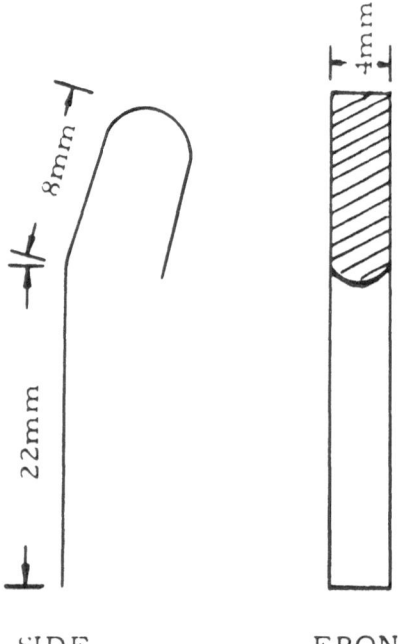

SIDE   FRONT

Fig. 1. Dimensions of electrode constructed of 1 mil gold-coated Mylar[TM] (GCM).

340

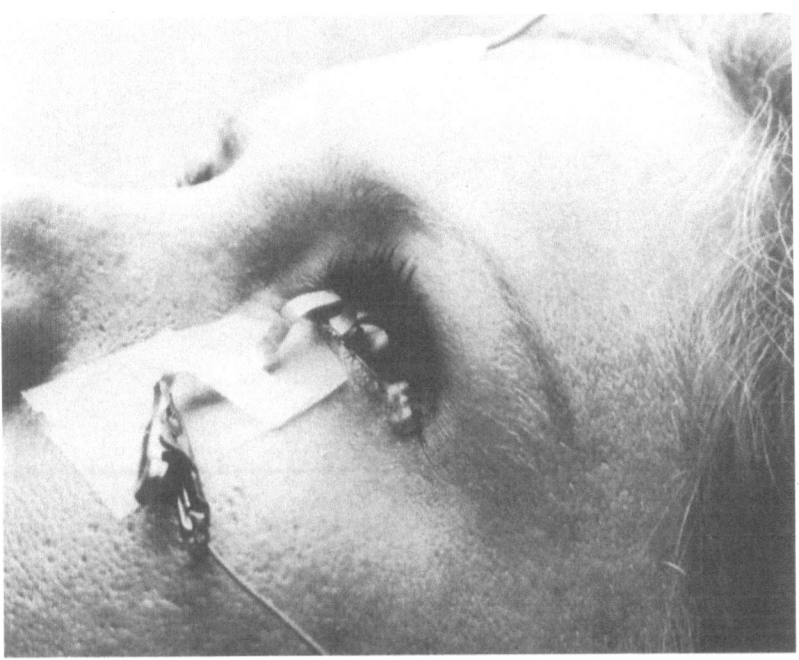

Fig. 2. GCM electrode inserted into lower cul-de-sac. Electrical contact is made through a small alligator clip, and electrode and clip taped to the skin.

More striking were the differences in the ocular irritation associated with use of the two electrodes. In rating the contact lens and GCM electrodes as to comfort during insertion, during the recording period, and ten minutes after completion of the recording (when the topical anesthetic was no longer effective), the eleven subjects reported the following:

| | | Degree of Discomfort | | | |
		None	Mild	Moderate	Marked
During insertion:	Contact lens	2	3	4	2
	GCM strip	5	5	0	1
During recording:	Contact lens	1	5	3	2
	GCM strip	5	2	3	1
After removal:	Contact lens	0	6	5	0
	GCM strip	11	0	0	0

All subjects actually slightly favored the GCM electrode, even those six who reported some discomfort with the GCM electrode during insertion and during the recording period and the two who were anesthetized in both eyes. The most marked differences in comfort were noted after the anesthetic was no longer effective – *none* of the subjects had residual discomfort in the eye

341

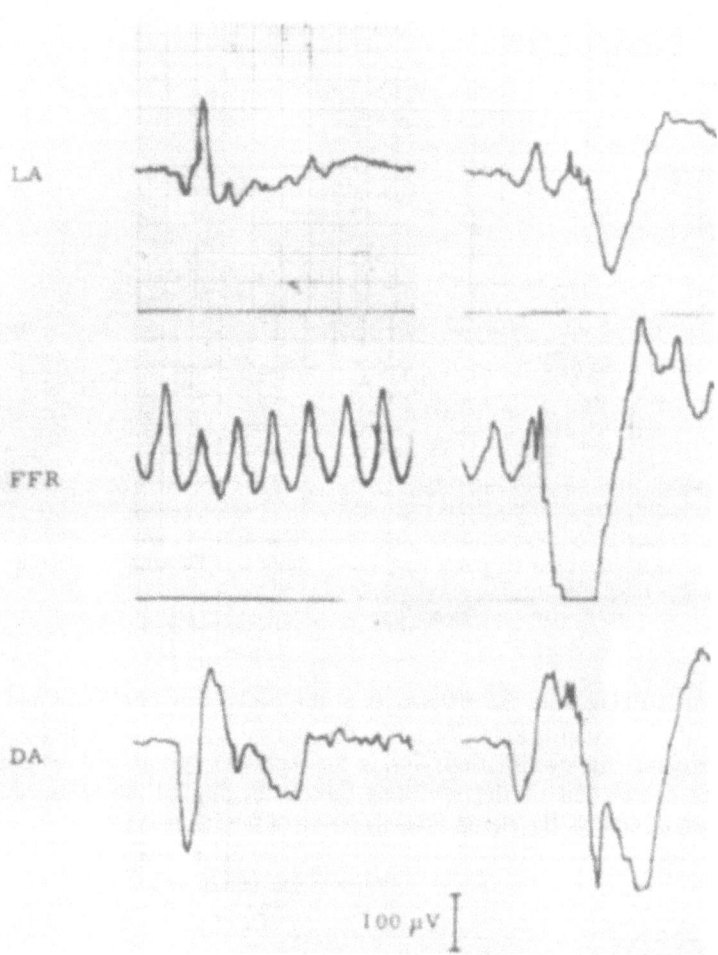

Fig. 3. Comparison of recordings obtained with a scleral contact lens electrode and the GCM electrode. LA = light-adapted (540 lux), FFR = flicker-following response to a 30/sec strobe, DA = dark adaptation for 10 min. All recordings were obtained with a Life-Tech Instruments Recorder, Model 7102, and Signal Averaging Computer, Model 7402. Stimuli consisted of flashes of approximately 5×10^{-3} lum. secs/cm^2 delivered by a Life-Tech Instruments Stimulator, Model 7310, with Parabolic Reflector, Model 7310M.

with the GCM electrode, whereas *all* eleven reported mild or moderate residual discomfort in the eye with the contact lens. These subjective reports correlated well with the findings of the post-recording slit-lamp examination, which are summarized below.

	Degree of Conjunctival Hyperemia			
	None	Mild	Moderate	Marked
Contact lens	0	3	7	1
GCM strip	10	1	0	0

	Degree of Corneal Epithelial Changes			
	None	Mild	Moderate	Marked
Contact lens	0	6	4	1
GCM strip	7	4	0	0

All eleven subjects evidenced some changes in the corneal epithelium of the eye tested by a lens, whereas the GCM electrode produced no changes in seven of the subjects and only minimal, focal changes in four.

In summary, electrodes constructed of metallic-coated Mylar apparently offer some advantages in clinical electroretinography, the primary advantages being:

1) good electrical contact with corneas of any curvature.
2) lack of optical distortion.
3) patient comfort (with topical anesthesia not required) and
4) low cost.

For these reasons, electrodes constructed of this material should be appropriate in testing such patients as children, apprehensive adults, those with corneal disease, and those with an allergy to topical anesthetics. This device should also be suitable for use in extended ERG recordings or recordings utilizing patterned stimuli. The only significant disadvantage noted was a tendency of the Mylar electrode to be more sensitive to eye movement artifacts. From our observation that the aluminum coating can 'unplate' from the plastic substrate at very low levels of applied current, we would caution against its use in clinical applications and would suggest that electrodes be constructed of gold-coated Mylar instead.

REFERENCES

Chase, W.W., N.E. Fradkin & S. Tauda. A new electrode for electroretinography. *Am. J. Optom. Physiol. Optics* 53: *668–671* (1976).

Authors' address:
Neurophysiology Dept.
Methodist Hospital
6516 Bertner Blvd.
Houston, Texas 77030
USA